Partha's
IMMUNIZATION DIGEST

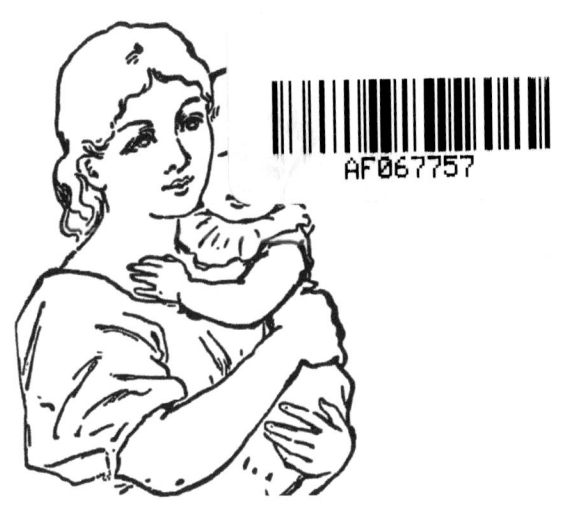

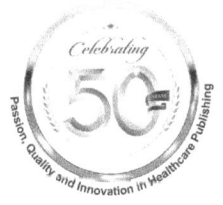

Partha's
IMMUNIZATION DIGEST

Fourth Edition

Editor-in-Chief
A Parthasarathy
MD (Ped) DCH DSc (Hon) FIAP
Senior Consultant Pediatrician
AP Child Care, Chennai
Former Distinguished Professor
Department of Pediatrics
The Tamil Nadu Dr MGR Medical University
Retired Senior Clinical Professor
Department of Pediatrics
Madras Medical College, Chennai
Deputy Superintendent
Institute of Child Health and Hospital for Children
Chennai, Tamil Nadu, India

Chief Academic Editor
Alok Gupta
MD (Ped) FIAP
Pediatrician and Counselor
Pediatric Specialties Clinic, Jaipur
Formerly Assistant Professor in Pediatric Medicine
Mahatma Gandhi Medical College and Hospital
Jaipur, Rajasthan, India

Academic Editor
Mohit Vohra
MBBS DNB (Ped) Fellow in Neonatology MHA
Consultant and Head
Department of Pediatrics
CKS Hospital
Jaipur, Rajasthan, India

Foreword
MKC Nair

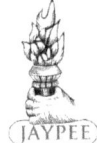

JAYPEE BROTHERS MEDICAL PUBLISHERS
The Health Sciences Publisher
New Delhi | London

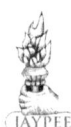 **Jaypee Brothers Medical Publishers (P) Ltd.**

Headquarters
Jaypee Brothers Medical Publishers (P) Ltd
4838/24, Ansari Road, Daryaganj
New Delhi 110 002, India
Phone: +91-11-43574357
Fax: +91-11-43574314
Email: jaypee@jaypeebrothers.com

Overseas Office
J.P. Medical Ltd
83 Victoria Street, London
SW1H 0HW (UK)
Phone: +44 20 3170 8910
Fax: +44 (0)20 3008 6180
Email: info@jpmedpub.com

Website: www.jaypeebrothers.com
Website: www.jaypeedigital.com

© 2020, Jaypee Brothers Medical Publishers

The views and opinions expressed in this book are solely those of the original contributor(s)/author(s) and do not necessarily represent those of editor(s) of the book.

All rights reserved. No part of this publication may be reproduced, stored or transmitted in any form or by any means, electronic, mechanical, photocopying, recording or otherwise, without the prior permission in writing of the publishers.

All brand names and product names used in this book are trade names, service marks, trademarks or registered trademarks of their respective owners. The publisher is not associated with any product or vendor mentioned in this book.

Medical knowledge and practice change constantly. This book is designed to provide accurate, authoritative information about the subject matter in question. However, readers are advised to check the most current information available on procedures included and check information from the manufacturer of each product to be administered, to verify the recommended dose, formula, method and duration of administration, adverse effects and contraindications. It is the responsibility of the practitioner to take all appropriate safety precautions. Neither the publisher nor the author(s)/editor(s) assume any liability for any injury and/or damage to persons or property arising from or related to use of material in this book.

This book is sold on the understanding that the publisher is not engaged in providing professional medical services. If such advice or services are required, the services of a competent medical professional should be sought.

Every effort has been made where necessary to contact holders of copyright to obtain permission to reproduce copyright material. If any have been inadvertently overlooked, the publisher will be pleased to make the necessary arrangements at the first opportunity. The **CD/DVD-ROM** (if any) provided in the sealed envelope with this book is complimentary and free of cost. **Not meant for sale.**

Inquiries for bulk sales may be solicited at: jaypee@jaypeebrothers.com

Partha's Immunization Digest

First Edition: 2005
Second Edition: 2011
Third Edition: 2017
Fourth Edition: **2020**

ISBN: 978-93-89776-36-2

Dedicated to
*The Underprivileged Children of India,
who miss the opportunity of Routine Immunization,
and need Special Campaigns for Catch-up Immunization*

Contributors

A Parthasarathy
MD (Ped) DCH DSc (Hon) FIAP
Senior Consultant Pediatrician
AP Child Care, Chennai
Former Distinguished Professor
Department of Pediatrics
The Tamil Nadu Dr MGR Medical University
Retired Senior Clinical Professor
Department of Pediatrics
Madras Medical College, Chennai
Deputy Superintendent
Institute of Child Health and Hospital for Children
Chennai, Tamil Nadu, India

Alok Gupta
MD (Ped) FIAP
Pediatrician and Counselor
Pediatric Specialties Clinic
Jaipur
Formerly Assistant Professor in Pediatric Medicine
Mahatma Gandhi Medical College and Hospital
Jaipur, Rajasthan, India

Mohit Vohra
MBBS DNB (Ped) Fellow in Neonatology MHA
Consultant and Head
Department of Pediatrics
CKS Hospital
Jaipur, Rajasthan, India

Srinivas G Kasi
MD (Ped)
Consultant Pediatrician
Kasi Clinic
Bengaluru, Karnataka, India

Suhas V Prabhu
MD DCH MNAMS
Consultant Pediatrician
PD Hinduja Hospital
Mumbai, Maharashtra, India

Foreword

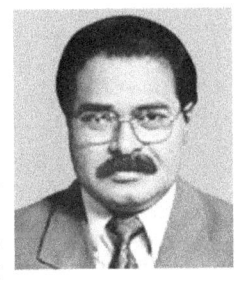

I am delighted to know that *Partha's Immunization Digest* the popular handbook on vaccines and immunization practices, written by my 'Guru', Professor A Parthasarathy is due for its 4th edition. The Internet era has revolutionized the Knowledge, Attitude and Practice (KAP) on Immunization of both parents as well as doctors. Day-in and day-out new information keeps on pouring in. So much so, the medical practitioner is in a dilemma as to which vaccine to prefer and how to schedule it.

Numerous guidebooks published on behalf of the Indian Academy of Pediatrics (IAP) and by private authors are available. A worthy addition to the existing collection, has now come in the form of this manual entitled *Partha's Immunization Digest*. The authors have taken pains to collect available useful literature on Immunization both from Indian and foreign sources and present the resume in a reader friendly, yet concise and informative manner. The text on development of various types of vaccine formulations is highly informative as also the text of future vaccines.

I compliment Professor (Dr) A Parthasarathy and his eminent team for their laudable effort and hope the new manual will be welcome by all those concerned with infant, child and adolescent immunization. I am happy to learn that the book is now being published in revised version which speaks of its popularity. I am sure that the revised version with updated information will benefit the reader to update his/her knowledge on changing concepts in immunization. I can say without hesitation that this is perhaps the one and the only digest of its kind available in Indian market, which incorporates concise, yet latest precise information on all aspects of globally available vaccines and immunization practices.

MKC Nair MD MMedSc PhD DSc MBA FIAP
Vice-Chancellor
Kerala University of Health Sciences, Thrissur
Founder Director
Child Development Center
Government Medical College
Thiruvananthapuram, Kerala, India
National President
Indian Academy of Pediatrics (IAP), 2004

Preface to the Fourth Edition

"Immunization is not a Business, But a Responsibility"
—**Professor M Indasekhar Rao**
National Conference of Pediatric Diseases (NCPID), 2019
Hyderabad, Telangana, India

Immunization has been regarded as the greatest success story of 20th century. With effective immunization of newborns, infants, children and adolescents, global eradication of smallpox was achieved in 1978. Similarly, poliomyelitis has been eradicated from the world except from three countries, viz. Afghanistan, Pakistan and Nigeria. Nevertheless, emerging and re-emerging infections are still posing a challenge.

Genetic engineering and molecular biology have further advanced, opening newer avenues in vaccine manufacturing. Nasal, oral, skin patch vaccines will ease vaccine delivery and safety. Syringes and needles have further improved in quality making vaccines more acceptable. Increasing vaccine awareness has reduced vaccine hesitancy in parents, adolescents, doctors and healthcare professionals. Global Polio Eradication Initiative (GPEI), Measles–Rubella Mass Vaccination Program, Vaccine Updates, Continuing Medical Education (CME) programs, Parent-School Vaccine Education and vigorous media campaigns have improved vaccine coverage and out-reach, making vaccine preventable diseases (VPD)—an easier target than in the past.

Increased need of eradication, elimination and containment of older diseases, re-emerging diseases and newer diseases has mobilized the research and development healthcare sectors. Newer vaccines are being rapidly developed and trials in various stages are in progress in India and world over. India has emerged as a leading country for vaccine research and manufacture. Vaccine stability is being improved for improving vaccine effectiveness and rural and remote outreach.

National Immunization Program (NIP) is designed by the Central Government for the masses. In office practice, when dealing with individuals, we need to offer all the available vaccine appropriately. Prenatal, natal, postnatal, under 5-year vaccination are needed but the older children, adolescents and even the adults should be protected by appropriate primary vaccines including the booster doses for continued lifelong protection.

We have in this manual incorporated the entire plethora of vaccines recommended in NIP, WHO, IAP and CDC immunization timetable. Available 'state-of-the-art' charts, tables and text of international and national authors and organizations have been included with necessary modifications with due acknowledgment.

We sincerely hope that this new revised 4th edition will get a warm welcome from you, the practicing pediatricians, adolescent and family physicians. Your comments and suggestions are most welcome to improve the quality of subsequent editions.

A Parthasarathy
Alok Gupta
Mohit Vohra

Preface to the First Edition

Immunization has been regarded as the greatest success story of 20th century. With effective immunization of newborns, infants, children and adolescents, global eradication of smallpox was achieved in 1978. Similarly, poliomyelitis has since been eradicated in developed countries; controlled in many countries and is in the process of elimination in developing countries, at the global scenario. Nevertheless, emerging and re-emerging infections are still posing a challenge.

Advances in molecular biology and genetic engineering are revitalizing the concept of immunization. Novel vaccine delivery systems have been developed. Auto-destruct/self-locking syringes have promoted the *Needle smart* message. Knowledge, attitude and practice (KAP) on immunization for doctors and parents have been enriched through continuing medical education (CME) of vaccine updates and parent health education, and through the vigorous media advertisements of the vaccine manufactures. Due to these awareness campaigns, demand generation has increased. Newer vaccines are being licensed in India, after their efficacies have been established at the global level.

In addition to the vaccines administered in the National Immunization Schedule, it has become necessary to recommend additional vaccines at different age groups. Apart from newborn, infant and childhood immunization practices, immunization of adolescents has also become a campaign by itself. In this manual, attempt has been made to present a *state-of-the art* information concerning issues related to vaccines and immunization. Existing *state-of-the art* tables and text of international and national authors have been included with necessary modifications with due acknowledgment. Hope, the new venture will be welcomed by practicing pediatricians and family physicians. Your comments and suggestion are most welcomed to improve the quality of future editions.

A Parthasarathy

Acknowledgments

Our grateful thanks to:
- M/s D Prakash, Mrs Padma, P Abhilash and Mrs Lakshmi of PharmaTech, Chennai and Mr Hariharputhran, Ajit Singh and Shukla of Serum Institute of India (SII), Chennai, for coordination and Mrs Uma Devi for assistance from time to time in fine tuning the revised manuscripts.
- Dr K Surendran, WHO Surveillance Medical Officer, National Polio Surveillance Project, Chennai Office, for providing latest maps and figures.
- Mrs Nirmala Parthasarathy, Dr Mrs Prathiba Janardhanan, Mrs Kavitha Balaji, Mr R Janarthanan, Mr P Balaji, Miss Shruthi Pavana, Miss Swathi Pavana, Miss Kavya Balaji, Miss Mahiya Balaji and Mr A Sriramulu for co-ordination.
- Indian Academy of Pediatrics (IAP) for the excerpts from IAP Guidebook on Immunization 2001, 2009, 2013–14 and 2018–19 edition.
- American Academy of Pediatrics (AAP) for the excerpts from Red Book 2009 and 2012 editions.
- Our sincere and grateful thanks go to Shri Jitendar P Vij (Group Chairman), Mr Ankit Vij (Managing Director), Mr MS Mani (Group President), Ms Chetna Malhotra Vohra (Associate Director-Content Strategy), Ms Pooja Bhandari (Production Head), and other members of M/s Jaypee Brothers Medical Publishers (P) Ltd, New Delhi, India, for their untiring coordination efforts in the production of the 4th edition.
- 'All sources' cited in the text where material has been collected in this digest.
- Dr Sweta Gupta, Dr Anant Gupta and Dr Khushbu Jain, for helping in editorial work.
- Professor K Nedunchelian, Senior Consultant in Pediatrics, Head (Research and Academics), Dr Mehta's Children Hospital, Chennai, Tamil Nadu, for critically reviewing the text of the 4th edition and suggesting valuable corrections which we have incorporated.

A Parthasarathy
Alok Gupta
Mohit Vohra

Contents

1. **The Vaccine Timeline** 1
   Suhas V Prabhu
   Smallpox: The First Target for Vaccination   *1*
   The Discovery of Bacterial Vaccines   *3*
   Determining Efficacy of Vaccines   *3*
   The Discovery of Toxoids   *4*
   New Methods of Production   *4*
   Mass Vaccination as a Public Health Programme   *6*
   Setbacks and Disasters from Vaccines Lead to
      Stronger Regulations   *7*
   Public Resistance to Immunization Programmes   *7*
   Notorious Vaccine Controversies   *8*

2. **Immunization: The Way Forward** 11
   A Parthasarathy
   GAVI, NTAGI, IEAG, IPEI Recommendations   *12*
   Development of New Vaccines and New Techniques for
      Vaccine Administration   *13*

3. **Basics of Vaccinology** 16
   Alok Gupta
   Terminologies   *16*
   Classification of Vaccines   *17*
   Characteristics of Vaccines   *21*
   Composition of Vaccines   *26*
   Common Misconceptions about Immunization   *27*

4. **Immunization Schedules** 29
   Alok Gupta
   National Immunization Schedule, 2019   *29*
   IAP Immunization Schedule, 2018–19   *34*
   General Instructions   *34*
   Specific Instructions   *43*
   IAP Recommended Vaccines for High-Risk Children   *56*
   Immunization of Adolescents   *59*
   WHO Immunization Timetable, 2019   *60*
   Summary   *64*
   You are Never too Old to Get Immunized   *66*
   Footnotes   *67*
   Travel-related Vaccines   *79*

Immunization Schedules FAQs by Parents
on Immunization *79*
FAQs Immunization Schedules *80*
FAQs Immunization of Adolescents *80*

5. Vaccines, Immunoglobulins and Antisera 83
A Parthasarathy

Vaccines Administered at Birth *84*
Vaccines Administered at 6, 10 and 14 Weeks *95*
Vaccines Administered at 9 Months *110*
Vaccine Administered at 15 Months *115*
Vaccines Administered at 18 Months (Booster) *119*
Vaccines Administered at 12 Months *120*
Vaccines Administered at 2 Years of Age *121*
Vaccines Administered at 5 Years *122*
Vaccines Administered at 10 Years *123*
Seasonal/Travel-related Vaccines *135*
Cholera Vaccine *143*
To Summarize *155*
Immunoglobulins *157*
Antisera *161*
Vaccines Licensed in India *162*

6. Immunization in Special Clinical Circumstances 171
Alok Gupta

Immunizations Required or Recommended
   Because of Risk of Diseases *171*
Recommended Schedule of Hepatitis B Immunoprophylaxis
   to Prevent Perinatal Transmission *171*
Recommendations for Postexposure Immune Prophylaxis of
   Hepatitis A Infection *173*
Recommended Immunization Schedules for Children not
   Immunized in the First Year of Life *173*
Simultaneous Administration of Multiple Vaccines *175*
Lapsed Immunizations *176*
Unknown or Uncertain Immunization Status *176*
Active Immunization of Persons Who Recently
   Received Immunoglobulin *176*
Pregnancy *178*
Children on Steroids *178*
Hodgkin's Disease *179*
Asplenic Children (Congenital Asplenia, Sickle Cell
   Disease, and Splenectomy) *179*
Children with HIV-AIDS *179*

Immunization in Bleeding Disorders *180*
Immunization in Children with
    History of Allergy *180*
Organ Transplant Individuals *180*
Vaccination of the Individual with
    Cancer/Chemotherapy *181*
Immunization in Relation to Antibody
    Containing Products *181*
Immunization for Travelers *181*

7. Adverse Events Following Immunization 183
Mohit Vohra

Vaccine Safety: A Universal Concern *183*
WHO Recommendations to Minimize AEFI *185*
Causes and Errors Leading to AEFI *185*
Vaccines and Contraindications *186*
Anaphylaxis and Drugs *187*
Threats to Immunization: Safety Concerns *189*
Adverse Events following Immunization:
    Practical Guidelines *191*
DCGI (Drugs Controller General of India) Suggested
    Surveillance: Adverse Event Reporting *192*
Common Adverse Events to Vaccines *193*

8. The Cold Chain for Vaccines 199
A Parthasarathy

Cold Chain *199*
Cold Chain Equipment *199*
Refrigerators *200*
Technical Specifications of Cold Chain Equipment *201*
Vaccine Vial Monitors *201*
Storage of Vaccines in Domestic Refrigerator *202*
Recommended Storage of Commonly Used Vaccines *204*
Power Failure *207*

9. Vaccine Development 209
Srinivas G Kasi

Vaccine Development Process *209*

10. Future Vaccines 213
Srinivas G Kasi

Newer Technologies in Vaccine Development *213*
Next Generation Technologies *216*
Future Trends in Immunization *227*
Vaccine Timeline 1780–2020 *228*

11. Vaccine Preventable Disease Surveillance 231
Mohit Vohra, Alok Gupta

Types of VPD Surveillance *231*
Acute Flaccid Paralysis Surveillance *232*
Endgame Strategic Plan: Milestones and Challenges *244*
Outcomes *245*
Integrated Disease Surveillance Program *252*
Reporting Requirement of IDSP *253*
Reporting Format for Sentinel Sites *254*
Private Sector Collaboration in Tuberculosis
   Control Program *255*
IAP Infectious Disease Surveillance Program *256*

12. WHO Position Papers on Vaccines in NIP and IAP Schedules 258
Alok Gupta

WHO Position Paper on BCG Vaccines:
   February, 2018 *258*
WHO Position Paper on Polio Vaccines:
   March, 2016 *261*
WHO Position Paper on Hepatitis B Vaccines:
   July, 2017 *263*
WHO Position Paper on Diphtheria Vaccines:
   August, 2017 *266*
WHO Position Paper on Pertussis Vaccines:
   September, 2015 *269*
WHO Position Paper on Tetanus Vaccines:
   February, 2017 *272*
WHO Position Paper on *Haemophilus Influenzae*
   Type B Vaccination: July, 2013 *274*
WHO Position Paper on Pneumococcal Conjugate
   Vaccines in Infants and Children Under
      5 Years of Age: February, 2019 *276*
WHO Position Paper on Rotavirus Vaccines *280*
WHO Position Paper on Measles Vaccine: April, 2017 *282*
WHO Position Paper on Rubella Vaccines Published in
   WER July, 2011 *285*
WHO Position Paper on Varicella and Herpes Zoster
   Vaccination: June, 2014 *288*
WHO Position Paper on Typhoid Vaccines:
   March, 2018 *290*
WHO Position Paper on Vaccines Against Influenza:
   November, 2012 *293*
WHO Position Paper on Hepatitis A Vaccines:
   July, 2012 *295*

Contents

WHO Position Paper on Vaccines Against Human
Papillomavirus: May, 2017 *299*
WHO Position Paper on Vaccination Against
Yellow Fever *301*
WHO Position Paper on Rabies Vaccines and
Immunoglobulins: April, 2018 *305*
WHO Position Paper on Vaccines Against Japanese
Encephalitis *309*
WHO Position Paper on Meningococcal, a Conjugate
Vaccine: Updated Guidance, February, 2015 *312*

ANNEXURES

I. Frequently Asked Questions on Immunization 315
Alok Gupta, Mohit Vohra

Immunization: General *315*
BCG Vaccine *318*
Oral Polio Vaccine *318*
Hepatitis B Vaccine *319*
DTP/DT/TT Vaccines *324*
Hib Vaccine *326*
Measles, MMR Vaccines *329*
Typhoid Vaccine *332*
Hepatitis A Vaccine *332*
Varicella Vaccine *334*
Pneumococcal Vaccine *337*
Rotavirus Vaccines *338*
HPV Vaccines *339*
Rabies Vaccines *340*
AEFI Guidelines *340*

II. Immunization Websites 343
Alok Gupta, Mohit Vohra

III. Immunization Techniques 346
Alok Gupta, Mohit Vohra

Immunization Techniques for Intramuscular,
Subcutaneous, and Intradermal Injections *346*
Administering Vaccines: Dose, Route,
Site, and Needle Size *349*
Comforting Restraint *364*

IV. Vaccine Formulations (Brands) Commonly Available in India for Office Practice (Vaccines in NIP—Government supply not included here) 366
Alok Gupta, Mohit Vohra

Index *371*

CHAPTER 1

The Vaccine Timeline

Suhas V Prabhu

Modern medicine has embraced immunization as an important arm in the fight against infectious diseases; but the practice is quite ancient, dating back to over a thousand years. Buddhist monks in the 7th century drank snake venom to confer immunity to snake bite; the first example of using the agent of the disease itself to help provide protection against it. But snake bite is of course not an infectious disease.

SMALLPOX: THE FIRST TARGET FOR VACCINATION

The first application of this principle to infectious disease was in the case of smallpox, a dreaded scourge in ancient times. The method involved grinding up smallpox scabs from a patient and blowing the matter into the nostril of the recipient. Inoculation may also have been practiced by scratching matter from the sore of a smallpox patient into the skin of the recipient, a process called variolation. This practice probably began in Central Asia as early as 200 BC and from there spread to China and India. The earliest documentation of this process includes several written accounts from the 16th century that describe variolation as practiced in China. One such account appears in Joseph Needham's *Science and Civilization in China*. When the Chinese Emperor Fu-lin died of smallpox, his third son K'ang Hsi became the Emperor. Having already survived a case of smallpox before he became Emperor, he was worried for his family members and so supported inoculation and wrote about it in a letter to his descendants:

"The method of inoculation having been brought to light during my reign, I had it used upon you, my sons and daughters, and my descendants, and you all passed through the smallpox in the happiest possible manner.... In the beginning, when I had it tested on one or two people, some old women taxed me with extravagance, and spoke very strongly against inoculation. The courage which I summoned up to insist on its practice has saved the lives and health of millions of men. This is an extremely important thing, of which I am very proud."

—**Ian Glynn and Jenifer Glynn**, *The Life and Death of Smallpox*

The practice gradually spread to the western World and the new World where it was sporadically practiced. It was, however, not without its risks as some recipients of variolation actually contracted severe diseases and some of them died of it!

In 1738, a smallpox epidemic struck the city of Charleston in present day South Carolina with 18% mortality. But comparatively, only 4% of those who were previously variolated died, proving that it did confer some amount of protection. These results encouraged the advocates of variolation despite its inherent risks. This included the renowned American scientist Benjamin Franklin who was a supporter of variolation.

"In 1736 I lost one of my Sons, a fine Boy of 4 years old, taken by the Smallpox in the common way. I long regretted that I had not given it to him by inoculation, which I mention for the sake of parents, who omit that operation on the supposition that they should never forgive themselves if a Child died under it; my example showing that the regret may be the same either way, and that therefore the safer should be chosen."

—**Benjamin Franklin**, quoted in *Franklin on Franklin* by Paul Zall

Much safer methods of protection from smallpox came to light only due to the sharp observations of a country doctor, Dr Edward Jenner of Gloucestershire, England, who noted that cowgirls who had suffered from cowpox were apparently immune to smallpox. He was the first person to vaccinate an individual (a 13-year-old boy) against smallpox by inoculating him with (the closely related) cowpox virus, in 1796. In 1798, the first smallpox vaccine was developed, and inoculations were carried out from one person to another; this marked the beginning of vaccine era. The term vaccination is derived from vaccine virus.

In 1836, the English physician Edward Ballard noted that cowpox transmitted from human to human seemed to decline in potency over time. He recommended re-introducing the pustule matter back into cows to boost its potency. This method was able to provide an enough supply of material for vaccination. It also eliminated the chance of transmitting other infections such as syphilis, if the vaccination was carried out directly from one human to another. Soon, the use of calves for vaccine material became widespread in Europe and the United States. Great Britain, however, did not adopt the practice in until 1881 and banned arm-to-arm transmission only as late as 1898.

THE DISCOVERY OF BACTERIAL VACCINES

However, all pathogens do not have a readily available closely related vaccine agent like the smallpox virus has. It required the genius of Louis Pasteur almost a century later to find a way out of this. He demonstrated that the harmful nature of disease-causing organisms could be weakened (or attenuated) in the laboratory. This first "vaccine made in the laboratory" was against chicken cholera which he successfully demonstrated in 1879. He showed the effectiveness of this vaccine (and another one against anthrax) in animals, before developing his vaccine against rabies for use in humans in 1885. Soon after, a vaccine for plague was also developed. Between 1890 and 1950, live bacterial vaccine development proliferated, including the Bacillus Calmette–Guérin (BCG) vaccination, which is still in use today.

Across the Atlantic, in 1886, Daniel Salmon and Theobald Smith demonstrated that killed pathogenic bacteria could be used to produce an immune response that was protective just like with live-attenuated organisms as demonstrated by Louis Pasteur. This discovery led to the development of several killed or inactivated vaccines against human diseases.

DETERMINING EFFICACY OF VACCINES

In 1893, Waldemar Haffkine arrived in India to conduct tests of his cholera vaccine. In his trials, he employed control and experimental groups, a relatively new practice for the time, and vaccinated more than 40,000 people. Though he was not always able to maintain rigorous controls, his methods would become useful models for future vaccine trials. His vaccine showed efficacy in many of the trial subgroups. These methods were then expanded by others into the strict vaccine trials that are the norm today.

THE DISCOVERY OF TOXOIDS

In the early 20th century, it was discovered that some diseases were not caused by the bacteria themselves but the chemicals (toxins) that they produced. These could be chemically inactivated and could then be administered like a vaccine to provide protection against these toxin-induced diseases. These vaccines came to be known as toxoids. In 1923, Alexander Glenny perfected a method to inactivate tetanus toxin using formaldehyde. The same method was applied to produce diphtheria toxoid in 1926.

NEW METHODS OF PRODUCTION

During the 20th century, several innovations led to the development of new methods of producing vaccines.

Viral tissue culture methods developed from 1950 onwards enabled the production of viral vaccines. This led to the advent of the Salk (inactivated) polio vaccine and the Sabin (live-attenuated oral) polio vaccine.

Merck acquired a licensed for a vaccine against *Pneumococcus* protecting against 14 types of bacteria based on their polysaccharide coating in 1977. In 1983, this was expanded to 23 types of pneumococcal bacteria. It was another challenge to conjugate these incomplete antigens (haptens) by combining them with proteins, to produce a vaccine that would induce lasting immunity even in infants where it as most needed. This feat was achieved by the licensing of the 7 valent Prevnar Vaccine by Pfizer in 1997 and its introduction in the US immunization schedule in the year 2000.

The past decades have seen the application of molecular genetics and its increased insights into immunology, microbiology and genomics applied to vaccinology. Current successes include the development of recombinant hepatitis B vaccines, the less reactogenic acellular pertussis vaccine, and new techniques for seasonal influenza vaccine manufacture.

The spurt of new vaccines comes at an important time when antibiotics are losing their sheen as first line defense against infections. As antimicrobial resistance spreads its tentacles and the pipeline for newer antibiotics is drying up, vaccines will continue to play a more and more important role in the fight against infectious diseases (**Fig. 1.1**).

Molecular genetics has set the scene for a bright future for vaccinology, including the development of new vaccine delivery systems (e.g. DNA vaccines, viral vectors, plant vaccines and topical formulations) and new adjuvants. Viral vaccines against cytomegalovirus (CMV), herpes simplex virus (HSV), respiratory syncytial virus (RSV), dengue and even HIV amongst others are works in progress. Research is ongoing on the development of more effective vaccine for tuberculosis. Other bacteria that are future targets for vaccines are *Staphylococcus*, *Streptococcus pyogenes* and *Shigella*. Vaccines have been produced for parasitic infections also. A few years ago, a vaccine for falciparum malaria from GSK underwent a phase III trial in 7 sub-Saharan countries with limited success. The World Health Organization (WHO) has not yet endorsed this vaccine for large scale use in national immunization programmes. The development of vaccines and trials of some vaccines such as HIV vaccine is depicted in **Figure 1.2**.

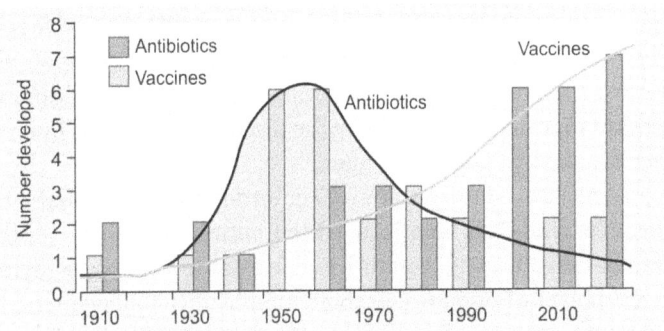

Fig. 1.1: Vaccines and antibiotics licensed during the last century, showing the golden era of antibiotics in 1950s and the present golden era of vaccines.

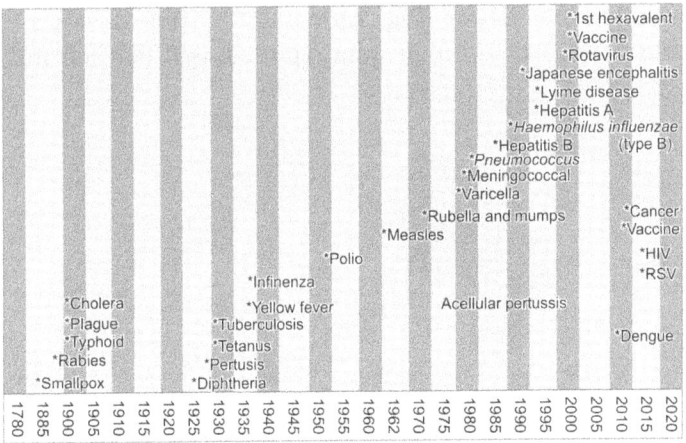

Fig. 1.2: The vaccine timeline (1780–2020).

MASS VACCINATION AS A PUBLIC HEALTH PROGRAMME

Governments recognized the power of immunization to protect its people and over the 18th and 19th centuries, systematic implementation of mass smallpox immunization was introduced. Other vaccines were also added to the immunization programmes of many countries leading to massive reduction in incidence of infectious diseases such as measles, whooping cough, rubella, polio and Hib meningitis.

President Roosevelt, himself stricken by polio, led his government's programme to fight polio in the US. In his broadcast to the nation on 29th of January 1944, he likened the fight against polio to the Second World War: "The dread disease that we battle at home, like the enemy we oppose abroad, shows no concern, no pity for the young. It strikes—with its most frequent and devastating force—against children. And that is why much of the future strength of America depends upon the success that we achieve in combating this disease." Government support for research was vital in the discovery of not one but two vaccines against polio soon after.

In the 20th century, the WHO co-ordinated an international effort to eradicate smallpox which culminated in its global eradication in 1979; a path-breaking achievement testifying to the power of vaccines. Emboldened by this achievement, in 1988, when polio was endemic in 125 countries, the WHO set its sights on eradicating polio through immunization by the end of the century. Great progress has been made but total eradication is still not achieved (**Fig. 1.3**). In 2017, only 22 cases of wild poliovirus infection were reported, and that too from

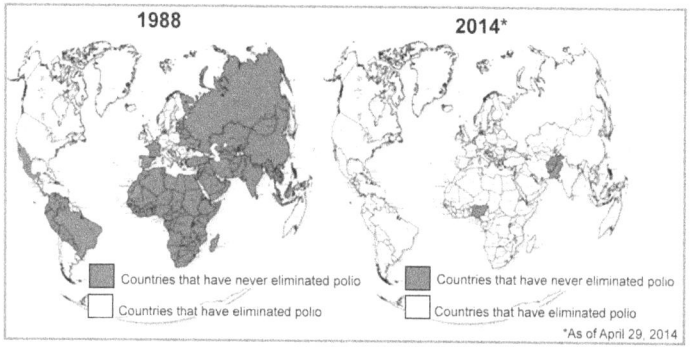

Fig. 1.3: Progress of polio elimination 1988 and 2014 (*Image Credit:* CDC).

only three countries: Afghanistan, Nigeria, and Pakistan. The Global Polio Eradication Initiative led by the Global Alliance Vaccine Initiative (GAVI), the WHO, the Bill and Melinda Gates Foundation, and other organizations continue their efforts to eradicate polio.

SETBACKS AND DISASTERS FROM VACCINES LEAD TO STRONGER REGULATIONS

In 1901, two outbreaks of tetanus occurred linked to vaccines; one in Camden, New Jersey linked to contaminated smallpox vaccine and one in Saint Louis, Missouri, traced to contaminated diphtheria antitoxin. The next year, the US government introduced stringent regulations of biologic products including vaccines.

In 1928, bacterial contamination of diphtheria toxin-antitoxin mixture in Bundaberg, Queensland, Australia, led to the deaths of 12 children. Five others became critically ill but recovered. The tragedy occurred when a multi-use bottle of the vaccine, containing no preservative, was improperly stored and reused. This came to be known as the Queensland disaster.

In 1955, some batches of polio vaccine administered to children were found to contain live polio virus, even though they had passed required safety testing. Over 250 cases of polio occurred (some of which resulted in paralysis) that were attributed to vaccines produced by the company: Cutter Laboratories. The vaccine was of course recalled as soon as cases of polio were detected. This "Cutter Incident" was a defining moment in the history of vaccine manufacturing and government oversight of vaccines. It led to the creation of a better system of regulating vaccines and polio vaccinations were resumed in the fall of 1955.

In more recent times, the first vaccine against rotavirus (called Rotashield), introduced in the US resulted in a substantial number of cases of intussusception in the recipients resulting in its withdrawal. Since then several new vaccines against rotavirus have been successfully introduced while keeping a close look out for this complication.

PUBLIC RESISTANCE TO IMMUNIZATION PROGRAMMES

Despite the overwhelming evidence of the health gains from immunization programmes, there has always been resistance to vaccines by some groups of people. Some of them were on religious grounds, but many were because of distrust and fear of possible complications of immunization. It was as early as 1882 that the Anti-Vaccination League of America held its first meeting in New York. Among the assertions made by the speakers at the meeting was the idea that smallpox was spread not by contagion, but by filth. This became a popular, though incorrect, argument of the anti-vaccinationists.

The late 1970s and 1980s marked a period of increasing litigation and decreased profitability for vaccine manufacture, which led to a decline in the number of companies producing vaccines. The decline was arrested in part by the implementation of the National Vaccine Injury Compensation programme by the US government in 1986 which indemnified vaccine companies. The legacy of this era of resistance to vaccination continues to this day fueled by media and social media sites and kept alive by a growingly vociferous anti-vaccination lobby.

NOTORIOUS VACCINE CONTROVERSIES

The measles, mumps, rubella (MMR) vaccine was introduced in UK in 1988 and by 1995 the vaccine uptake rate reached 95%; enough for herd immunity for these three diseases. In 1998, Andrew Wakefield, et al. published a paper in the Lancet suggesting a link between autism and MMR. The very next year, research published in the Lancet from the Royal Free, where Wakefield did his research, found no evidence for a link between MMR and autism. Further on, between 2002 and 2004 many scientific studies found no evidence for a link between MMR and autism and suggested that the benefits of MMR vaccination far outweighed the risks. Some of this research was published in prestigious journals such as the British Medical Journal, New England Journal of Medicine, Pediatrics and the Lancet itself. In 2004, 10 co-authors of the 1998 Wakefield Lancet paper issued a retraction and editors of the Lancet said, with hindsight, that they should not have published the paper. But the damage was done and by next year the uptake of MMR vaccine in the UK fell to 81%. This resulted in an outbreak of measles and, in 2006, the first death from measles in the UK in 13 years. Various other studies have confirmed the safety of MMR vaccine and several government campaigns to inspire public trust in this vaccine have taken place. But confidence of its safety is still shaky, and the Wakefield paper of 1998 still provides good fodder for the anti-vaccine lobbyists.

Another controversy was ignited in 2010 when the Morbidity and Mortality Weekly Report (MMWR) report of the Center for Diseases Control (CDC) noted that cases of pertussis reported to the Department of Health of the state of California in the first half of that year had increased by 418% over those reported during the same period in 2009. Most of these were in infants less than six months of age, who were too young to be fully immunized against pertussis and included 5 deaths. The debate about whether this outbreak was as a result of fading immunity due to the use of the acellular pertussis vaccine rather than the whole cell vaccine has not been resolved satisfactorily till today and has had repercussions even in our country.

A quadrivalent vaccine against dengue from Sanofi Pasteur was marketed in 2015. Philippines was the first country to introduce it in the national vaccination programme in April 2016. Within a year of introduction, after about 700,000 doses had been administered, surveillance noted almost 600 deaths following immunization with this vaccine. Although the causality of these deaths was not ascertained, the vaccine programme was rescinded in December 2017. There has been a diatribe against conductors of the vaccine trial and accusations of using Philipino children as "guinea pigs". Court cases against the "perpetrators" are still in progress.

These controversies have confused both the public and some clinicians. They have raised doubts on the efficacy of vaccines for protection against disease and honesty of the vaccine trial data from various vaccine companies. Efforts are needed to convince both the layman and the professionals that the advantages of vaccines outweigh the risks so that the anti-vaccine lobby does not derail vaccination programmes and deprive the human population of the great benefits of vaccination in the fight against infectious diseases. Today, advocacy for vaccines and vaccinations and successful counseling for the same are a vital part of many conferences on vaccines and there is a deep need for all who desire the welfare of humankind in general and children in particular to become crusaders for this wonderful weapon against infections.

BIBLIOGRAPHY

1. Children's Hospital of Philadelphia; Vaccine Developments by Year. https://www.chop.edu/centers-programs/vaccine-education-center/vaccine-history/developments-by-year.
2. Glynn I, Glynn J. The Life and Death of Smallpox. Cambridge University Press; 2004.
3. Kinch M. Between Hope and Fear: A History of Vaccines and Human Immunity. Pegasus Books; 2018
4. Link K. The Vaccine Controversy: The History, Use and Safety of Vaccinations. Praeger; 2005.
5. Needham J. Science and Civilization in China. Cambridge University Press, 1956.
6. Plotkin SA (Ed). History of Vaccine Development. Springer, 2011.
7. The History of Vaccines: An Educational Resource by the College of Physicians of Philadelphia. https://www.historyofvaccines.org/timeline/all.
8. Zall PM (Ed). Franklin on Franklin. University Press of Kentucky; 2001.

CHAPTER 2

Immunization: The Way Forward

A Parthasarathy

INTRODUCTION

When Edward Jenner first administered smallpox vaccine in 1796, the process was known as variolation. Later came the use of the term *vaccination*, which was widely accepted. The term *immunization* came into vogue in due course to emphasize the importance of active immunity induced by various antigens. The Greek word *Immune* means to be protected. Whereas the protection offered by vaccines is *active*, passive protection is achieved by the administration of antisera or immunoglobulins. So, certain terminologies need to be defined carefully. Today both the terms *vaccination* and *immunization* are used interchangeably. However, the global practice is to use the term *immunization* more frequently, viz. Expanded Program on Immunization (EPI), Universal Child Immunization (UCI), Global Alliance on Vaccines and Immunization (GAVI), etc.

After the discovery of smallpox vaccine in the year 1796, it took 79 years, for Louis Pasteur to develop the killed rabies vaccine in 1885 followed by the discovery of many more monovalent childhood antigens and the discovery of the first combination vaccine DTP in 1945 and measles, mumps and rubella combined vaccine, MMR, in 1971. With advances in genetic engineering and molecular biology the future will witness the development of more new antigens and perhaps most of these new antigens will be in combination formulation.

Immunization has rightly been claimed as the greatest success story in the history of mankind in the 20th century. Eradication of smallpox in 1978 had paved the way for the elimination/eradication of similar vaccine preventable diseases in several developed countries. Many developing countries such as India too, have achieved outstanding success in eliminating vaccine preventable diseases (VPDs) such as neonatal tetanus, diphtheria, pertussis, measles, poliomyelitis, etc. Global eradication of poliomyelitis by eradicating the circulation of wild as well as vaccine-derived polioviruses is expected to be achieved by 2020.

Vaccines not only save lives; they help children learn and grow, they mean more days in school, they avert many debilitating risks from childhood diseases, and they reduce healthcare costs, protecting families and communities from sliding into poverty.

GAVI, NTAGI, IEAG, IPEI RECOMMENDATIONS

Following repeated representations from the Indian Academy of Pediatrics (IAP), the Government of India has constituted a National Technical Advisory Group on Immunization (NTAGI) and India Experts Advisory Group (IEAG), which considers the exiting immunization practices and India Polio Eradication Initiative (IPEI) and AFP surveillance respectively and suggest introduction of a few more vaccines into the National Immunization Schedule and Strategies to be adopted for polio eradication. It is fervently hoped that the laudable objective of *All Vaccines for the Entire World's Children* will become a reality soon.

The National Technical Advisory Group on Immunization since recommended the introduction of measles-rubella (MR) vaccine in the National Immunization Schedule in place of measles vaccine as well as DTwP Booster in place of diphtheria-tetanus (DT) at 5 years. Apart from introducing the pentavalent fully liquid DTwP-HB-Hib vaccine throughout the country, introduction of rotavirus vaccine, one dose of IPV along with 3rd dose of PENTA and the switch to bivalent OPV, viz. bOPV1 and bOPV3, replacing the conventional trivalent OPV, viz. tOPV are in place already.

The Government of India has in principle approved the introduction of pneumococcal conjugate vaccine (PCV) in the National Immunization Program (NIP), with GAVI subsidy. Introduction of the rotavirus vaccine using the indigenous monovalent 116E strain is also being contemplated. Annual campaign with a single dose of JE vaccine in JE hyperendemic areas has been successfully implemented. Introduction of MR vaccine at 16–24 months along with DTwP booster and rubella vaccine at 10 years for adolescent girls are also in the agenda. A single dose of IPV along the 3rd dose of DTwP to enhance mucosal immunity is also being considered as strategy towards Polio End Game. Switch from tOPV to bOPV for routine immunization and NIDs has already taken place.

DEVELOPMENT OF NEW VACCINES AND NEW TECHNIQUES FOR VACCINE ADMINISTRATION

Apart from the currently available toxin based, subunit, live organisms, inactivated organisms, polysaccharide, glycol conjugate vaccines, etc. We will be having additional or replacement vaccines, viz. anti-idiotype vaccines, re-assorted genomes, temperature sensitive mutants, recombinant viruses and bacteria, recombinant viral or bacterial vectors, genetic (DNA), plant (edible) vaccines, and transcutaneous vaccines which will revolutionize the concept of immunization.

In addition to development of new vaccines, new vaccine implementation and delivery strategies along with new developments in basic and applied immunology, including those directly related to vaccine biotechnology applied implementation, research and the bioethics of clinical trials promise to make the 21st century exciting for vaccinology. Developments such as whole genome sequencing may reveal entirely new paradigms for vaccine development. With molecular medicine's exorable advances, parallel research must progress to ensure that the scientific advances of developed countries are available in developing countries, as well.

LEARNING POINTS

Pediatric and Adolescent Immunization—yesterday, today and tomorrow:

Yesterday

Handful of vaccines, Expanded Program on Immunization (EPI), Targeted universal coverage of under 5 children and pregnant mothers, development of combination vaccine formulations, elimination and eradication of VPDs, smallpox eradication achieved.

Today

Pocketful of vaccines, EPI, UCI, Stress on Adolescent and Adult Immunization, more antigens for immunization during pregnancy, Global Program on Vaccines (GPV), GAVI, development of more combination vaccine formulations, newer adjuvants, newer technologies for vaccine development and administration, vaccine vial monitors to assess cold chain maintenance, elimination and eradication of VPDs, viz. Eradication of poliomyelitis, control and elimination of neonatal and maternal tetanus, diphtheria, pertussis, and measles have been achieved.

Only 30 years ago for instance, wild poliovirus was widespread across 125 countries, causing millions to endure lifelong paralysis. Last year, there were wild poliovirus infections in just two countries—Afghanistan and Pakistan—with only 33 confirmed cases reported worldwide.

Maternal and neonatal tetanus, an often-fatal disease, has been eliminated in all but 13 countries because of vaccination of women before or during pregnancy. And promising results from nations that have introduced the human papillomavirus vaccine early, suggests that cervical cancer is set to decline.

Tomorrow

Bag full of vaccines, all vaccines for all the world's children with GAVIs subsidy, more sophisticated combination vaccine formulations, needle-free vaccine patches, more antigens for universal coverage, improved cold chain equipment, elimination and eradication of more VPDs, global eradication of poliomyelitis, neonatal and maternal tetanus, measles and many more.

The new vaccines are on the horizon to protect against some of our most dangerous known pathogens. The rVSV-ZEBOV Ebola vaccine has already played a critical role in controlling the spread of the current outbreak in the Democratic Republic of the Congo, while RTS, S, the world's first ever malaria vaccine is soon going to be piloted in routine immunization programs.

BIBLIOGRAPHY

1. https://www.who.int 2019
2. John T J. National Technical Advisory Group on Immunization. Indian Pediatr. 2002;39:327-30.
3. John TJ. Towards an Ideal Vaccination Schedule in India. Indian J Pediatr. 1998;65:S8-12.

4. National Rural Health Mission GOI document Brief overview of Universal Immunization Program in India, ASOV workshop course material, IAP, 2009.
5. Universal Immunization Program in India. Breaking New Ground. Ministry of Health and Family Welfare, Government of India; 2002;1-25.
6. Widdus R. The potential to control or eradicate infectious diseases through immunization. Vaccine. 1999;17:S6-12.
7. Yewale VN, Gupta A, Parthasarathy A. Rationale of Selection of Vaccines in National Immunization Program and IAP Immunization Timetable. In: Parthasarathy A, Nair MKC, Menon PSN, Kundu R (Eds). IAP Textbook of Pediatrics (6th edn). Jaypee Brothers Medical Publishers, New Delhi; 2010. pp. 205-17.

CHAPTER 3

Basics of Vaccinology

Alok Gupta

INTRODUCTION

Understanding basics of vaccinology and certain terminologies is important as we practice immunization.

TERMINOLOGIES

Principles of Immunization

Immunity

- Self vs. non-self
- Protection from infectious disease
- Usually indicated by the presence of antibody
- Very specific to a single organism

Active immunity
- Protection produced by the person's own immune system
- Usually permanent

Passive immunity
- Protection transferred from another human or animal
- Temporary protection that wanes with time

Antigen

A live or inactivated substance (e.g. protein, polysaccharide) capable of producing an immune response.

Antibody

Protein molecules (immunoglobulin) produced by B-lymphocytes to help eliminate an antigen.
- Transfer of antibody produced by one human or another animal to another
- Temporary protection
- Transplacental transfer is the most common source in infancy

Sources of passive immunity
- Almost all blood or blood products
- Homologous pooled human antibody (immunoglobulin)
- Homologous human hyperimmune globulin
- Heterologous hyperimmune serum (antitoxin)

Monoclonal Antibody

- Derived from a single type, or clone, of antibodyproducing cells (B cells)
- Antibody is specific to a single antigen or closely related group of antigens.
- Used for diagnosis and therapy of certain cancers and autoimmune and infectious diseases.

Vaccination

- Active immunity produced by vaccine
- Immunity and immunologic memory similar to natural infection but without risk of disease.

CLASSIFICATION OF VACCINES (FIG. 3.1)

Live-attenuated Vaccines

- Attenuated (weakened) form of the wild virus or bacterium
- Must replicate to be effective
- Immune response similar to natural infection
- Usually produce immunity with one dose*
- Severe reactions possible
- Interference from circulating antibody
- Fragile—must be stored and handled carefully
- Viral—measles, mumps, rubella, vaccine, varicella, zoster, yellow fever, rotavirus, intranasal influenza, hepatitis A, oral polio, Japanese encephalitis (JE) vaccine and dengue
- Bacterial—BCG, oral typhoid

Inactivated Vaccines

- Cannot replicate
- Less interference from circulating antibody than live vaccines

---
* Except those administered orally

- Generally require 3–5 doses
- Immune responses mostly humoral
- Antibody titer diminishes with time

Whole Cell Vaccines

- Viral—polio, hepatitis A, rabies, influenza and JE vaccine
- Bacterial—pertussis, typhoid, cholera, plague

Fractional Vaccines

- Subunit—hepatitis B, influenza, acellular pertussis, human papillomavirus, anthrax
- Toxoid—diphtheria, tetanus

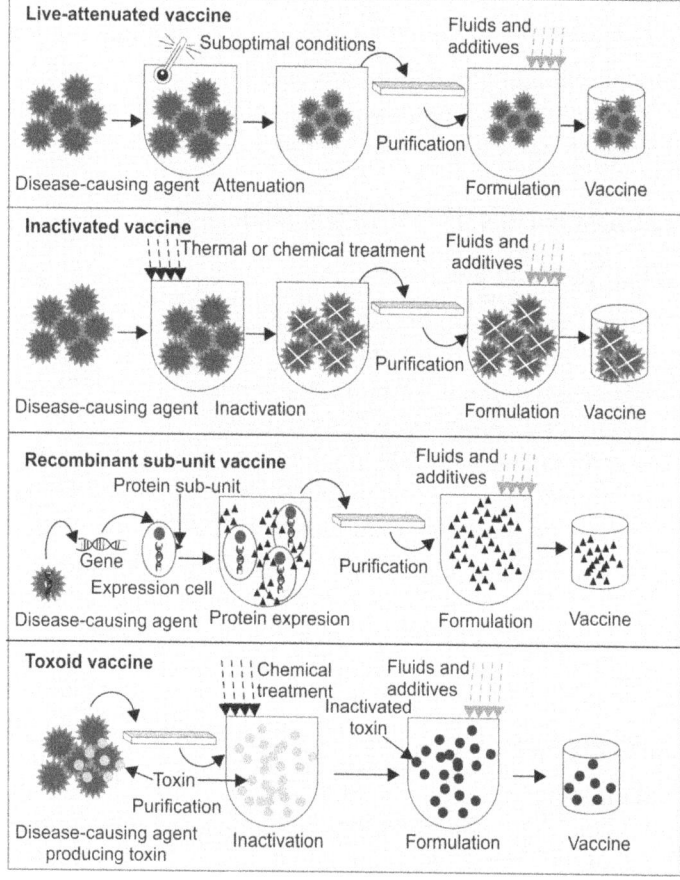

Fig. 3.1: Classification of vaccines *(Contd...)*

Contd...

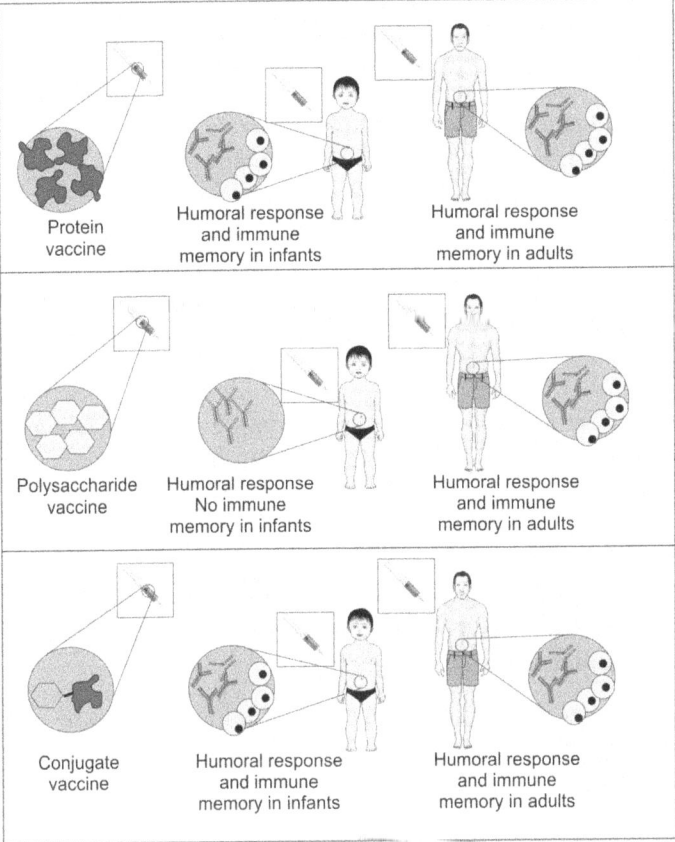

Fig. 3.1: Classification of Vaccines.

Polysaccharide Vaccines

Pure Polysaccharide

- Pneumococcal
- Meningococcal
- *Salmonella typhi* (VI)

Conjugate Polysaccharide

- *Haemophilus influenzae* type B
- Pneumococcal
- Meningococcal
- *Salmonella typhi*

Pure Polysaccharide Vaccines

- Not consistently immunogenic in children younger than 2 years of age
- No booster response
- Antibody with less functional activity
- Immunogenetically improved by conjugation

Immune Response

Process by which antibodies are evolved against a specific antigen.

Primary Response

Response resulting in specific antibody formation following administrating the antigen for the first time. It consists of:

Latent period: The lag period varies from 24 hours to 2 weeks after which antibodies appear.

Peak period: At the end of the latent period (lag), the measurable amount of antibody is detected and the amount reaches peak levels and then maintains a plateau.

Period of decline: Antibodies start declining after a time—IgM type declining more rapidly than IgG. The period of decline is variable.

Secondary Response

Response which occurs when the antigen is repeated. When some antigen is introduced over a period of time (usually 1 year, 5 years, 10 years or 16 years say in the case of Tetanus Toxoid), there is a rapid appearance of antibodies in large numbers may even reach higher proportion than initial response. This is called 'booster effect' or 'memory response' of both B- and T-cells.

Immune response is influenced by the following factors: Maternal antibodies, nature and dose of vaccine, route of administration, immunological adherents, nutritional status, genetic control of immune response, immune suppressants. Maternal antibodies may persist for as long as 6–9 months, e.g. measles.

CHARACTERISTICS OF VACCINES

The characteristics of an ideal vaccine and those of inactivated, live-attenuated and genetic (DNA) vaccines and main pediatric vaccines are described in **Tables 3.1 to 3.5**.

Table 3.1: Characteristics of the ideal vaccines.

- Good immunity at all ages
- Long-lasting protection
- Easy delivery system, e.g. oral
- Both short- and long-term
- Minimal or no adverse effects
- Easy to manufacture
- Maintains potency under variable field conditions
- Affordable

Table 3.2: Characteristics of inactivated (killed) vaccines.

- Unable to replicate in the host
- *Advantages:*
  - Will not multiply or revert to pathogenicity
  - Less reactogenic in general
  - Not transmissible
  - Easier to produce
- *Disadvantages:*
  - Little cellular immunity produced (although humoral immunity is produced)
  - Need multi-dose (booster) series for full protection

Table 3.3: Characteristics of live-attenuated vaccines.

- Replicate in the host, but attenuated in pathogenicity
- *Advantages:*
  - Humoral plus cellular
  - Fewer doses required in general
  - Long-lasting protection
- *Disadvantages:*
  - Rarely may revert to pathogenicity
  - May be more reactogenic antigens
  - Infection may be transmissible from vaccine
  - More complex production

Table 3.4: Characteristics of genetic (DNA) vaccines.

- Leads to antigen synthesis by host cells, in-turn evoking immunity
- *Advantages:*
    - Cellular plus humoral immunity produced
    - Standardized production, good field stability predicted
- *Disadvantages:*
    - Difficult to produce for multigene products, e.g. carbohydrate capsular
    - Theoretical safety risks (autoimmunity, oncogenesis)

Table 3.5: Characteristics of main pediatric vaccines.

Nature	Vaccines	Adjuvants	Major protective mechanisms
Toxin-based	• Diphtheria toxoid • Tetanus toxoid	Aluminum salts	Antitoxin antibodies
Subunit	• Hepatitis B • Pertussis (acellular)	Aluminum salts	Anti-HBsAg antibodies (+role of memory)
	Influenza (split, subunit)		?Antibodies (type? titers?) T-cell Antibodies; T-cells?
Live organisms	Oral polio vaccine, measles, mumps, rubella varicella vaccine	None	Antibodies+ T-cells?
Inactivated organisms	• Pertussis (whole-cell) • Inactivated polio vaccine (IPV) • Influenza (whole virions) • Hepatitis A	• Aluminum salts • None • None • Aluminum salts	• Antibodies (type? titers?) T-cells? • Antibodies +T-cells Antibodies; T-cells? • Antibodies to viral antigens
Polysaccharides	Pneumococcal PS Meningococcal PS	None	Antibodies to capsular PS
Glycoconjugates	Hib conjugates	Lactose	Antibodies to capsular PS

Note: General indication; may differ depending on vaccine manufacturer.

Immune Response to Protein Vaccines (Fig. 3.2)

Why so many vaccine doses?

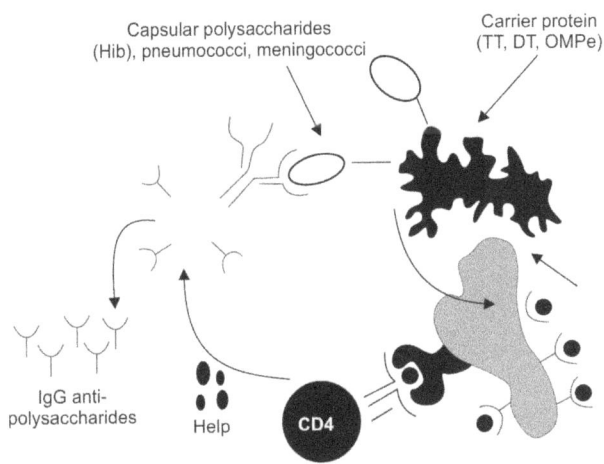

Fig. 3.2: Immune responses to protein vaccines (diphtheria, tetanus toxoids). Vaccine antigens are recognized directly by B-lymphocytes bearing antigen-specific surface immunoglobulins (Ig). They are phagocytosed also by antigen-presenting cells (APC) such as macrophages and dendritic cells, by which they are processed into small peptides. These antigenic peptides bind to nascent HLA class II molecules and reach the cell surface as peptide-HLA complexes. CD4 T-lymphocytes bearing the appropriate T-cell receptors are able to bind to these complexes, are activated and produce a panel of cytokines. These cytokines (mainly IL-4, IL-5, IL-10, IL-13) help B-lymphocytes to complete their activation process into/differentiation process into antigen-specific antibody secreting plasma cells.

Immune Memory and the Booster Requirements (Fig. 3.3)

Why booster doses are not required for hepatitis B vaccine?

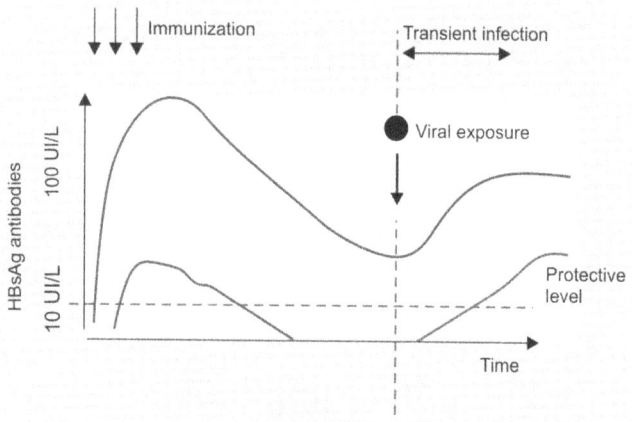

Fig. 3.3: Immune responses to hepatitis B immunization. Three vaccine doses induce in most individuals a strong increase in hepatitis B surface antigen (HBsAg) specific antibodies. These antibodies persist for a period of time. The duration of this protection is directly correlated to their initial levels. Initial levels progressively decline and disappear. If exposure to hepatitis B occurs in a vaccinated subject, vaccine antibodies neutralize the virus and memory B-cells are reactivated readily. This results in a boosting of HBsAg specific antibodies. Should exposure occur after the disappearance of HBsAg antibodies below protective levels, a transient infection will occur? However, rapid memory responses will allow the clearance of the viral infection without the development of chronic hepatitis and its complications.

Response to Polysaccharide Vaccines (Fig. 3.4)

The recognition of the importance of T helper cells in the induction of optimal antibody responses led to the design of novel vaccines against encapsulated bacteria. These vaccines are based on the conjugate of the bacterial polysaccharides, or its derivative.

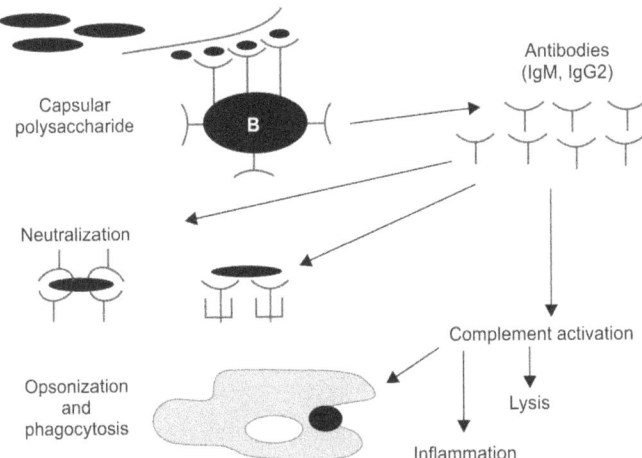

Fig. 3.4: Immune responses to polysaccharides. Capsular poly- saccharides (PS) are recognized directly by B-lymphocytes bearing antigen specific surface immunoglobulins. These B-cells produce IgM and IgG antibodies allowing bacterial neutralization, opsono-phagocytosis and complement activation that all contribute to bacterial clearance T-cells do not play a major role in responses to PS.

The Response to Glycoconjugate Vaccines (Fig. 3.5)

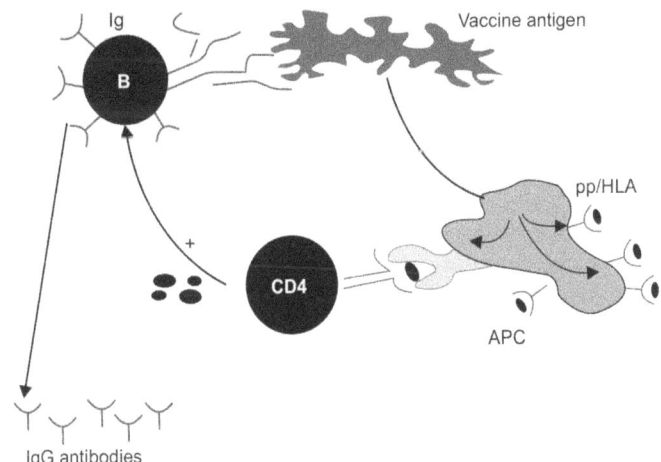

Fig. 3.5: Glycoconjugate vaccine—from B-cell to B- and T-cell responses. Conjugation of a bacterial PS to a carrier protein allows this protein to be processed and presented at the surface of antigen presenting cells (APC). This allows the activation of carrier specific CD4 T-cells that are capable of providing T-cell help to PS specific B-cells. As a result, B-cell differentiation is supported strongly and results in significantly higher antibody responses.

COMPOSITION OF VACCINES

Immunizing Antigens

Physicians should be familiar with the major constituents of the products they use. The major constituents are listed in the package inserts. If a vaccine is produced by different manufacturers, some differences may exist in the active and inert ingredients contained in the various products. The major constituents of vaccines include the following:

Active Immunizing Antigens

Some vaccines consist of a single antigen that is a highly defined constituent (e.g. tetanus or diphtheria toxoid); in other vaccines, the antigens are complex of less welldefined, e.g. live viruses or killed bacteria.

Suspending Fluid

The suspending fluid frequently is as simple as sterile water for injection or saline, but it may be a complex tissue-culture fluid. This fluid may contain proteins or other constituents derived from the medium and biologic system in which the vaccine is produced, e.g. egg antigens, gelatin, or tissue culture-derived antigens.

Preservatives, Stabilizers and Antibiotics

Trace amounts of chemicals, e.g. mercurial (such as thimerosal in some vaccines and immunoglobulin preparations) and certain antibiotics (such as neomycin or streptomycin) frequently are included to prevent bacterial growth onto stabilize the antigen. Allergic reactions may occur if the recipient is sensitive to one or more in identifying known host hypersensitivity to specific vaccine components.

Adjuvants

An aluminum salt is frequently used to increase immunogenicity and to prolong the stimulatory effect, particularly for vaccines containing inactivated bacteria or virus, toxoids). Investigational adjuvants are under evaluation.

Basics of Vaccinology

COMMON MISCONCEPTIONS ABOUT IMMUNIZATION

Claims	Facts
Natural methods of enhancing immunity are better than vaccinations	The only "natural way" to be immune is to have the disease. Immunity from a preventive vaccine provides protection against disease when a person is exposed to it in the future. That immunity is usually similar to what is acquired from natural infection, although several dose of a vaccine may have to be given for a child to develop a full immune response.
Epidemiology—often used to establish vaccine safety—is not science but number crunching	Epidemiology is a well-established scientific discipline that among other things, identifies the cause of diseases and factors that increase a person's risk for a disease.
Giving multiple vaccine at the same time causes an "overload" of the immune system.	Vaccination does not overburden a child's immune system; the recommended vaccines use only a small portion of the immune system's "memory".
Vaccines are ineffective.	Vaccines have spared millions of people the effects of devastating diseases.
Prior to the use of vaccination, these diseases had begun to decline because of improved nutrition and hygiene.	In the 19th and 20th centuries, some infectious diseases began to be better controlled because of improvements in sanitation, clean water, pasteurized milk, and pest control. However, vaccine-preventable diseases decrease dramatically after the vaccines for those diseases were licensed and were given to large numbers of children.
Vaccines cause poorly understood illnesses or disorders, such as autism, sudden infant death syndrome (SIDS), immune dysfunction, diabetes, neurologic disorders, allergic rhinitis, eczema, and asthma.	Scientific evidence does not support these claims. See Institute of Medicine (IOM) reports
Vaccines weaken the immune system.	If vaccines weakened the immune system, vaccinated children would be at greater risk from diseases not prevented by vaccines. Several studies have shown that this is not the case. Importantly, natural infections such as influenza, measles, and chickenpox do weaken the immune system, increasing the risk of other infections.

Contd...

Contd...

Claims	Facts
Giving many vaccines at the same time is untested.	Concomitant use studies require all new vaccines to be tested with existing vaccines. These studies are performed to ensure that new vaccines do not affect the safety or effectiveness of existing vaccines given at the same time and that existing vaccines administered at the same time do not affect the safety or effectiveness of new vaccines.

Source: Red Book 2018 AAP Publication.

LEARNING POINTS

- Immunity is of two types—Active and passive
- Vaccines act by inducing active immunity
- Vaccines are classified into live-attenuated, inactivated, polysaccharide, conjugate, subunit and toxoids.
- Each category of vaccine has its own characteristics.
- Misconceptions about immunization are baseless.

BIBLIOGRAPHY

1. American Academy of Pediatrics, Active Immunization. In: Pickering LK (Ed). 2009 Red Book: Report of the committee on Infectious Diseases, 28th edn. American Academy of Pediatrics, 2009. pp.52.
2. Centers for Disease Control and Preventions Epidemiology and Preventions of Vaccine Presentable Diseases. Atkinson W, Wolfe S, Hamborsky J, McIntyre L (Eds), 11th edn. Washington DC: Public Health Foundation, 2009.
3. Claire-Anne, Siegrist: Understanding immune response to Vaccines: Annales Nestle'. 2000;58:75-81.
4. Weinberg GA. Development of new vaccines. Annales Nestle'. 2000;58:96.
5. www.pharma-jp.org

CHAPTER 4

Immunization Schedules

Alok Gupta

INTRODUCTION

The most important aspect in immunization is scheduling the vaccine administration. A vaccine is selected based on its necessity, safety and efficacy. Vaccines are licensed only when they have passed three important tests in humans, viz. immunogenicity and safety, tolerance and safety, and field efficacy and safety which are known as phase I, phase II, and phase III trials, respectively. The vaccine also passes through sterility, purity and immunogenicity tests before it is marketed. The extensive literature supplied along with the vaccine packs contain details about the vaccine ingredients, their pharmacokinetics, contraindications, complications and the most important aspects of dose, route and schedule of vaccine administration which must be gone through carefully by every practitioner before administrating a vaccine/serum/immunoglobulin.

The World Health Organization (WHO) recommended Expanded Program on Immunization (EPI) schedule may be modified by the Ministries of health of individual countries based on local consideration. A National Schedule in which the vaccines are given free of cost should satisfy the following five criteria viz. epidemiological relevance, immunological appropriateness, technical feasibility, economic viability, and sociocultural acceptability.

NATIONAL IMMUNIZATION SCHEDULE, 2019

National immunization schedule for infants, children, and pregnant women are illustrated in **Table 4.1**.

Notes

- Introduction of rotavirus vaccine at 6, 10, and 14 weeks, pneumococcal vaccine at 14 weeks, 9 months and 18–24 months, measles and rubella (MR) vaccine in place of measles vaccine at 9 months and 15–18 months in a phased

Table 4.1: National Immunization Schedule for infants, children and pregnant women.

For pregnant women

Vaccine	Due age	Max age	Dose	Diluent	Route	Site
TT1/Td1	Early in pregnancy	Give as early as possible in pregnancy	0.5 mL	No	Intramuscular	Upper arm
TT2*/Td2*	4 weeks after TT-1/Td1*		0.5 mL	No	Intramuscular	Upper arm
TT/Td- Booster	If received two TT/Td doses in a pregnancy within the last 3 years*		0.5 mL	No	Intramuscular	Upper arm

For infants

Vaccine	Due age	Max age	Dose	Diluent	Route	Site
BCG	At birth	Till 1 year of age	(0.05 mL until 1 month) 0.1 mL beyond age 1 month	Yes Manufacturer supplied diluent (sodium chloride)	Intradermal	Upper arm (left)
Hepatitis B—birth dose	At birth	Within 24 hours	0.5 mL	No	Intramuscular	Anterolateral side of midthigh (left)

Contd...

Immunization Schedules

Contd...

Vaccine	Due age	Max age	For infants Dose	Diluent	Route	Site
OPV0	At birth	Within the first 15 days	2 drops	–	Oral	Oral
OPV 1, 2, and 3	At 6, 10, and 14 weeks	Till 5 years of age	2 drops	–	Oral	Oral
Pentavalent 1, 2, and 3** (Diphtheria + Pertussis + Tetanus + Hep B + Hib)	At 6, 10, and 14 weeks**	1 year of age	0.5 mL	No	Intramuscular	Anterolateral side of midthigh (left)
Fractional inactivated polio vaccine (IPV)	At 6 and 14 weeks	1 year of age	0.1 mL	No	Intradermal	Upper arm (right)
Rotavirus‡ (where applicable)	At 6, 10, and 14 weeks	1 year of age	5 drops	No	Oral	Oral
Pneumococcal conjugate vaccine (PCV) (where applicable)	At 6 and 14 weeks At 9 completed months—booster	1 year of age	0.5 mL	No	Intramuscular	Anterolateral side of midthigh (right)
Measles-rubella (MR) 1st dose#	At 9 completed months to 12 months	5 years of age	0.5 mL	Yes Manufacturer supplied diluent (sterile water)	Subcutaneous	Upper arm (right)

Contd...

Contd...

For infants

Vaccine	Due age	Max age	Dose	Diluent	Route	Site
Japanese encephalitis (JE)1@ (where applicable)	At 9–12 months@	15 years of age	0.5 mL	Yes Manufacturer supplied diluent (phosphate buffer solution)	Subcutaneous	Upper arm (left)
Vitamin A (1st dose)	At 9 months	5 years of age (1 lakh IU)	1 mL	-	Oral	Oral

For children

Vaccine	When to give	Max age	Dose	Diluent	Route	Site
DPT (diptheria, tetanus toxoids and pertussis) Booster-1	16–24 months	7 years of age	0.5 mL	No	Intramuscular	Anterolateral side of midthigh (left)
Measles-rubella 2nd dose##	16–24 months	5 years of age	0.5 mL	Yes Manufacturer supplied diluent (sterile water)	Subcutaneous	Upper arm (right)
OPV (oral polio vaccine) booster	16–24 months	5 years	2 drops	No	Oral	Oral

Contd...

Contd...

For children

Vaccine	When to give	Max age	Dose	Diluent	Route	Site
Japanese encephalitis 2@ (where applicable)	16–24 months@	Till 15 years of age	0.5 mL	Yes Manufacturer supplied diluent (phosphate buffer solution)	Subcutaneous	Upper arm (left)
Vitamin A$ (2nd– 9th dose)	At 16 months. Then, one dose every 6 months	Up to the age of 5 years	2 mL (2 lakh IU)	-	Oral	Oral
DPT Booster-2	5–6 years	7 years of age	0.5 mL	No	Intramuscular	Upper arm
TT/Td	10 and 16 years	16 years	0.5 mL	No	Intramuscular	Upper arm

*Give TT2/Td2 or booster doses before 36 weeks of pregnancy. However, give these even if more than 36 weeks have passed. Give TT/Td to a woman in labor, if she has not previously received TT/Td.

**Pentavalent vaccine is introduced in place of DPT and Hep B 1, 2, and 3.

‡Rotavirus vaccine is being introduced in phases.

##MR vaccine introduced in phases replacing measles vaccine in the Universal Immunization Program (UIP) schedule. If first dose delayed beyond 12 months ensure minimum 1 month gap between two MR doses.

@JE vaccine has been introduced in select endemic districts. If first dose delayed beyond 12 months ensure minimum 3 months gap between two JE doses.

$The 2nd–9th doses of Vitamin A can be administered to children 1–5 years old during biannual rounds, in collaboration with ICDS.

Note: Human papillomavirus (HPV) vaccine—presently not in schedule; Td— tetanus diphtheria to replace; TT— to be added in schedule.

manner throughout India have also been recommended by the National Technical Advisory Group on Immunization (NTAGI).
- Pregnant woman should receive two doses of tetanus toxoid at 4–6 weeks' interval. Three doses are recommended if not immunized till this age.
- Changes include introduction of hepatitis B (Hep B) vaccine, PENTA VAC and MR vaccine as incorporated in the modified UIP schedule.
- Introduction HPV vaccine, etc. are also in the cards.
- Single dose of Japanese encephalitis (JE) vaccine is administered to children below 10 years of age annually in a campaign mode in JE hyperendemic regions.

IAP IMMUNIZATION SCHEDULE, 2018–19

Refer to **Tables 4.2 to 4.5**.

GENERAL INSTRUCTIONS

- Vaccination at birth means as early as possible within 24–72 hours after birth or at least not later than 1 week after birth.
- Whenever multiple vaccinations are to be given simultaneously, they should be given within 24 hours if simultaneous administration is not feasible due to some reasons.
- The recommended age in weeks/months/years mean completed weeks/months/years.
- Any dose not administered at the recommended age should be administered at a subsequent visit, when indicated and feasible.
- The use of a combination vaccine generally is preferred over separate injections of its equivalent component vaccines.
- When two or more live parenteral/intranasal vaccines are not administered on the same day, they should be given at least 28 days (4 weeks) apart; this rule does not apply to live oral vaccines.
- Any interval can be kept between live and inactivated vaccines.
- If given <4 weeks apart, the vaccine given 2nd should be repeated.
- The minimum interval between 2 doses of same inactivated vaccines is usually 4 weeks (exception rabies). However, any

Table 4.2: IAP recommended immunization schedule for children aged 0–18 years (with range), 2018–19.

	Birth	6 weeks	10 weeks	14 weeks	6 months	9 months	12 months	13 months	15 months	16–18 months	2–3 years	4–6 years	9–14 years	15–18 years
BCG	BCG													
Hepatitis B	HB 1	HB 2	HB 3	HB* 4										
Polio	OPV 0	IPV** 1	IPV** 2	IPV** 3						IPV*** 1				
DTwP/DTaP		DTP 1	DTP 2	DTP 3						DTP B1		DTP B2		
HiB		HiB 1	HiB 2	HiB 3						HIB B1				
Pneumococcal		PCV 1	PCV 2	PCV 3					PCV B1				PCV	
Rotavirus		Rota1	Rota2	Rota3****										
MMR						MMR 1			MMR 2			MMR3/MMRV		
Varicella									Varicella 1			Varicella 2		
Hepatitis A							Hep A1			Hep. A2*****				
Typhoid					TCV#									
Influenza							Influenza (yearly)******							
Meningococcal						MCV 1	MCV 2				MCV			

Contd...

Contd...

	Birth	6 weeks	10 weeks	14 weeks	6 months	9 months	12 months	13 months	15 months	16–18 months	2–3 years	4–6 years	9–14 years	15–18 years
JE							JE 1	JE 2						
Tdap													Tdap	Td
HPV##													HPV 1 and 2	HPV 1, 2, and 3
Cholera									Cholera 1 and 2					

- Range of recommended age for all children
- Range of recommended age for high-risk children / area
- Range of recommended age for catch-up immunization
- Not recommended

*Fourth dose of Hep B permissible for combination vaccines only
**In case IPV is not available or feasible, the child should be offered bOPV (three doses). In such cases, give two fractional doses of IPV at 6 weeks and 14 weeks
***bOPV, if IPV booster (standalone or combination) not feasible
****Third dose not required for RV1. Catch-up up to 1 year of age in UIP schedule
*****Live attenuated Hep A vaccine: single dose only
******Begin influenza vaccination after 6 months of age, about 2–4 weeks before season; give two doses at the interval of 4 weeks during first year and then single dose yearly till 5 years of age
#TCV: Typhoid conjugate vaccine, ##HPV: human papillomavirus
Meningococcal vaccine (MCV): 9 months through 23 months: two doses, at least 3 months apart; 2 years through 55 years: single dose only
Japanese encephalitis (JE): For individuals living in endemic areas and for travelers to JE endemic areas provided their expected stay is for a minimum period of 4 weeks

HPV: two doses at 6 months interval 9–14 years age; Three doses (as 0, 1–2 and 6 month schedule) 15 years or older and immunocompromised
Cholera vaccine: Two doses 2 weeks apart for >1 year old; for individuals living in high endemic areas and travelling to areas where risk of transmission is very high.

Immunization Schedules

Table 4.3: IAP recommended vaccines for routine use.

Age (completed weeks/months/years)	Vaccines	Comments
Birth	BCG bOPV 0 Hep B1	• Administer these vaccines to all newborn within 7 days • Hepatitis B vaccine preferably within 24 hours
6 weeks	DTwP 1/DTaP 1 IPV1* Hep B2 Hib 1 Rotavirus 1 PCV 1	*DTP:* • Both DTwP and DTaP or their combinations can be used in primary series. • Immunogenicity and longevity of immune response is better with DTwP • DTaP/DTwP combination vaccines may be offered as an alternative in view of non-availability of standalone IPV preparations in the private sector. DTaP combination vaccines may be offered in view of parental anxiety of increased reactogenicity with DTwP. *Polio:* • No child should leave the facility without polio immunization (IPV* or OPV) • Continue birth dose OPV, and OPV on SIAs • Ideally IPV should replace OPV completely as early as possible. • Three doses of IM IPV in primary series is the best option. • Two doses of IM IPV instead of three for primary series if started at 8 weeks, with an interval of at least 8 weeks between two doses • In case IPV is not available or feasible, the child should be offered bOPV (three doses). In such cases, two fractional doses of IPV at a Government facility or at least one dose of a IM IPV either standalone or as a combination at least at 14 weeks of age.

Contd...

Partha's Immunization Digest

Contd...

Age (completed weeks/ months/years)	Vaccines	Comments
		Rotavirus: Two doses of RV1 or three doses of RV5 and RV 116E and BRV-PV RV1 can be given at 6 and 10 weeks. *PCV:* • Minimum age—6 weeks • Both PCV10 and PCV13 are licensed for children from 6 weeks to 5 years of age (although the exact labeling details may differ by country). • Additionally, PCV13 is licensed for the prevention of pneumococcal diseases in adults >50 years of age. • Primary schedule (for both PCV10 and PCV13)—three primary doses at 6, 10, and 14 weeks with a booster at age 12 through 15 months
10 weeks	DTwP 2/DTaP2 Hep B3 IPV2 Hib2 Rotavirus 2 PCV 2	*Rotavirus:* • Only two doses of RV1 are recommended. • If RV1 is chosen, the 2nd dose should be given at 10 weeks.
14 weeks	DTwP 3/DTaP3 Hep B4** IPV3 Hib3 Rotavirus3 PCV 3	• If any dose in series was RV 5 or RV 116E or BRV-P a total of three doses of RV vaccine should be administered. • **Fourth dose of Hep B permissible for combination vaccines only
6 months	Influenza vaccine (FLU vaccine)	*Influenza vaccine:* • IIV is recommended for routine immunization of children 6–59 months of age • Children 6–59 months are grouped as "high risk" and should be offered routine influenza vaccine • Beyond 5 years age only high-risk group • Both TIIV and QIIV are licensed in India.

Contd...

Immunization Schedules

Contd...

Age (completed weeks/ months/years)	Vaccines	Comments
		• QIIV is preferred if available. • *Minimum age:* 6 months for trivalent/quadrivalent IIV • *First time vaccination:* 6 months to below 9 years—two doses 1 month apart; 9 years and above—single dose • Annual revaccination with single dose, 2–4 weeks before flu season
6 months onwards	Typhoid conjugate vaccine (TCV)	• Single dose of any of the licensed TCV can be administered. • Can be administered with MMR vaccine if started at 9 months. • Sufficient data on safety and immunogenicity available for 25 µg TCV. • Currently available data is insufficient for making any recommendation for 5 µg TCV.
9 Months	*MMR1/MR*	*MMR/MR:* • Standalone measles will no more be available • Measles-containing vaccine (MMR/MR) ideally should not be administered after completing 9 months of age. • The 2nd dose must follow in 2nd year of life. • MR is not available in private sector as on date. If available, it should be offered instead of MMR. • Additional dose during MR campaign for children 9 months to 15 years, irrespective of previous vaccination status.
12 months	Hep A1 Japanese encephalitis (JE) vaccine [for endemic areas]	*Hepatitis A:* • Single dose for live-attenuated H2-strain Hep A vaccine • Two doses for all inactivated Hep A vaccines are recommended. *JE vaccine:* • Any of the licensed JE vaccine can be administered

Contd...

Contd...

Age (completed weeks/ months/years)	Vaccines	Comments
		• Two doses to be given 1 month apart • Live-attenuated SA-14-14-2 is not available in private market.
15 months	MMR 2 Varicella 1 PCV booster	*MMR:* • The 2nd dose must follow in 2nd year of life. • However, it can be given at any time 4–8 weeks after the 1st dose. *Varicella:* • The risk of breakthrough varicella is lower if given 15 months onwards. • MMRV as a combination is more reactogenic at 15–18 months.
16–18 months	DTwP B1/ DTaP B1 IPVB1*** Hib B1	• The first booster (4th dose) may be administered as early as age 12 months, provided at least 6 months after the third dose • Both DTwP and DTaP as combination vaccine can be offered. • No child should leave the facility without booster dose of IPV (standalone or combination) or bOPV vaccination.
18 months	Hep A2	*Hepatitis A:* 2nd dose for inactivated vaccines only
4–6 years	DTwP B2/ DTaP B2 MMRV or MMR3 + Varicella 2	*Tdap* is not recommended here. *Varicella:* • A total of two doses of varicella vaccine should be administered. • The second dose of varicella vaccine should be given at 4–6 years of age or at 3 months after the first dose. • MMRV can be used without increased risk of adverse reactions at this age. • MMR 3rd dose is recommended at 4–6 years of age.

Contd...

Contd...

Age (completed weeks/ months/years)	Vaccines	Comments
9–12 years	Tdap/Td HPV	*Tdap:* • Recommended age is 10 years. • Tdap is preferred to Td followed by Td every 10 years. • Minimum age for Tdap is 7 years. *HPV:* • Only two doses of either of the two HPV vaccines for girls aged 9–14 years. • For girls 15 years and older, and immunocompromised individuals three doses are recommended. • For two-dose schedule, the minimum interval between doses should be 6 months. • For three dose schedule, the doses can be administered at 0, 1, or 2 (depending on brand) and 6 months.

*In case IPV is not available or feasible, the child should be offered bOPV (three doses). In such cases, two fractional doses of IPV at a Government facility.
**Fourth dose of Hepatitis B permissible for combination vaccines only.
***bOPV, if IPV booster (standalone or combination) not feasible.
(Hep B: hepatitis B; IPV: inactivated polio vaccine; OPV: oral polio vaccine; PCV: pneumococcal conjugate vaccine; MMR: measles, mumps, and rubella; MR: measles-rubella; HPV: human papillomavirus)

Table 4.4: Major changes in IAP immunization timetable (2018–19).

Hepatitis B vaccine
- One dose of hepatitis B vaccine within 24 hours of birth
- In case of use of a combination vaccines a total of four doses of hepatitis B vaccine are justified.

DTwP, DTaP and DTP combination vaccines
- DTwP or DTaP can be offered in primary series.

Polio vaccines
- Ideally IPV should replace OPV as early as possible.
- Three doses of intramuscular IPV in primary series is the best option.
- Two doses of intramuscular IPV instead of three for primary series if started at 8 weeks, with an interval of 8 weeks between two doses is an alternative.
- In case IPV is not available or feasible, the child should be offered three doses of bOPV. In such cases, the child should be referred for two fractional doses of IPV at a Government facility at 6 and 14 weeks or at least one dose of intramuscular IPV, either standalone or as a combination vaccine, at 14 weeks of age.

Contd...

Contd...

Rotavirus vaccine
- In case of Rotavirus vaccine, RV1 can be used in 6 and 10 weeks schedule.

Influenza vaccine
- Inactivated influenza vaccine (either trivalent or quadrivalent) is recommended routinely to all children below 5 years of age starting from 6 months of age annually (2–4 weeks before influenza season).

Measles-containing vaccines
- Measles-containing vaccine (MMR/MR) should be administered after 9 months of age.
- MR vaccine as part of the national campaign is to be administered irrespective of previous vaccination.

Typhoid vaccines
- Single dose of any of typhoid conjugate vaccine (TCV 25 mg) is recommended from 6 months onwards and can be administered with MMR also.
- Booster dose of typhoid conjugate vaccine not recommended in subsequent years.

Rabies vaccines
- ACVIP IAP endorses administration of a 4-dose schedule of rabies vaccine recommended by WHO 2018 for postexposure prophylaxis.
- ACVIP also endorses administration of rabies monoclonal antibody as an alternative to rabies immunoglobulin for category-III bites.

(ACVIP: Advisory Committee on Vaccines and Immunization Practices; IAP: Indian Academy of Pediatrics; IPV: injectable polio vaccine; OPV: oral polio vaccine; bOPV: bivalent oral polio vaccine; MR: measles-rubella vaccine; MMR: measles, mumps, and rubella vaccine)

Table 4.5: Catch-up vaccination schedule (for an unimmunized child).

Visit	Suggested vaccines
First visit	- MMR if 9 months' plus - DTwP1/DTaP1 (Tdap if 7 years or more) - bOPV1/IPV1 (only if less than 5 years) - Hib 1 (only if less than 5 years) - Hep B1
Second visit (after 1 month of first visit)	- BCG (only in less than 5 years) - DTwP2/DTaP2 (Td if 7 years or more) - bOPV2 (if OPV given earlier) - Hep B2 - Hib 2 (if less than 15 months)
Third visit (after 1 month of second visit)	- bOPV3/IPV2 - MMR2 (if more than 12 months) - TCV if age 9–12 months - Typhoid (TCV or Vi) (if more than 2 years)
Fourth visit (6 months after first visit)	- DTwP3/DTaP3 (Td/Tdap if 7 years or more) - bOPV4/IPVB1 - Hep B3

interval can be kept between doses of different inactivated vaccines.
- Vaccine doses administered up to 4 days before the minimum interval or age can be counted as valid (exception rabies). If the vaccine is administered >5 days before minimum period it is counted as invalid dose.
- Any number of antigens can be given on the same day.
- Changing needles between drawing vaccine into the syringe and injecting it into the child is not necessary.
- Once the protective cap on a single-dose vial has been removed, the vaccine should be discarded at the end of the immunization session because it may not be possible to determine if the rubber seal has been punctured.
- Different vaccines should not be mixed in the same syringe unless specifically licensed and labeled for such use.
- Patients should be observed for an allergic reaction for 15-20 minutes after receiving immunization(s).
- When necessary, two vaccines can be given in the same limb at a single visit.
- The anterolateral aspect of the thigh is the preferred site for two simultaneous intramuscular (IM) injections because of its greater muscle mass.
- The distance separating the two injections is arbitrary but should be at least 1 inch so that local reactions are unlikely to overlap.
- Although most experts recommend *aspiration* by gently pulling back on the syringe before the injection is given, there are no data to document the necessity for this procedure. If blood appears after negative pressure, the needle should be withdrawn and another site should be selected using a new needle.
- A previous immunization with a dose that was less than the standard dose or one administered by a nonstandard route should not be counted, and the person should be re-immunized as appropriate for age.

SPECIFIC INSTRUCTIONS

Bacillus Calmette–Guérin (BCG) Vaccine

Routine Vaccination

Should be given at birth or at first contact.

Catch-up Vaccination

May be given up to 5 years.

Hepatitis B (Hep B) Vaccine

Routine Vaccination

- Minimum age— birth
- Administer monovalent Hep B vaccine to all newborn within 48 hours of birth
- Monovalent Hep B vaccine should be used for doses administered before age 6 weeks.
- Administration of a total of four doses of Hep B vaccine is permissible when a combination vaccine containing Hep B is administered after the birth dose.
- Infants who did not receive a birth dose should receive 3 doses of a Hep B containing vaccine starting as soon as feasible.
- The ideal minimum interval between dose 1 and dose 2 is 4 weeks, and between dose 2 and dose 3 is 8 weeks. Ideally, the final (3rd or 4th) dose in the Hep B vaccine series should be administered no earlier than age 24 weeks and at least 16 weeks after the first dose, whichever is later.
- *Hep B vaccine may also be given in any of the following schedules:* Birth, 1, and 6 months; birth, 6 and 14 weeks; 6, 10, and 14 weeks; birth, 6 ,10, and 14 weeks, etc. All schedules are protective.

Catch-up vaccination

- Administer the 3-dose series to those not previously vaccinated.
- In catch-up vaccination use 0, 1, and 6 months' schedule.

Poliovirus Vaccines

Routine Vaccination

- Inactivated polio vaccine (IPV) should replace oral polio vaccine (OPV) as soon as possible.
- Birth dose of OPV usually does not lead to vaccine-associated paralytic polio (VAPP).
- OPV in place of IPV, if IPV is unfeasible, minimum three doses.

- Additional doses of OPV on all supplementary immunization activities (SIAs).
- *IPV:* Minimum age—6 weeks
- *IPV:* Two instead of three doses can be also used if primary series started at 8 weeks and the interval between the doses is kept 8 weeks.
- No child should leave your facility without polio immunization (IPV or OPV), if indicated by the schedule!
- *Intradermal vaccination:* Advisory Committee on Vaccines and Immunization Practices (ACVIP) does not approve the use of *intradermal fractional-dose IPV* (ID-fIPV) for office-practice. However, considering the extreme shortage of IPV and the urgent need of providing immunity against type-2 poliovirus, the committee has now provisionally accepted the immune-protection accorded by two ID-fIPV doses given at 6- and 14-week as moderately effective against type-2 polioviruses. However, another full dose of IM-IPV should be offered at least at 8 weeks' interval of the second dose of ID-fIPV.
- If a child has received one dose of ID-fIPV at 6 weeks, two more full doses of IM-IPV should be offered at least 8 weeks after the first dose.
- The minimum interval between the 2nd and 3rd dose should also be at least 8 weeks.

Catch-up Vaccination

IPV catch-up schedule: 2 doses at 2 months apart followed by a booster after 6 months of previous dose.

Diphtheria and Tetanus Toxoids and Pertussis (DTP) Vaccine

Routine Vaccination

- Minimum age—6 weeks
- The first booster (4th dose) may be administered as early as age 12 months, provided at least 6 months have elapsed since the third dose.
- DTaP or DTwP can be offered in primary series.
- DTaP may be preferred to DTwP in children with history of severe adverse effects after previous dose(s) of DTwP or children with neurologic disorders.

- First and second boosters may also be of DTwP. However, considering a higher reactogenicity, DTaP can be considered for the boosters.
- ACVIP does not approve the use of Tdap as second booster of DTP schedule!
- If any *acellular pertussis* containing vaccine is used, it must at least have three or more components in the product.
- No need of repeating/giving additional doses of whole-cell pertussis (wP) vaccine to a child who has earlier completed their primary schedule with acellular pertussis (aP) vaccine-containing products.

Catch-up Vaccination

- *Catch-up schedule:* The 2nd childhood booster is not required if the last dose has been given beyond the age of 4 years.
- *Catch-up below 7 years*: DTwP/DTaP at 0, 1 and 6 months
- *Catch-up above 7 years:* Tdap, diphtheria toxoids (Td), and Td at 0, 1, and 6 months.

Tetanus and Diphtheria Toxoids and Acellular Pertussis (TDAP) Vaccine

Routine Vaccination

- Minimum age—7 years (Adacel® is approved for 11–64 years by ACIP and 4–64 years old by Food and Drugs Administration (FDA), while Boostrix® for 10 years and older by ACIP and 4 years of age and older by FDA in US).
- Administer one dose of Tdap vaccine to all adolescents aged 11 through 12 years.
- *Tdap during pregnancy:* One dose of Tdap vaccine to pregnant mothers/adolescents during each pregnancy (preferred during 27 through 36 weeks' gestation) regardless of number of years from prior Td or Tdap vaccination.

Catch-up Vaccination

- Catch-up above 7 years—Tdap, Td, at 0, 1 and 6 months.
- Persons aged 7 through 10 years who are not fully immunized with the childhood DTwP/DTaP vaccine series, should receive Tdap vaccine as the first dose in the catch-up series; if additional doses are needed, use Td vaccine. For these children, an adolescent Tdap vaccine should not be given.

- Persons aged 11 through 18 years who have not received Tdap vaccine should receive a dose followed by tetanus and diphtheria toxoids (Td) booster doses every 10 years thereafter.
- Tdap vaccine can be administered regardless of the interval since the last tetanus and diphtheria toxoid—containing vaccine.
- Tdap vaccine should not be used as second booster for DTP series.

Haemophilus Influenzae Type B (Hib) Conjugate Vaccine

Routine Vaccination

- Minimum age—6 weeks
- Primary series includes Hib conjugate vaccine at ages 6, 10, 14 weeks with a booster at age 12 through 18 months.

Catch-up Vaccination

- Catch-up is recommended till 5 years of age
- 6–12 months—two primary doses 4 weeks apart and 1 booster
- 12–15 months—one primary dose and 1 booster
- Above 15 months—single dose
- If the first dose was administered at age 7 through 11 months, administer the second dose at least 4 weeks later and a final dose at age 12–18 months at least 8 weeks after the second dose.

Pneumococcal Conjugate Vaccines (PCVs)

Routine Vaccination

- Minimum age—6 weeks
- Both PCV10 and PCV13 are licensed for children from 6 weeks to 5 years of age (although the exact labeling details may differ by country). Additionally, PCV13 is licensed for the prevention of pneumococcal diseases in adults >50 years of age.
- Primary schedule (for both PCV10 and PCV13)—three primary doses at 6, 10, and 14 weeks with a booster at age 12 through 15 months.

Catch-up Vaccination

- Administer one dose of PCV13 or PCV10 to all healthy children aged 24 through 59 months who are not completely vaccinated for their age.
  - *For PCV13:* Catch-up in 6–12 months—two doses 4 weeks apart and 1 booster; 12–23 months—two doses 8 weeks apart; 24 months and above—single dose.
  - *For PCV10:* Catch-up in 6–12 months—two doses 4 weeks apart and 1 booster; 12 months to 5 years—two doses 8 weeks apart.
- *Vaccination of persons with high-risk conditions:*
  - PCV and pneumococcal polysaccharide vaccine (PPSV) both are used in certain high-risk group of children.
  - For children aged 24 through 71 months with certain underlying medical conditions, administer one dose of PCV13 if three doses of PCV were received previously, or administer two doses of PCV13 at least 8 weeks apart if fewer than three doses of PCV were received previously.
  - A single dose of PCV13 may be administered to previously unvaccinated children aged 6 through 18 years who have anatomic or functional asplenia (including sickle cell disease), HIV infection or an immunocompromising condition, cochlear implant or cerebrospinal fluid leak.
  - Administer PPSV23 at least 8 weeks after the last dose of PCV to children aged 2 years or older with certain underlying medical conditions.

Pneumococcal Polysaccharide Vaccine (PPSV23)

- Minimum age—2 years
- Not recommended for routine use in healthy individuals. Recommended only for the vaccination of persons with certain high-risk conditions.
- Administer PPSV at least 8 weeks after the last dose of PCV to children aged 2 years or older with certain underlying medical conditions like anatomic or functional asplenia (including sickle cell disease), HIV infection, cochlear implant or cerebrospinal fluid leak.
- An additional dose of PPSV should be administered after 5 years to children with anatomic/functional asplenia or an immunocompromising condition.

Immunization Schedules

- PPSV should never be used alone for prevention of pneumococcal diseases amongst high-risk individuals.
- Children with following medical conditions for which PPSV23 and PCV13 are indicated in the age group 24 through 71 months:
  - Immunocompetent children with chronic heart disease (particularly cyanotic congenital heart disease and cardiac failure); chronic lung disease (including asthma if treated with high-dose oral corticosteroid therapy), diabetes mellitus; cerebrospinal fluid leaks; or cochlear implant.
  - Children with anatomic or functional asplenia (including sickle cell disease and other hemoglobinopathies, congenital or acquired asplenia, or splenic dysfunction);
  - Children with immunocompromising conditions: HIV infection, chronic renal failure and nephrotic syndrome, diseases associated with treatment with immunosuppressive drugs or radiation therapy, including malignant neoplasms, leukemias, lymphomas and Hodgkin's disease; or solid organ transplantation, congenital immunodeficiency.

Rotavirus (RV) Vaccines

Routine Vaccination

- Minimum age—6 weeks for all available brands [RV1 (Rotarix), RV5 (RotaTeq) and RV116E (Rotavac)].
- *Only two doses of RV1 are recommended:*
  1. RV1 should preferably be employed in 10- and 14-week schedule, instead of 6 and 10 week; the former schedule is found to be far more immunogenic than the later.
  2. If any dose in series was RV5 or RV116E or vaccine product is unknown for any dose in the series, a total of three doses of RV vaccine should be administered.

Catch-up Vaccination

- The maximum age for the first dose in the series is 14 weeks, 6 days.
- Vaccination should not be initiated for infants aged 15 weeks, 0 days or older.
- The maximum age for the final dose in the series is 8 months, 0 days.

Measles, Mumps, and Rubella (MMR) Vaccine

Routine Vaccination

- Minimum age—9 months or 270 completed days
- Administer the first dose of MMR vaccine at age 9 through 12 months, the second dose at age 15 through 18 months, and final (the 3rd) dose at age 4 through 6 years.
- The 2nd dose must follow in 2nd year of life. However, it can be given at any time 4–8 weeks after the 1st dose.
- No need to give standalone measles vaccine.

Catch-up Vaccination

- Ensure that all school-aged children and adolescents have had at least two doses of MMR vaccine (three doses if the 1st dose is received before 12 months).
- The minimum interval between the two doses is 4 weeks.
- One dose if previously vaccinated with one dose (two doses if the 1st dose is received before 12 months).
- *Standalone* measles/any measles-containing vaccine or MMR can be administered to infants aged 6 through 8 months during outbreaks. However, this dose should not be counted.

Varicella Vaccine

Routine Vaccination

- Minimum age—12 months
- Administer the first dose at age 15 through 18 months and the second dose at age 4 through 6 years.
- The second dose may be administered before age 4 years, provided at least 3 months have elapsed since the first dose. If the second dose was administered at least 4 weeks after the first dose, it can be accepted as valid.
- The risk of breakthrough varicella is lower, if given 15 months onwards.

Catch-up Vaccination

- Ensure that all persons aged 7 through 18 years without *evidence of immunity* have two doses of the vaccine.

- For children aged 12 months through 12 years, the recommended minimum interval between doses is 3 months. However, if the second dose was administered at least 4 weeks after the first dose, it can be accepted as valid.
- For persons aged 13 years and older, the minimum interval between doses is 4 weeks.
- For persons without evidence of immunity, administer two doses if not previously vaccinated or the second dose if only one dose has been administered.
- Evidence of immunity to varicella includes any of the following:
  - Documentation of age-appropriate vaccination with a varicella vaccine
  - Laboratory evidence of immunity or laboratory confirmation of disease
  - Diagnosis or verification of a history of varicella disease by a health-care provider
  - Diagnosis or verification of a history of herpes zoster by a healthcare provider.

Hepatitis A (Hep A) Vaccines

Routine Vaccination

- Minimum age—12 months
- *Inactivated Hep A vaccine:* Start the two-dose Hep A vaccine series for children aged 12 through 23 months; separate the two doses by 6–18 months.
- *Live attenuated H2-strain Hep A vaccine:* Single dose starting at 12 months and through 23 months of age.

Catch-up Vaccination

- Either of the two vaccines can be used in "catch-up" schedule beyond 2 years of age.
- Administer two doses of inactivated vaccine at least 6 months apart to unvaccinated persons.
- Only single dose of live attenuated H2-strain vaccine.
- For catch-up vaccination, pre-vaccination screening for Hepatitis A antibody is recommended in children older than 10 years as at this age the estimated seropositive rates exceed 50%.

Typhoid Vaccines

Routine Vaccination

- Both Vi-PS conjugate and Vi-PS (polysaccharide) vaccines are available.
- *Minimum ages:*
  - Vi-PS conjugate (Typbar-TCV®)—6 months
  - Vi-PS conjugate (PedaTyph®)—6 months
  - Vi-PS (polysaccharide) vaccines—2 years, booster every 3 years.
- *Vaccination schedule:*
  - Single dose of any of typhoid conjugate vaccine (TCV 25 mg) is recommended from 6 months onwards and can be administered with MMR also.
  - Booster dose of typhoid conjugate vaccine not recommended in subsequent years.
  - No evidence of hyporesponsiveness on repeated revaccination of Vi-polysaccharide vaccine so far. However, typhoid conjugate vaccine should be preferred over unconjugated Vi-PS vaccine.

Catch-up Vaccination

Recommended throughout the adolescent period, i.e. up to 18 years of age.

Influenza Vaccine

Routine Vaccination

- *Minimum age:*
  - 6 months for trivalent or quadrivalent IIV
  - 2 years for live-attenuated influenza vaccine (LAIV).
- *IIV:* IAP recommends routine vaccination of all children from 6 months to 5 years of age and to children at high risk above 5 years of age.
- *For most healthy children LAIV:* Recommended for only healthy children aged 2–18 years.
- LAIV should not be administered to following category of children:
  - WHO have experienced severe allergic reactions to LAIV, any of its components, or to a previous dose of any other influenza vaccine
  - Children 2 through 17 years receiving aspirin or aspirin-containing products

- Children with immunodeficiency
- Children 2 through 4 years of age with asthma or who had wheezing in the past 12 months
- Children who have taken influenza antiviral medications in the previous 48 hours
- Children who have experienced severe allergic reactions to LAIV, any of its components.

- *IIV—first time vaccination:* 6 months to below 9 years—two doses 1 month apart; 9 years and above—single dose.
- Annual revaccination with single dose
- *LAIV:* 2–9 years—one or two doses as per the ACVIP annual recommendations; 9 years and above—single dose.
  Dosage:
- *IIV:* Aged 6–35 months—0.25 mL; 3 years and above—0.5 mL
- *LAIV:* See product insert of the available formulation
- *Best time to vaccinate:*
  - As soon as the new vaccine is released and available in the market
  - Just before the onset of rainy season
  - Some regions may consider vaccination just prior to onset of winters based on local epidemiology data.

Human Papillomavirus (HPV) Vaccines

Routine Vaccination

- Minimum age—9 years
- HPV4 [Gardasil®] and HPV2 [Cervarix®] are licensed and available.
- Only two doses of either of the two HPV vaccines (HPV4 and HPV2) for adolescent/preadolescent girls aged 9–14 years.
- For girls 15 years and older, and immunocompromised individuals three doses are recommended.
- For two-dose schedule, the minimum interval between doses should be 6 months.
- Either HPV4 (0, 2, 6 months) or HPV2 (0, 1, 6 months) is recommended in a three-dose series for females aged 15 years and older.
- HPV4 can also be given in a three-dose series for males aged 11 or 12 years, but not yet licensed for use in males in India.
- The vaccine series can be started beginning at age 9 years.
- For three-dose schedule, administer the 2nd dose 1–2 months after the 1st dose and the 3rd dose 6 months after the 1st dose (at least 24 weeks after the first dose).

Catch-up Vaccination

- Administer the vaccine series to females (either HPV2 or HPV4) at age 14 through 45 years if not previously vaccinated.
- Use recommended routine dosing intervals (as above) for vaccine series catch-up.

Meningococcal Vaccine

- Recommended only for certain high-risk group of children, during outbreaks, and international travelers, including students going for study abroad and travelers to Hajj and sub-Sahara Africa.
- Both meningococcal conjugate vaccines (Quadrivalent MenACWY-D, Menactra® by Sanofi Pasteur and monovalent group A, PsA-TT, MenAfriVac® by Serum Institute of India) and polysaccharide vaccines (bi- and quadrivalent) are licensed in India. PsA-TT is not freely available in market.
- Conjugate vaccines are preferred over polysaccharide vaccines due to their potential for herd protection and their increased immunogenicity, particularly in children <2 years of age.
- *MCV can be administered:*
  - 9 months through 23 months—two doses at least 3 months apart
  - 2 years through 55 years—single dose.

Cholera Vaccine

- Minimum age—1 year [inactivated whole cell *Vibrio cholera* (Shanchol®)]
- Not recommended for routine use in healthy individuals; recommended only for the vaccination of persons residing in highly endemic areas and traveling to areas where risk of transmission is very high such as Kumbh mela, etc.
- Two doses 2 weeks apart for >1-year-old.

Japanese Encephalitis (JE) Vaccine

Routine Vaccination

- Recommended only for individuals living in endemic areas till 18 years of age.

- The vaccine should be offered to the children residing in rural areas only and those planning to visit endemic areas (depending upon the duration of stay).
- Three types of new generation JE vaccines are licensed in India: one, live-attenuated, cell culture derived SA-14-14-2, and two inactivated JE vaccines, namely *"vero cell culture-derived SA 14-14-2 JE vaccine' (JEEV® by BE India) and "vero cell culture-derived, 821564XY, JE vaccine" (JENVAC® by Bharat Biotech).*
- *Live-attenuated, cell culture derived SA-14-14-2:*
  - Minimum age—8 months
  - Two dose schedule, first dose at 9 months along with measles vaccine and second at 16–18 months along with DTP booster
  - Not available in private market for office use.
- *Inactivated cell culture derived SA-14-14-2 (JEEV® by BE India):*
  - Minimum age—1 year (US FDA—2 months)
  - Primary immunization schedule: 2 doses of 0.25 mL each administered intramuscularly on days 0 and 28 for children aged ≥1 to ≤3 years
  - 2 doses of 0.5 mL for children >3 years and adults aged ≥18 years
  - Need of boosters still undetermined
- *Inactivated Vero cell culture-derived Kolar strain, 821564XY, JE vaccine (JENVAC® by Bharat Biotech)*
- Minimum age—1 year.
- Primary immunization schedule—2 doses of 0.5 mL each administered intramuscularly at 4 weeks interval.
- Need of boosters still undetermined.

Catch-up Vaccination

All susceptible children up to 18 years should be administered during disease outbreak/ahead of anticipated outbreak in campaigns.

Rabies Vaccine

- Pre-exposure prophylaxis (Pre-EP) is recommended in following two situations:
  1. Children exposed to pets in home

2. Children identified to have a higher risk of being bitten by dogs.
- WHO recommends a "1-site vaccine administration on Days 0 and 7 for intramuscular administration" for pre-exposure prophylaxis (9).
- For post-exposure prophylaxis (PEP), recently the WHO [9] has recommended a new 4-dose schedule of either of the following: (i) 1-site intramuscular administration of vaccine on Days 0, 3, 7 and between Day 14 and 28, or (ii) 2-sites intramuscular administration on Days 0 and 1-site on days 7, 21 (intramuscular).
- Not given in the gluteal region
- Rabies monoclonal antibody is as effective as rabies immunoglobulin (Ig) and is a cost-effective option in category 3 bites.

IAP RECOMMENDED VACCINES FOR HIGH-RISK* CHILDREN

Vaccines under Special Circumstances

1. Influenza vaccine
2. Meningococcal vaccine
3. Japanese encephalitis vaccine
4. Cholera vaccine
5. Rabies vaccine
6. Yellow fever vaccine
7. Pneumococcal polysaccharide vaccine (PPSV 23).

- The IAP endorses the continued use of whole-cell pertussis vaccine because of its proven efficacy and safety. Acellular

---

* High-risk Category of Children
- Congenital or acquired immunodeficiency (including HIV infection)
- Chronic cardiac, pulmonary (including asthma if treated with prolonged high-dose oral corticosteroids), hematologic, renal (including nephrotic syndrome), liver disease and diabetes mellitus
- Children on long-term steroids, salicylates, immunosuppressive or radiation therapy
- Diabetes mellitus, cerebrospinal fluid leak, cochlear implant, malignancies
- Children with functional/anatomic asplenia/hyposplenia
- During disease outbreaks
- Laboratory personnel and healthcare workers
- Travelers
- Children having pets in home
- Children perceived with higher threat of being bitten by dogs such as hostellers, risk of stray dog menace while going outdoor.

pertussis vaccines may have fewer side-effects (such as fever, local reactions at injection site irritability etc.), but this minor advantage does not justify the high cost involved in the routine use of this vaccine.
- If the mother is known to be HBsAg negative, HB vaccine can be given along with DTPw at 6, 10, 14 weeks/6 months. If the mother's HBsAg status is not known, it is advisable to start vaccination soon after birth to prevent perinatal transmission of the disease. If the mother is HBsAg positive (and especially HBeAg positive), the baby should be given Hepatitis B immune globulin (HBIG) within 12 hours of birth, along with HB vaccine.
- Varicella, hepatitis A and pneumococcal conjugate vaccines should be offered to children of affordable parents.
- Combination vaccines can be used to reduce the number of pricks and to decrease the number of clinic visits. The manufacturer's instructions should be followed strictly whenever extemporal mixing of vaccines is done in the same syringe prior to injection.
- At present, the typhoid vaccine available in our country is the Vi polysaccharide vaccine (Both conjugate and unconjugated vaccine formulations are available). Revaccination may be carried out every 3–4 years.
- Under special circumstances (e.g. epidemics), measles vaccine may be given earlier than 9 months, followed by routine measles vaccine dose at 9 months and MMR vaccine dose at 15 months.
- During pregnancy, the interval between the two doses of TT should be at least 1 month.
- We should continue to use OPV (in future bOPV will be used for routine and pulse polio immunization replacing tOPV) to sustain mucosal immunity as recommended by IEAG. Sequential bOPV-IPV use will help eradication of polio due to cVDPV.
- OPV must be given to children less than 5 years of age at the time of each supplementary immunization activity.

Points to Note

- To prevent perinatal transmission, birth dose of Hep B vaccine within 12 hours is essential.
- BCG and OPV vaccines, if missed at birth can be given within first 2 weeks after birth.

- Combined DTPw-HB-Hib vaccine formulation can be given at 6, 10, and 14 weeks for babies born to HBs Ag negative mothers.
- For babies who receive monovalent hepatitis B vaccine at birth combined DTPw—HB vaccine can be given at 6 and 14 weeks for the 2nd and 3rd doses. No boosters are recommended.
- In addition to "Routine OPV doses", the recommended "Pulse OPV doses" are also mandatory during PPI campaigns.
- For typhoid immunization, earliest age recommended: Typhoid conjugate vaccine at 9 months' Vi antigen (1st dose)/TCV booster at 2 years and Booster every 3 years only if Ty-ViPS vaccine used.
- Apart from the earliest age indicated, MMR, typhoid, varicella and hepatitis A vaccines can be given at any age, relevant to local epidemiology. MMR vaccine can be started at 9 months earliest.
- Td (tetanus/diphtheria toxoid) can be preferred to TT (tetanus toxoid) where available and Tdap if adolescent pertussis is endemic in your region.
- Varicella and Hep A are additional vaccines as recommended by Indian Academy of Pediatrics.
- Indigenous combined DTPw/HB/Hib vaccine (Pentavalent) when available can be given at 6, 10, and 14 weeks.
- For aluminium salt adjuvanted vaccines where multiple primary doses are needed, they should be administered preferably at the recommended interval of 4 weeks, however, care should be taken to complete the 3rd dose within 1 year of starting the first dose.
- The booster dose for Hep A should be completed at 6–12 months.
- The booster for DTP, OPV and Hib are best completed between 15 and 18 months of age.
- The second dose of varicella vaccine for children aged 4–6 years should be completed at 4–8 weeks interval after the 1st dose.
- National immunization schedule prefers DT whereas IAP recommends DTP at 5 years.

The recommended route and site of vaccination should be strictly adhered to as in guidelines. In general, aluminum adjuvanted vaccines should not be given SC/ID for fear of local reaction and poor immunogenicity. They should always be given by the IM route, e.g. DTP, DT, TT, Hib, HB, hepatitis A, all DTP combination vaccines, etc. Subcutaneous route is recommended for measles, MMR, varicella (live-attenuated virus) and intradermal route is recommended for BCG (live-attenuated bacteria). The preferred site for injection is anterolateral thigh in newborns and infants and deltoid in older children and adolescents.

Adolescent immunization schedule is currently picking up in India. Even though the government of India recommends only TT vaccine, IAP recommends MMR, typhoid, varicella, Hep B and Hep A, Tdap, HPV vaccines apart from TT, for those who are not already immunized during childhood. Countries like USA warrant that adolescents seeking admission to their educational institutions should have been immunized with two doses of MMR, Hep A, and varicella vaccines apart from other recognized vaccines before the student enters the United States meningococcal vaccine is mandatory for entrants to UK.

IMMUNIZATION OF ADOLESCENTS (TABLE 4.6)

Adolescence should be considered an appropriate age for *catch-up* immunization for administration of certain vaccines which might not have been available earlier or missed (**Table 4.6**). Preferred age for administration is at 10–12 years but catch-up may be done till 18 years. Vaccines to be considered for adolescents if not received earlier are detailed in **Table 4.6**.

Table 4.6: Immunization schedule for adolescents.

Tdap/Td	Tdap preferred and then Td every 10 years
MMR	Two doses at 4–8 weeks' interval
Hepatitis B	Three doses at 0, 1 and 6 months
Typhoid	One dose every three years if Ty Vi used else only one dose of TCV when given after 2 years of age
HPV	Three doses at 0, 1–2 and 6 months, 2 doses 0–6 months if given to girls aged 9–14 years
Hepatitis A*	Two doses at 0, 6 months (prior check for Anti-HAV IgG is likely to be cost effective)
Varicella*	Two doses at 4–8 weeks' interval

*After one to one discussion with parents.
Source: IAP Guidebook on Immunization. IAP Publication; 2018.

WHO IMMUNIZATION TIMETABLE, 2019 (TABLE 4.7)

Table 4.7: Summary of WHO Position Papers—recommendations for routine immunization.

Antigen		Children	Adolescents	Adults	Considerations
Recommendations for all immunization programs					
BCG		1 dose			• Birth dose and HIV; Universal vs selective vaccination; • Co-administration; Vaccination of older age groups • Pregnancy
Hepatitis B		3–4 doses	3 doses (for high-risk groups if not previously immunized)		• Birth dose • Premature and low birth weight • Co-administration and combination vaccine • Definition high-risk
Polio		3–4 doses (at least one dose of IPV) with DTPCV			• bOPV birth dose • Type of vaccine • Transmission and importation risk criteria
DTP-containing vaccine (DTPCV)		3 doses	2 boosters 12–23 months (DTPCV) and 4–7 years (Td/ DT containing vaccine)	1 booster 9–15 years (Td)	• Delayed/interrupted schedule • Combination vaccine • Maternal immunization
Haemophilus influenzae type b	Option 1	3 doses, with DTPCV			• Single dose if >12 months of age • Not recommended for children >5 years old • Delayed/interrupted schedule • Co-administration and combination vaccine
	Option 2	2 or 3 doses, with booster at least 6 months after last dose			

Immunization Schedules

Contd...

Antigen		Children	Adolescents	Adults	Considerations
Pneumococcal (Conjugate)	Option 1	3 doses (3p+0) with DTPCV			• Schedule options (3p+0 vs 2p+1) • Vaccine options • HIV + and preterm neonate booster
	Option 2	2 doses before 6 months of age, plus booster dose at 9–15 months of age (2p+1) with DTPCV			
Rotavirus		2–3 doses depending on product with DTPCV			• Vaccine options • Not recommended if >24 months old
Measles		2 doses			• Combination vaccine • HIV early vaccination • Pregnancy
Rubella		1 dose	1 dose (adolescent girls and women of child-bearing age if not previously vaccinated)		• Achieve and sustain 80% coverage • Combination vaccine and Co-administration • Pregnancy
HPV			2 doses (females)		• Target 9–14 year old girls; Multiage cohort vaccination; • Pregnancy • Older age groups ≥15 years 3 doses • HIV and immunocompromised

Contd...

Contd...

Antigen		Children	Adolescents	Adults	Considerations
Recommendations for certain regions					
Japanese encephalitis		*Inactivated Vero cell-derived vaccine:* Generally 2 doses *Live attenuated vaccine:* 1 dose *Live recombinant vaccine:* 1 dose			• Vaccine options and manufacturer's recommendations • Pregnancy • Immunocompromised
Yellow fever		1 dose, with measles containing vaccine			
Tick-Borne encephalitis		3 doses (>1 year FSME-Immun and Encepur; >3 years TBE-Moscow and EnceVir) with at least 1 booster dose (every 3 years for TBE-Moscow and EnceVir)			• Definition of high-risk • Vaccine options • Timing of booster
Recommendations for some high-risk populations					
Typhoid		*Typhoid conjugate vaccine (Typbar-TCV®):* 1 dose; *Vi polysaccharide (ViPS):* 1 dose; *Ty21a live oral vaccine:* 3–4 doses; *Revaccination for ViPS & Ty21a;* every 3–7 years			• Definition of high-risk • Vaccine options
Cholera		*Dukoral (WC-rBS):* 3 doses ≥2–5 years, booster every 6 months; 2 doses adults/children ≥6 years, booster every 2nd year; *Shanchol, Euvchol & mORCVAX:* 2 doses ≥1 years, booster dose after 2 years			• Minimum age • Definition of high-risk
Meningococcal	MenA conjugate	1 dose 9–18 months (5μg)			2 doses if < 9 months with 8 week interval
	MenC conjugate	2 doses (2–11 months) with booster 1 year after 1 dose (≥12 months)			Schedule options (3p+0 vs 2p+1)
	Quadrivalent conjugate	2 doses (9–23 months) 1 dose (≥2 years)			

Contd...

Immunization Schedules

Contd...

Antigen	Children	Adolescents	Adults	Considerations
Hepatitis A	At least 1 dose ≥1 year of age			• Level of endemicity • Vaccine options; • Definition of high-risk groups
Rabies	2 doses			• PrEP vs PEP • Definition of high risk • Booster
Dengue (CYD-TDV)	3 doses 9–45 years of age			• Minimize risk of vaccine among seronegative individuals by pre-vaccination screening • Pregnancy and lactation
Recommendations for immunization programmes with certain characteristics				
Mumps	2 doses, with measles containing vaccine			• Coverage criteria > 80% • Combination vaccine
Seasonal influenza (inactivated tri- and quadrivalent)	First vaccine use: 2 doses Revaccinate annually: 1 dose only	Priority for pregnant women 1 dose ≥9 years of age Revaccinate annually		• Priority risk groups • Lower dosage for children 6–35 months
Varicella	1–2 doses	2 doses		• Achieve and sustain ≥ 80% coverage • Pregnancy • Co-administration with other live vaccines

Refer to *http://www.who.int/immunization/documents/positionpapers/* for most recent version of this table and position papers.

This table summarizes the WHO child vaccination recommendations. It is designed to assist the development of country specific schedules and is not intended for direct use by healthcare workers. Country specific schedules should be based on local epidemiologic, programmatic, resource and policy considerations. While vaccines are universally recommended, some children may have contraindications to particular vaccines.

SUMMARY (TABLE 4.8)

Table 4.8: Recommended and minimum ages and intervals between vaccine doses.

Vaccine and dose no.	Recommended age for this dose	Minimum age for this dose	Recommended interval to next dose	Minimum interval to next dose
Hepatitis B (Hep B)-1	Birth	Birth	1–4 months	4 weeks
Hep B2	1–2 months	4 weeks	2–17 months	8 weeks
Hep B3	6–18 months	24 weeks	–	–
Diphtheria-tetanus-acellular pertussis (DTap)–1	2 months	6 weeks	2 months	4 weeks
DTaP-2	4 months	10 weeks	2 months	4 weeks
DTaP-3	6 months	14 weeks	6–12 months	6 months
DTaP-4	15–18 months	12 months	35 months	6 months
DTaP-5	4–6 years	4 years	–	–
Haemophilus influenzae type b (Hib)-1	2 months	6 weeks	2 months	4 weeks
Hib-2	4 months	10 weeks	2 months	4 weeks
Hib-3	6 months	14 weeks	6–9 months	8 weeks
Hib-4	12–15 months	12 months	–	–
Inactivated poliovirus (IPV)-1	2 months	6 weeks	2 months	4 weeks
IPV-2	4 months	10 weeks	2–14 months	4 weeks
IPV-3	6–18 months	14 weeks	3–5 years	4 weeks
IPV-4	4–6 years	18 weeks	–	–
Pneumococcal conjugate (PCV)-1	2 months	6 weeks	2 months	4 weeks
MMR-2	4–6 years	13 months	–	–
Varicella (Var)-1	12–15 months	12 months	3–5 years	12 weeks
Var-2	4–6 years	15 months	–	–
Hepatitis A (Hep A)-1	12–23 months	12 months	6–18 month	6 month

Contd...

Contd...

Vaccine and dose no.	Recommended age for this dose	Minimum age for this dose	Recommended interval to next dose	Minimum interval to next dose
HepA-2	18–41 months	18 months	–	–
Influenza inactivated (TIV)	6 months–18 years	6 months	1 months	4 weeks
Influenza live-attenuated (LAIV)	24 months–18 years	24 months	1 months	4 weeks
Meningococcal conjugate (MCV)	11–12 years	2 years	–	–
Meningococcal polysaccharide (MPSV)-1	–	2 years	5 years	5 years
MPSV-2	–	7 years	–	–
Td	11–12 years	7 years	10 years	5 years
Tdap	11 years	10 years	–	–
Pneumococcal polysaccharide (HPV)-1	–	2 years	5 years	5 years
PPV-2	–	7 years	–	–
Human papillomavirus (HPV)-1	11–12 years	9 years	2 months	4 weeks
HPV-2	11–12 years (+2 months)	109 months	4 months	12 weeks
HPV-3	11–12 years (+6 months)	114 months	–	–
Rotavirus (RV)-1	2 months	6 weeks	2 months	4 weeks
RV-2	4 months	10 weeks	2 months	4 weeks

Source: Red Book 2018, AAP Publication.

YOU ARE NEVER TOO OLD TO GET IMMUNIZED (FIG. 4.1)

Vaccine	19–21 years	22–26 years	27–49 years	50–64 years	≥65 years
Influenza inactivated (IIV) or Influenza recombinant (RIV) **or** Influenza live attenuated (LAIV)	1 dose annually **or** 1 dose annually				
Tetanus, diphtheria, pertussis (Tdap or Td)	1 dose Tdap, then Td booster every 10 years				
Measles, mumps, rubella (MMR)	1 or 2 doses depending on indication (if born in 1957 or later)				
Varicella (VAR)	2 doses (if born in 1980 or later)				
Zoster recombinant (RZV) (preferred) **or** Zoster live (ZVL)					2 doses **or** 1 dose
Human papillomavirus (HPV) Female	2 or 3 doses depending on age at initial vaccination				
Human papillomavirus (HPV) Male	2 or 3 doses depending on age at initial vaccination				
Pneumococcal conjugate (PCV13)					1 dose
Pneumococcal polysaccharide (PPSV23)	1 or 2 doses depending on indication				1 doses
Hepatitis A (Hep A)	2 or 3 doses depending on Vaccine				
Hepatitis B (Hep B)	2 or 3 doses depending on Vaccine				
Meningococcal A, C, W, Y (MenACWY)	1 or 2 doses depending on indication, then booster every 5 years if risk remains				
Meningococcal B (MenB)	2 or 3 doses depending on vaccine and indication				
Haemophilus influenzae type b (Hib)	1 or 3 doses depending on indication				

Recommended vaccination for adults who meet age requirement, lack documentation of vaccination, or lack evidence of past infection

Recommended vaccination for adults with an additional risk factor or another indication

No recommendation

Fig. 4.1: Recommended immunization schedule for adults by age group.

FOOTNOTES

Recommended immunization schedule for adults aged 19 years or older: United States, 2019 additional information.

1. *Influenza vaccination*

   Annual vaccination against influenza is recommended for all persons aged ≥6 months. A list of currently available influenza vaccines can be found at http://www.cdc.gov/flu/protect/vaccine/vaccines.htm.

   Persons aged ≥6 months, including pregnant women, can receive the inactivated influenza vaccine (IIV). An age-appropriate IIV formulation should be used.
   - Intradermal IIV is an option for persons aged 18 through 64 years.
   - High-dose IIV is an option for persons aged ≥ 65 years.
   - Live attenuated influenza vaccine [LAIV (FluMist)] is an option for healthy, non-pregnant persons aged 2 through 49 years.
   - Recombinant influenza vaccine [RIV (Flublok)] is approved for persons aged ≥18 years.
   - RIV, which does not contain any egg protein, may be administered to persons aged ≥18 years with egg allergy of any severity; IIV may be used with additional safety measures for persons with hives-only allergy to eggs.
   - Health care personnel who care for severely immunocompromised persons who require care in a protected environment should receive IIV or RIV; health care personnel who receive LAIV should avoid providing care for severely immunosuppressed persons for 7 days after vaccination.

2. *Tetanus, diphtheria, and acellular pertussis (Td/Tdap) vaccination*
   - Administer one dose of Tdap vaccine to pregnant women during each pregnancy (preferably during 27–36 weeks' gestation) regardless of interval since prior Td or Tdap vaccination.
   - Persons aged ≥11 years who have not received Tdap vaccine or for whom vaccine status is unknown should receive a dose of Tdap followed by tetanus and diphtheria toxoids (Td) booster doses every 10 years thereafter. Tdap can be administered regardless of interval since the most recent tetanus or diphtheria- toxoid-containing vaccine.

- Adults with an unknown or incomplete history of completing a 3-dose primary vaccination series with Td-containing vaccines should begin or complete a primary vaccination series including a Tdap dose.
- For unvaccinated adults, administer the first two doses at least 4 weeks apart and the third dose 6–12 months after the second.
- For incompletely vaccinated (i.e. less than three doses) adults, administer remaining doses.
- Refer to the ACIP statement for recommendations for administering Td/Tdap as prophylaxis in wound management (see footnote 1).

3. *Varicella vaccination:*
   - All adults without evidence of immunity to varicella (as defined below) should receive two doses of single-antigen varicella vaccine or a second dose if they have received only one dose.
   - Vaccination should be emphasized for those who have close contact with persons at high-risk for severe disease (e.g. healthcare personnel and family contacts of persons with immunocompromising conditions) or are at high-risk for exposure or transmission (e.g. teachers; child care employees; residents and staff members of institutional settings, including correctional institutions; college students; military personnel; adolescents and adults living in households with children; non-pregnant women of childbearing age; and international travelers).
   - Pregnant women should be assessed for evidence of varicella immunity. Women who do not have evidence of immunity should receive the first dose of varicella vaccine upon completion or termination of pregnancy and before discharge from the health care facility. The second dose should be administered 4–8 weeks after the first dose.
   - Evidence of immunity to varicella in adults includes any of the following: documentation of two doses of varicella vaccine at least 4 weeks apart:
     - US-born before 1980, except health care personnel and pregnant women;
     - History of varicella based on diagnosis or verification of varicella disease by a healthcare provider;

- History of herpes zoster based on diagnosis or verification of herpes zoster disease by a healthcare provider; or
- Laboratory evidence of immunity or laboratory confirmation of disease.

4. *Human papillomavirus (HPV) vaccination:*
    - Three HPV vaccines are licensed for use in females [bivalent HPV vaccine (2vHPV), quadrivalent HPV vaccine (4vHPV), and 9-valent HPV vaccine (9vHPV)] and two HPV vaccines are licensed for use in males (4vHPV and 9vHPV).
    - For females, 2vHPV, 4vHPV, or 9vHPV is recommended in a 3-dose series for routine vaccination at age 11 or 12 years and for those aged 13 through 26 years, if not previously vaccinated.
    - For males, 4vHPV or 9vHPV is recommended in a 3-dose series for routine vaccination at age 11 or 12 years and for those aged 13 through 21 years, if not previously vaccinated. Males aged 22 through 26 years may be vaccinated.
    - HPV vaccination is recommended for men who have sex with men through age 26 years who did not get any or all doses when they were younger.
    - Vaccination is recommended for immunocompromised persons (including those with HIV infection) through age 26 years who did not get any or all doses when they were younger.
    - A complete HPV vaccination series consists of three doses. The second dose should be administered 4–8 weeks (minimum interval of 4 weeks) after the first dose; the third dose should be administered 24 weeks after the first dose and 16 weeks after the second dose (minimum interval of 12 weeks).
    - HPV vaccines are not recommended for use in pregnant women. However, pregnancy testing is not needed before vaccination. If a woman is found to be pregnant after initiating the vaccination series, no intervention is needed; the remainder of the 3-dose series should be delayed until completion or termination of pregnancy.

5. *Zoster vaccination:*
    - A single dose of zoster vaccine is recommended for adults aged ≥60 years regardless of whether they report a prior episode of herpes zoster. Although, the vaccine is licensed by the US Food and Drug Administration (FDA) for use among and can be administered to persons aged ≥50 years, ACIP recommends that vaccination begin at age 60 years.
    - Persons aged ≥60 years with chronic medical conditions may be vaccinated unless their condition constitutes a contraindication, such as pregnancy or severe immunodeficiency.
6. *Measles, mumps, and rubella (MMR) vaccination:*

    Adults born before 1957 are generally considered immune to measles and mumps. All adults born in 1957 or later should have documentation of one or more doses of MMR vaccine unless they have a medical contraindication to the vaccine or laboratory evidence of immunity to each of the three diseases. Documentation of provider-diagnosed disease is not considered acceptable evidence of immunity for measles, mumps, and rubella.

    Measles component:
    - A routine second dose of MMR vaccine, administered a minimum of 28 days after the first dose, is recommended for adults who:
        - Are students in postsecondary educational institutions,
        - Work in a health care facility, or
        - Plan to travel internationally.
    - Persons who received inactivated (killed) measles vaccine or measles vaccine of unknown type during 1963–1967 should be revaccinated with two doses of MMR vaccine.

    Mumps component:
    - A routine second dose of MMR vaccine, administered a minimum of 28 days after the first dose, is recommended for adults who:
        - Are students in a postsecondary educational institution,
        - Work in a healthcare facility, or
        - Plan to travel internationally.

- Persons vaccinated before 1979 with either killed mumps vaccine or mumps vaccine of unknown type who are at high-risk for mumps infection (e.g. persons who are working in a health care facility) should be considered for revaccination with two doses of MMR vaccine.

Rubella component:
For women of child-bearing age, regardless of birth year, rubella immunity should be determined. If there is no evidence of immunity, women who are not pregnant should be vaccinated. Pregnant women who do not have evidence of immunity should receive MMR vaccine upon completion or termination of pregnancy and before discharge from the health care facility.

Healthcare personnel born before 1957:
For unvaccinated health care personnel born before 1957 who lack laboratory evidence of measles, mumps, and/or rubella immunity or laboratory confirmation of disease, healthcare facilities should consider vaccinating personnel with two doses of MMR vaccine at the appropriate interval for measles and mumps or one dose of MMR vaccine for rubella.

7. *Pneumococcal vaccination*
   - *General information:*
     - Adults are recommended to receive one dose of 13-valent pneumococcal conjugate vaccine (PCV13) and 1, 2, or 3 doses (depending on indication) of 23-valent pneumococcal polysaccharide vaccine (PPSV23).
     - PCV13 should be administered at least 1 year after PPSV23.
     - PPSV23 should be administered at least 1 year after PCV13, except among adults with immunocompromising conditions, anatomical or functional asplenia, cerebrospinal fluid leak, or cochlear implant, for whom the interval should be at least 8 weeks; the interval between PPSV23 doses should be at least 5 years.
     - No additional dose of PPSV23 is indicated for adults vaccinated with PPSV23 at age ≥65 years.
     - When both PCV13 and PPSV23 are indicated, PCV13 should be administered first; PCV13 and PPSV23 should not be administered during the same visit.

- When indicated, PCV13 and PPSV23 should be administered to adults whose pneumococcal vaccination history is incomplete or unknown.
- *Adults aged ≥65 years (immunocompetent) who:*
  - Have not received PCV13 or PPSV23: Administer PCV13 followed by PPSV23 at least 1 year after PCV13.
  - Have not received PCV13 but have received a dose of PPSV23 at age ≥65 years: Administer PCV13 at least 1 year after PPSV23.
  - Have not received PCV13 but have received 1 or more doses of PPSV23 at age <65 years: Administer PCV13 at least 1 year after the most recent dose of PPSV23. Administer a dose of PPSV23 at least 1 year after PCV13 and at least 5 years after the most recent dose of PPSV23.
  - Have received PCV13 but not PPSV23 at age <65 years: Administer PPSV23 at least 1 year after PCV13.
  - Have received PCV13 and 1 or more doses of PPSV23 at age <65 years: Administer PPSV23 at least 1 year after PCV13 and at least 5 years after the most recent dose of PPSV23.
- Adults aged ≥19 years with immunocompromising conditions or anatomical or functional asplenia (defined below) who have not received PCV13 or PPSV23: Administer PCV13 followed by PPSV23 at least 8 weeks after PCV13. Administer a second dose of PPSV23 at least 5 years after the first dose of PPSV23.
  - Have not received PCV13 but have received 1 dose of PPSV23: Administer PCV13 at least 1 year after the PPSV23. Administer a second dose of PPSV23 at least 8 weeks after PCV13 and at least 5 years after the first dose of PPSV23.
  - Have not received PCV13 but have received 2 doses of PPSV23: Administer PCV13 at least 1 year after the most recent dose of PPSV23.
  - *Have received PCV13 but not PPSV23:* Administer PPSV23 at least 8 weeks after PCV13. Administer a second dose of PPSV23 at least 5 years after the first dose of PPSV23.
  - *Have received PCV13 and 1 dose of PPSV23:* Administer a second dose of PPSV23 at least 8 weeks

after PCV13 and at least 5 years after the first dose of PPSV23.
- If the most recent dose of PPSV23 was administered at age <65 years, at age ≥65 years, administer a dose of PPSV23 at least 8 weeks after PCV13 and at least 5 years after the last dose of PPSV23.
- Immunocompromising conditions that are indications for pneumococcal vaccination are congenital or acquired immunodeficiency (including B- or T-lymphocyte deficiency, complement deficiencies, and phagocytic disorders excluding chronic granulomatous disease), HIV infection, chronic renal failure, nephrotic syndrome, leukemia, lymphoma, Hodgkin's disease, generalized malignancy, multiple myeloma, solid organ transplant, and iatrogenic immunosuppression (including long-term systemic corticosteroids and radiation therapy).
- Anatomical or functional asplenia that are indications for pneumococcal vaccination are: Sickle cell disease and other hemoglobinopathies, congenital or acquired asplenia, splenic dysfunction, and splenectomy. Administer pneumococcal vaccines at least 2 weeks before immunosuppressive therapy or an elective splenectomy, and as soon as possible to adults who are newly diagnosed with asymptomatic or symptomatic HIV infection.

- *Adults aged ≥19 years with cerebrospinal fluid leaks or cochlear implants:* Administer PCV13 followed by PPSV23 at least 8 weeks after PCV13; no additional dose of PPSV23 is indicated if aged <65 years. If PPSV23 was administered at age <65 years, at age ≥65 years, administer another dose of PPSV23 at least 5 years after the last dose of PPSV23.
- Adults aged 19 through 64 years with chronic heart disease (including congestive heart failure and cardiomyopathies, excluding hypertension), chronic lung disease (including chronic obstructive lung disease, emphysema, and asthma), chronic liver disease (including cirrhosis), alcoholism, or diabetes mellitus, or who smoke cigarettes: Administer PPSV23. At age ≥65 years, administer PCV13 at least 1 year after PPSV23,

followed by another dose of PPSV23 at least 1 year after PCV13 and at least 5 years after the last dose of PPSV23.
- Routine pneumococcal vaccination is not recommended for American Indian/Alaska Native or other adults unless they have an indication as above; however, public health authorities may consider recommending the use of pneumococcal vaccines for American Indians/Alaska Natives or other adults who live in areas with increased risk for invasive pneumococcal disease.

8. *Hepatitis A vaccination:*
   - Vaccinate any person seeking protection from hepatitis A virus (HAV) infection and persons with any of the following indications: men who have sex with men:
     - Persons who use injection or non-injection illicit drugs;
     - Persons working with HAV-infected primates or with HAV in a research laboratory setting;
     - Persons with chronic liver disease and persons who receive clotting factor concentrates;
     - Persons traveling to or working in countries that have high or intermediate endemicity of hepatitis A (see footnote 1)
     - Unvaccinated persons who anticipate close personal contact (e.g. household or regular babysitting) with an international adoptee during the first 60 days after arrival in the United States from a country with high or intermediate endemicity of hepatitis A (see footnote 1). The first dose of the 2-dose hepatitis A vaccine series should be administered as soon as adoption is planned, ideally 2 or more weeks before the arrival of the adoptee.
   - Single-antigen vaccine formulations should be administered in a 2-dose schedule at either 0 and 6–12 months (Havrix), or 0 and 6–18 months (Vaqta).

     If the combined hepatitis A and hepatitis B vaccine (Twinrix) is used, administer three doses at 0, 1, and 6 months; alternatively, a 4-dose schedule may be used, administered on Days 0, 7, and 21–30 followed by a booster dose at 12 months.

9. *Hepatitis B vaccination:*
    - Vaccinate any person seeking protection from hepatitis B virus (HBV) infection and persons with any of the following indications:
        - Sexually active persons who are not in a long-term, mutually monogamous relationship (e.g. persons with more than 1 sex partner during the previous 6 months); persons seeking evaluation or treatment for a sexually transmitted disease (STD); current or recent injection drug users; and men who have sex with men;
        - Healthcare personnel and public safety workers who are potentially exposed to blood or other infectious body fluids;
        - Persons who are aged <60 years with diabetes as soon as feasible after diagnosis; persons with diabetes who are aged ≥60 years at the discretion of the treating clinician based on the likelihood of acquiring HBV infection, including the risk posed by an increased need for assisted blood glucose monitoring in long-term care facilities, the likelihood of experiencing chronic sequelae if infected with HBV, and the likelihood of immune response to vaccination;
        - Persons with end-stage renal disease (including patients receiving hemodialysis), persons with HIV infection, and persons with chronic liver disease;
        - Household contacts and sex partners of hepatitis B surface antigen–positive persons, clients and staff members of institutions for persons with developmental disabilities, and international travelers to regions with high or intermediate levels of endemic HBV infection (see footnote 1); and
        - All adults in the following settings: STD treatment facilities, HIV testing and treatment facilities, facilities providing drug abuse treatment and prevention services, health care settings targeting services to injection drug users or men who have sex with men, correctional facilities, end-stage renal disease programs and facilities for chronic hemodialysis patients, and institutions and nonresidential day care facilities for persons with developmental disabilities.

- Administer missing doses to complete a 3-dose series of hepatitis B vaccine to those persons not vaccinated or not completely vaccinated. The second dose should be administered at least 1 month after the first dose; the third dose should be administered at least 2 months after the second dose (and at least 4 months after the first dose). If the combined Hep A and Hep B vaccine (Twinrix) is used, give three doses at 0, 1, and 6 months; alternatively, a 4-dose Twinrix schedule may be used, administered on days 0, 7, and 21–30, followed by a booster dose at 12 months.
- Adult patients receiving hemodialysis or with other immunocompromising conditions should receive 1 dose of 40 µg/mL (Recombivax HB) administered on a 3-dose schedule at 0, 1, and 6 months or two doses of 20 µg/mL (Engerix-B) administered simultaneously on a 4-dose schedule at 0, 1, 2, and 6 months.

10. *Meningococcal vaccination:*
    - *General information:*
        - Serogroup A, C, W, and Y meningococcal vaccine is available as a conjugate [MenACWY (Menactra, Menveo)] or a polysaccharide [MPSV4 (Menomune)] vaccine.
        - Serogroup B meningococcal (MenB) vaccine is available as a 2-dose series of MenB-4C vaccine (Bexsero) administered at least 1 month apart or a 3-dose series of MenB-FHbp (Trumenba) vaccine administered at 0, 2, and 6 months; the two MenB vaccines are not interchangeable, i.e. the same MenB vaccine product must be used for all doses.
        - MenACWY vaccine is preferred for adults with serogroup A, C, W, and Y meningococcal vaccine indications who are aged ≤55 years, and for adults aged ≥56 years: (1) who were vaccinated previously with MenACWY vaccine and are recommended for revaccination or (2) for whom multiple doses of vaccine are anticipated; MPSV4 vaccine is preferred for adults aged ≥56 years who have not received MenACWY vaccine previously and who require a single dose only (e.g. persons at risk because of an outbreak).

- Revaccination with MenACWY vaccine every 5 years is recommended for adults previously vaccinated with MenACWY or MPSV4 vaccine who remain at increased risk for infection (e.g. adults with anatomical or functional asplenia or persistent complement component deficiencies, or microbiologists who are routinely exposed to isolates of Neisseria meningitidis).
- MenB vaccine is approved for use in persons aged 10 through 25 years; however, because there is no theoretical difference in safety for persons aged >25 years compared to those aged 10 through 25 years, MenB vaccine is recommended for routine use in persons aged ≥10 years who are at increased risk for serogroup B meningococcal disease.
- There is no recommendation for MenB revaccination at this time.
- MenB vaccine may be administered concomitantly with MenACWY vaccine but at a different anatomic site, if feasible.
- HIV infection is not an indication for routine vaccination with MenACWY or MenB vaccine; if an HIV-infected person of any age is to be vaccinated, administer two doses of MenACWY vaccine at least 2 months apart.

- Adults with anatomical or functional asplenia or persistent complement component deficiencies: administer two doses of MenACWY vaccine at least 2 months apart and revaccinate every 5 years. Also administer a series of MenB vaccine.
- Microbiologists who are routinely exposed to isolates of *Neisseria meningitidis*: Administer a single dose of MenACWY vaccine; revaccinate with MenACWY vaccine every 5 years if remain at increased risk for infection. Also administer a series of MenB vaccine.
- Persons at risk because of a meningococcal disease outbreak: If the outbreak is attributable to serogroup A, C, W, or Y, administer a single dose of MenACWY vaccine; if the outbreak is attributable to serogroup B, administer a series of MenB vaccine.

- Persons who travel to or live in countries in which meningococcal disease is hyperendemic or epidemic: Administer a single dose of MenACWY vaccine and revaccinate with MenACWY vaccine every 5 years if the increased risk for infection remains (see footnote 1); MenB vaccine is not recommended because meningococcal disease in these countries is generally not caused by serogroup B.
- *Military recruits:* Administer a single dose of MenACWY vaccine.
- First-year college students aged ≤21 years who live in residence halls: Administer a single dose of MenACWY vaccine if they have not received a dose on or after their 16th birthday.
- Young adults aged 16 through 23 years (preferred age range is 16 through 18 years): May be vaccinated with a series of MenB vaccine to provide short-term protection against most strains of serogroup B meningococcal disease.

11. *Haemophilus influenzae type b vaccination:*
    - One dose of Hib vaccine should be administered to persons who have anatomical or functional asplenia or sickle cell disease or are undergoing elective splenectomy if they have not previously received Hib vaccine. Hib vaccination 14 or more days before splenectomy is suggested.
    - Recipients of a hematopoietic stem cell transplant (HSCT) should be vaccinated with a 3-dose regimen 6–12 months after a successful transplant, regardless of vaccination history; at least 4 weeks should separate doses.
    - Hib vaccine is not recommended for adults with HIV infection since their risk for Hib infection is low.

12. *Immunocompromising conditions:*
    - Inactivated vaccines (e.g. pneumococcal, meningococcal, and inactivated influenza vaccines) generally are acceptable and live vaccines generally should be avoided in persons with immune deficiencies or immunocompromising conditions. Information on specific conditions is available at www.cdc.gov/vaccines/hcp/acip-recs/index.html.

TRAVEL-RELATED VACCINES (TABLE 4.9)

Table 4.9: IAP recommended travel related vaccines schedule.

Vaccine	Place of travel	Dose recommended
Meningococcal vaccine	USA/UK/endemic areas Saudi Arabia and Africa[#]	One dose
Yellow fever[^]	Yellow fever endemic zones**	10 days before travel
Oral cholera vaccine	Endemic area or area with an outbreak	Two doses 1 week apart
Japanese B encephala's	Endemic areas for JE	Single dose up to 15 years
Rabies vaccine (Pre-exposure prophylaxis)	For adolescents going on trekking	0 and 7 days

[#]Meningococcal quadrivalent vaccine for those traveling to the US and bivalent (A + C) or quadrivalent for those traveling to the UK.
[^]Mandatory for all travelers to yellow fever endemic zones as per International Health Regulations.
**The list of endemic countries can be obtained at http://wwwn.cdc.gov/travel Yellow Book ch 4,Yellow Fever.aspx currently available only at select government controlled centers in India. For more information on travelers vaccination, visit http://wwwnc.cdc.qov/travel/default.as:
Source: IAPCOI updated immunization timetables, 2011 (Courtesy: Dr Vijay Yewle) More detailed country specific information regarding vaccination required can be seen at: http://wwwnc.cdc.gov/travel/destinations/list.

IMMUNIZATION SCHEDULES FAQS BY PARENTS ON IMMUNIZATION

- If my child misses the primary schedule—What to do?
- Are booster doses necessary for all vaccines?
- Is cough, cold, mild fever, loose motions—contraindications for immunization?
- Is it necessary to give MMR, Hep B, Hib, Hep A and varicella vaccine to my child?
- Will extra doses of polio drops administered during NIDs harm the child?
- What vaccines we should give for older children/adolescents?
- Should we, adults also take some vaccines?

FAQS IMMUNIZATION SCHEDULES
FAQs by Doctors
- What is the National Immunization Schedule?
- Is WHO schedule meant only for developing countries?
- Is there a separate schedule for immunization by the Indian Academy of Pediatrics?
- Can you suggest an ideal schedule for the practitioners?
- What is the schedule for missed opportunities?

FAQS IMMUNIZATION OF ADOLESCENTS
FAQs by Parents
- My son/daughter has not received many of the newer vaccines, at >2 years of age.
  Do they also need these vaccines?
- My son/daughter is leaving abroad for higher studies.
- We do not have documentary evidence of immunization. What to do?
- Some universities in US want specific vaccines and some of the vaccines in 2 doses. Kindly advice?
- What if my son/daughter has missed/discontinued the appropriate doses, for example Hep B vaccine?
- Are 2 doses of MMR vaccine mandatory for adolescent boys and girls?
- And many more...???

FAQs by Doctors
- My client is going abroad; Can I give different vaccines at the same time?
- What to do for vaccines requiring two doses if the boy/girl is flying abroad urgently?
- Can I give chickenpox and MMR vaccines together?
- Will there be immunological overload if I give too many vaccines at the same time?
- Is documentary evidence mandatory for immunization?

LEARNING POINTS
- Immunization schedules keep on changing based on epidemiological relevance/availability of newer vaccines.

Immunization Schedules

- Recommended schedules for infants, children, adolescents, travelers, under special clinical situations should be followed for better benefits of immunization.
- ALL registered vaccines are recommended by IAP ACVIP.
- National Immunization Schedule is based on Epidemiological relevance, immunological appropriateness, technical competence, sociocultural accept- ability and economic viability as recommended by National Technical Advisory Group on Immunization (NTAGI).
- ACVIP IAP Immunization Time Table is "revised on evidence based' information whenever new concepts are emerging and newer vaccines are registered.
- Keep all vaccines at +2°C to +8°C. Do not freeze. DTPw/DTPa, DT, TT, HB, Hib, and HA+HB aluminium salt adjuvanted vaccines. If VVM is used do not use OPV if the color of the square and circle match with each other. For such vaccines requiring multiple doses, e.g. DTPa, DT, TT, HB,Hib, MMR, OPV, varicella, maintain minimum 4 weeks' interval between the recommended doses.
- Two viral vaccines such as MMR, varicella can be given together; but if given separately 4 weeks' interval is mandatory between the two vaccines.
- DTPw/HB vaccine can also be used as a solvent to dissolve the pellet of Hib vaccine.
- When extemporal mixing is done, make sure that the antigen of the same manufacturer is used and insist on approved vaccine information certification.
- For low birth weight and preterm babies a rule of two approaches may be adopted, viz. baby must be 2 months old, weigh 2 kg and healthy otherwise. Irrespective of the period of gestation/birth weight, all vaccines can thus be given as per schedule of a normal baby.
- Position the child properly as per oral or injectable vaccine(s).
- Clean the site of immunization with an alcohol/warm water swab from medial to lateral aspect and allow the surface to dry before administering the vaccine.
- Always use autodestruct syringes where available. Pre-filled syringes are safer.
- Do not rub the site of injection vigorously. Gentle pressure for a period of 10–20 seconds is sufficient. Place a wet cloth

soaked in potable water for about 10 minutes and repeat the procedure 2-3 times about 10 minutes each time if necessary in case the baby develops redness/indurations at the vaccination site.

BIBLIOGRAPHY

1. Adult Immunization Schedule, https://www.cdc.gov/vaccines/schedules/hcp/adult.html (Accessed on Dec, 2016).
2. Bhave SY, Yadav S. EPI vaccines. In: Bhave SY, Yadav S, Parthasarathy A (Eds). A ready reckoner for vaccinations adult, adolescent and pediatric. Jaypee Brothers Medical Publishers, New Delhi; 2009. [online] Available at: UIP. http://mohfw.nic.in/WriteReadData/l892s/5628564789562315.pdf (Accessed on Dec, 2016).
3. https://apps.who.int/iris/bitstream/handle/10665/272371/WER9316.pdf?ua=1(accessed on Dec 5, 2019).
4. https://www.cdc.gov/vaccines/schedules/hcp/imz/adult.html (Accessed on Dec 5, 2019).
5. https://www.indianpediatrics.net/dec2018/1066.pdf accessed on Dec 5, 2019.
6. IAP Guidebook on Immunization. In: Parthasarathy A, Dutta AK, Bhave S (Eds). Committee on Immunization. IAP Publication; 2001.
7. Parthasarathy A, Gupta A. Adolescent vaccines. In: Parthasarathy A, Gupta A (Eds). Handbook on Adolescent Immunization. Jaypee Brothers Medical Publishers, New Delhi; 2014.
8. Thacker N, Thacker D. Immunization. In: Parthasarathy A, Gupta A (Eds). Frequently asked Questions in Pediatric and Adolescent Practice. Jaypee Brothers Medical Publishers, New Delhi; 2015.
9. Vasishtha VM, Choudhary J, Jog P, Yadav S, Unni JC, Kamath SS, et al. Indian Academy of Pediatrics (IAP) recommended immunization schedule for children aged 0 through 18 years—India, 2016 and Updates on Immunization. Indian Pediatrics; 2016.

CHAPTER 5

Vaccines, Immunoglobulins and Antisera

A Parthasarathy

INTRODUCTION

In this chapter, a brief resume is given about the vaccines, immunoglobulins and antisera available in our country. Standard recommended routes of administration of the various vaccines has been included. At the end of the chapter, you will also find a 'Ready Reckoner' for vaccines:

Vaccines

- Vaccines administered at birth—BCG, bOPV, HB
- Vaccines administered at 6, 10 and 14 weeks—DTwP/ DTaP, HB, Hib, bOPV, IPV, pneumococcal, rotavirus vaccines
- Vaccines administered at 6 months—HB (3rd/4th dose), bOPV, influenza (2 doses 1 month apart then every year)
- Vaccines administered at 9 months—Measles/MMR, TCV
- Vaccines administered at 12 months—Hepatitis A
- Vaccines administered at 15 months—MMR, Varicella, PCV
- Vaccines administered at 18 months—(Boosters) DTwP/ DTaP, bOPV/eIPV, Hib, Hep A (2 doses of inactivated vaccine).
- Vaccines administered at 24 months—Typhoid (TCV booster or TyVi 1st dose).
- Vaccines administered at 4-6 years—(Boosters) bOPV, DTwP/DTaP
- Vaccines administered at 10 years—(Booster) Td/Tdap, HPV (age appropriate 2 or 3 dose schedule)
- Seasonal/area of residence/travel-related vaccines—Influenza, meningococcal, Japanese encephalitis, yellow fever, hepatitis A
- Pre-exposure and post-exposure prophylaxis vaccines—Rabies, hepatitis B
- Combination vaccines—DTwP/DTaP, HB, Hib, IPV (in various combinations), hepatitis A-hepatitis B, MMR-Varicella (DPT, MMR are also combination vaccines)

Immunoglobulins
- Hepatitis B immunoglobulin (HBIG)
- Tetanus immunoglobulin (TIG)
- Rabies immunoglobulin (RIG)
- Gamma-globulin
- Human immunoglobulin
- Human anti-D immunoglobulin

Antisera
- Anti-snake venom
- Diphtheria antitoxin

VACCINES ADMINISTERED AT BIRTH

BCG Vaccine

The BCG vaccine is named after the strain *Bacillus Calmette-Guérin*. This is a live-attenuated bovine vaccine. WHO recommends the 'Danish 1331' strain for production of BCG vaccine. This comes as a freeze-dried powder with a diluent. Protection offered varies from 0 to 80%.

Indications: To reduce morbidity from primary tuberculosis. Induces a benign, artificial primary infection, which will stimulate an acquired resistance to possible subsequent infections with the virulent tubercle bacilli. Variable protection against serious forms of TB, e.g. TBM.

Dosage: Usual strength is 0.1 mg in 0.1 mL volume. Infants <4 weeks: 0.05 mL intradermally using a 'Tuberculin' syringe. Site of injection should be just above the insertion of the deltoid muscle of left arm. May be given at birth along with the bOPV '0' dose and hepatitis B—1st dose or at 6 weeks along with DPT-1st dose and bOPV-1st dose. BCG can be given on the same day with MCV if not given earlier, else should be given one month before or after MCV.

Contraindications: In patients with generalized eczema, infective dermatosis, hypogammaglobulinemia and history of deficient immunity.

Special features: Dilution with distilled water can cause irritation. It should be diluted with normal saline. The reconstituted vaccine must be used within 4 hours. Any leftover vaccine should be discarded.

After 2-3 weeks, a papule develops. Grows to about 4-8 mm in about 5 weeks. This subsides or breaks into a shallow ulcer, usually with a crust. Sometimes open. Spontaneous healing within 6-12 weeks. Leaves behind a permanent, tiny, round scar, typically 4-8 mm in diameter. Normally, the child becomes Mantoux positive after a period of 8 weeks.

Adverse effects: Prolonged severe ulceration at the site of injection—suppurative lymphadenitis. Rarely osteomyelitis of humerus, if inoculated deep, disseminated BCG infection.

To summarize:
- Developed by Calmette and Guerin in 1921. It has been found to be efficacious over the period; efficacy rated 0-80% in various studies all over the world, few countries recommend booster doses to improve efficacy and obtain sustained protection.
- *Recent meta-analysis:* It has revealed that BCG now protects >50% of pulmonary lesions also both in adults and children.
- *BCG controls hematogenous spread:* Thus, preventing miliary TB, disseminated TB, TB meningoencephalitis, etc.
- Every year 24th March is observed as World Tuberculosis Day.
- Control of TB is based on 5Cs concepts, viz. case detection, chemotherapy short course, contact elimination, chemoprophylaxis and control with BCG vaccination.
- *Case detection:* Conventional TST, radiology, newer technologies in microbiological investigation
- *Chemotherapy short course:* Revised National Tuberculosis Control Program (RNTCP) for adults and children, Directly Observed Treatment Short Course (DOTS)
- BCG vaccine is supplied in multi-dose freeze-dried powder form in brown-colored vials (heat and light sensitive) to be reconstituted with the recommended diluent (reconstituted BCG vaccine should be used within 4 hours): *Dose:* 0.1 mL ID; over left deltoid muscle.
- *New DNA-BCG vaccine is on trial:* Currently recombinant modified BCGs (rBCG) that have shown promise in animal TB disease model testing and other new TB vaccines are

under trails, viz. attenuation and modification of MTb for replacing BCG–recombinant MTb proteins and fusion proteins combined with new adjuvants, MTb antigens vectored by viruses (non-replicating adenovirus, modified *vaccinia Ankara*), and a bacterial phage capsid delivery system which has potential for oral administration.

Oral Polio Vaccine (Sabin)

This is a live-attenuated vaccine containing: (i) Over 3,00,000 TCID50 (Median Tissue Culture Infectious Dose) of type 1 poliovirus; (ii) Over 1,00,000 TCID50 of type 2 poliovirus; and (iii) Over 3,00,000 TCID50 of type 3 polio virus dose. Currently only bOPV containing Polioviruses type 1 and 3 is the Global recommendation instead of tOPV which has been replaced by bOPV, Wild Polio Virus type 2 having been eradicated globally.

2.1.IPV (SALK) Inactivated Polio Vaccine containing Polioviruses type 1, 2 and 3 was used in developed countries to control and eradicate poliomyelitis. Currently available enhanced potency inactivated polio vaccine (eIPV) has enhanced potency and better vaccine stability than classical IPV. The eIPV is now recommended in NIP as a single dose along with DPT-3 at 14 weeks, as strategy towards POLIO endgame.

Indications: In prophylaxis against poliomyelitis—not just the paralysis, but also to intercept reinfection.

Dosage: Course of 3 doses of bOPV given at 1-month interval. 1st dose starting at 6 week and 1 booster given at 12–18 months of age. 1st dose is 2 drops using dropper supplied with vial containing bOPV. For hospital delivery, '0'-dose if bOPV is advised immediately after birth. eIPV can be given in 3 doses at 6, 10 and 14 weeks, if available or single dose along with DPT 3rd dose or 2 doses of ID factional (fIPV) at 6 and 14 weeks in selected states in the National Immunization Program.

Contraindications: Acute infectious diseases, high fever, severe diarrhea and dysentery, leukemia and other malignancy.

Special features: Breastfeeding does not decrease effectiveness of OPV. However, avoid hot milk or hot fluids immediately after the administration. OPV is given concurrent with DTP. BCG can be given along with the '0' dose of OPV.

Adverse effects: Rare cases of vaccine-associated polio in recipients of the vaccine and their contact.

Oral Polio Vaccine

- tOPV contained 3 serotypes of vaccine virus
- Grown on monkey kidney (Vero) cells
- Contains neomycin and streptomycin
- Shed in stool for up to 6 weeks following vaccination
- Highly effective in producing immunity to polio virus
- Approximately 50% immune after 1 dose
- More than 95% immune after 3 doses
- Immunity probably lifelong
- bOPV contains only Polio virus type 1 and 3.

Vaccine-associated Paralytic Polio Following OPV

- Increased risk in persons 18 years and older
- Increased risk in persons with immunodeficiency
- No procedure available for identifying persons at risk of paralytic disease
- 5–10 cases per year with exclusive use of OPV. cVDP mostly due to circulating vaccine-derived Poliovirus.
- Most cases in healthy children and their household contacts, may occur.

Polio Vaccine: Adverse Reactions

- Rare local reactions (IPV)
- No serious reactions to IPV have been documented
- Paralytic poliomyelitis (OPV)

Polio Eradication

- Last case in United States in 1979
- Western hemisphere certified polio-free in 1994
- Last isolate of type 2 poliovirus in India at Howdah, Kolkata, West Bengal in October 1999
- Global eradication goal is evading because of endemicity of polio virus, especially type 1 in 2 countries, viz. Afghanistan and Pakistan as of 2019.
- *WHO declared global eradication of WPV2 in 2015 and WPV3 in Oct 2019.*

What exactly is polio eradication?

	AFP due to non-polios	Infection: OPV virus	Infection: Wild virus
Endemicity	+	+	+
Eradication phase "w"	+	+	0
Eradication phase "v"	+	0	0

AFP: acute flaccid paralysis; OPV: oral polio vaccine

Role of OPV and IPV

- Without OPV, polio eradication is impossible!
  - Proven track-record
  - Needed where wild polio viruses circulate
  - Necessary to control outbreaks.
- Without IPV, polio eradication is also impossible!
  - *To prevent virus circulation:*
    - Vaccine-derived polioviruses
    - Wild viruses from remote locations, laboratory samples, or bioterrorism.
  - To facilitate detection of re-emerging polioviruses
  - To ensure protection until definitive eradication
- OPV and IPV are not contradictory but complementary!

WHO Position Strategic Plan (2016–2030)

- tOPV stopped after certification and instead bOPV introduced
- WHO-GPEI developed guidelines and strategies on OPV and IPV usage, which has since commenced in India also, to assist countries in the Global Polio Eradication Initiative (GPEI).

Post-polio Scenario

- Vaccine-associated paralytic polio
- Risk of VAPP ~ 1 per 1 million OPV doses
- In 2006: 1,228 cases of wild polio vs. 250–500 cases of VAPP are reported at the global level.

VDPV (Vaccine-derived Polio Viruses)

- Definition (WHO): Sabin virus with >1% drift in VP1

- cVDPV = Circulating in population
- iVDPV = Immunodeficient long-term excretors (may excrete virus for years)
- Both can be neuro-virulent/entero-virulent and can cause outbreaks.

What has VDPV changed?
- *OPV perception before VDPV:*
  - OPV causes rare, isolated, cases of vaccine associated paralytic polio (VAPP)
  - OPV circulation is short-lived and overall beneficial.
- *OPV perception after VDPV:*
  - Circulating cVDPV can cause polio outbreaks
  - iVDPV can be excreted for many years by immunodeficient individuals.

India reported 20 cases in the year 2009 from 3 states, viz. Assam (1), Bihar (3), UP (16), due to CVDPV, 18 due to P_2 and 2 due to P_3.

Seroconversion rates following administration of OPV-only, IPV-only, and IPV–OPV sequential vaccination schedules

Poliovirus serotype (after dose 3)				
Schedule	Study size (N)	P_1	P_2	P_3
OPV only	337	97%	100%	100%
IPV only	332	100%	100%	100%
Sequential	96	100%	100%	100%

Inactivated Polio Vaccine
- Highly effective in producing immunity to poliovirus
- 90% or more immune after 2 doses
- At least 99% immune after 3 doses
- Duration of immunity not known with certainty.

Ideally, IPV should replace OPV as early as possible:
- Three doses of intramuscular IPV in primary series is the best option.
- Two doses of intramuscular IPV instead of three for primary series if started at 8 weeks, with an interval of 8 weeks between two doses is an alternative.
- In case IPV is not available or feasible, the child should be offered three doses of bOPV. In such cases, the child should be referred for two fractional doses of IPV at a Government

facility at 6 and 14 weeks or at least one dose of intramuscular IPV, either stand-alone or as a combination vaccine, at 14 weeks of age.

Polio Vaccine: Contraindications and Precautions

- Severe allergic reaction to a vaccine component or following a prior dose of vaccine
- Moderate or severe acute illness.

Hepatitis B Vaccine

This is an inactivated subunit viral vaccine. Each 1 mL contain 20 µg of hepatitis B surface antigen formulated in an alum adsorbent. Effective antibody response is seen in about 95% of vaccines after 3 doses. Protection continues for 20 years following which natural boosting occurs when viral exposure challenges in the vaccinated individual **(Fig. 5.1)**.

Indications: Pre-exposure prophylaxis is given along with the childhood vaccination schedule. Post-exposure prophylaxis to newborns of carrier mothers, individuals accidentally exposed parenterally to HBV infection.

Dosage: Three doses at birth, 6 weeks and 6 months or birth, 6 weeks and 14 weeks or 6, 10, 14 weeks (0-1-6 is the most accepted schedule). *Children <20 years:* 0.5 mL IM. *Children >20 years:* 1 mL IM. No booster dose after 3 valid doses.

Contraindications: Severe febrile illness. Hypersensitivity to any of the components.

Special features: The vaccine has no effect on the HBsAg carriers. Unnecessary in children with surface antibody from previous infection.

Adverse effects: Mild transient soreness, erythema and induration at the injection site. Occasional low-grade fever and fatigue.
- Composition—Recombinant HBsAg
- Efficacy—95% (Range, 80–100%)
- Duration of immunity at least for 20 years
- Schedule—3 doses
- Booster is not routinely recommended.

Protective antibody titers: The proportion of recipients who respond to each dose varies by age.

Anti-HBs antibody titer of 10 mlU/m or higher is considered protective.

Preterm infants less than 2 kg have been shown to respond less to vaccination.

Factors that may lower vaccine response rates are age 40 years or older, male gender, smoking, obesity, and immune deficiency.

Hepatitis B Vaccine: Long-term Efficacy

- Immunologic memory established following vaccination
- Exposure to HBV results in anamnestic anti-HBs response
- Chronic infection rarely documented among vaccine responders.

Third Dose of Hepatitis B Vaccine

- Minimum of 8 weeks after second dose
- At least 16 weeks after first dose
- 3rd or final dose—at least 24 weeks of age.

Preterm Infants

- Birth dose and HBIg, if mother HBsAg-positive
- Preterm infants <2,000 g have a decreased response to vaccine administered before 1 month of age.
- Delay first dose until chronologic age 1 month if mother is HBsAg negative.

Prevention of Perinatal Hepatitis B Virus Infection

- Begin treatment within 12 hours of birth
- Hepatitis B vaccine (first dose) and HBIg at different sites
- Complete vaccination series at 6 months of age
- Test for response at 9–18 months of age.

Pre-vaccination Serologic Testing

- Not indicated before routine vaccination of infants or children
- *Recommended for:*
  - All persons born in Africa, Asia, the Pacific Islands and other regions with HBsAg prevalence of 8% or higher
  - Household, sex and needle-sharing contacts of HBsAg positive persons
  - HIV-infected persons.

- *Consider for:*
  - Groups with high risk of HBV infection (laboratory worker medical and nursing faculty).

Adults at Risk for HBV Infection

- *Sexual exposure:*
  - Sex partners of HBsAg-positive persons
  - Sexually active persons not in a long-term, mutually monogamous relationship*
  - Persons seeking evaluation nor treatment for asexually transmitted disease
  - Men who have sex with men.

Adults at Risk for HBV Infection

- *Percutaneous or mucosal exposure to blood:*
  - Current or recent intravenous drug usage (IDU)
  - Household contacts of HBsAg-positive persons
  - Residents and staff or facilities for developmentally disabled persons
  - Health care and public safety workers with risk for exposure to blood or blood-contaminated body fluids
  - Persons with end-stage renal disease.
- *Other groups:*
  - International travelers to regions with high or intermediate levels (HBsAg prevalence of 2% or higher of endemic HBV infection)
  - Persons with HIV infection.

Persistent Nonresponse to Hepatitis B Vaccine

- <5% of vaccinees do not develop anti-HBsAg after 6 valid doses
- May be non-responder or "hypo-responder"
- Check HBsAg status
- If exposed, treat as non-responder with post-exposure prophylaxis.

Hepatitis B Vaccine: Contraindications and Precautions

- Severe allergic reaction to a vaccine component or following a prior dose
- Moderate or severe acute illness.

---

*persons with more than one sex partner during the previous 6 months.

Hepatitis B Vaccine: Adverse Reactions

	Adults	Infants and Children
Pain at injection site	13–29%	3–9%
Mild systemic complaints (fatigue, headache)	11–17%	0–20%
Temperature ≤99.9°F (37.7°C)	1%	0.4–6%
Severe systemic reactions	rare	rare

Recommended post-exposure prophylaxis for occupational exposure to hepatitis B virus

	Vaccination and antibody status of exposed person*	Treatment — Source HBsAg Positive	Source HBsAg Negative	Source unknown or not available for testing
	Unvaccinated	HBIg × 1 and initiate HB vaccine series	Initiate HB vaccine series	Initiate HB vaccine series
Previously Vaccinated	Known Responder	No treatment	No treatment	No treatment
	Known non-responder	HBIg × 1 and initiate re-vaccination or HBIg × 2	No treatment	If known high-risk source, treat as if source were HBsAg positive
	Antibody response unknown	Test exposed person for anti-HBs • If adequate, no treatment is necessary • If inadequate Administer HBIg × 1 and vaccine booster	No treatment	Test exposed person for anti-HBs • If adequate, no treatment is necessary • If inadequate, administer vaccine booster and recheck titer in 1–2 months

- Hepatitis B vaccine is the only vaccine in infant immunization given in different schedules/doses.
- *For routine immunization:* Birth, 6 and 14 weeks is valid. For babies born to HBsAg +ve mothers, HBIg within 12–24 hours of birth along with birth dose of HB vaccine.

- Mercury (thiomersal) and cesium chloride free Hepatitis B vaccine formulation since registered in India: Best suited for birth dose especially in preterm and low-birth weight babies.
- *For babies born to HBsAg –ve mothers:* 6, 10- and 14-weeks schedule may be followed.
- *Immunogenicity of 6, 10- and 14-weeks' schedule:* Is now nearly comparable with the immunogenicity of 0, 1- and 6-months schedule: Seroconversion and sero-protection excellent—96%.
- *0, 1- and 6-months' schedule:* Ideally for children ≥1 year, adolescents, adults and when combined hepatitis A and hepatitis B vaccine is administered.
- *Government of India has introduced HB vaccine:* In select pilot project areas in 2002 (15 major cities/32 districts) at 6-, 10- and 14-weeks' schedule. The project since expanded to the entire states in 2007.
- In case of use of a combination vaccine a total of four doses of hepatitis B vaccine are justified.

Why Booster Doses are not Required for Hepatitis B Vaccine?

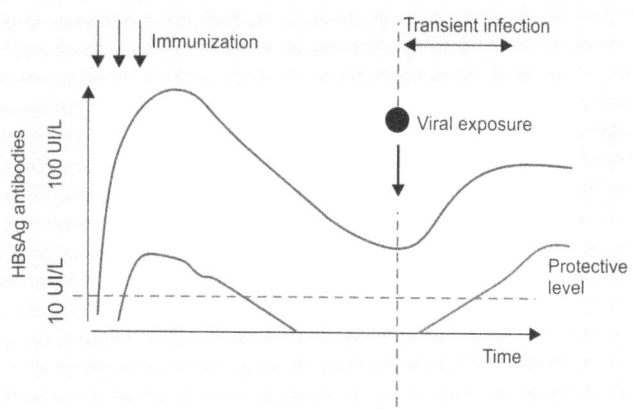

Fig. 5.1: Hepatitis B antibody titer levels after HB vaccination.
Source: Centers for Disease Control and Prevention. In: Atkinson W, Wolfe S, Hamborsky J, McIntyre L (Eds). Epidemiology and Prevention of Vaccine: preventable diseases, 11th edition. Washington DC: Public Health Foundation; 2009.

- Immunogenicity at different schedules are comparable.

0, 1, and 6 months	96–98%
0, 1, and 2 months	96%
0, 6, and 14 weeks	95–96%
6, 10, and 14 weeks	97%
2, 4, and 6 months	99%

VACCINES ADMINISTERED AT 6, 10 AND 14 WEEKS

Diphtheria, Pertussis, Tetanus, DTwP/DTaP Vaccines

This is a combination of diphtheria pertussis and tetanus toxoid adsorbed on aluminum phosphate and suspended in isotonic sodium chloride solution. Adsorption increases the immunological effectiveness. 3 doses provide more than 80% protection.

Indications: In primary immunization of infants against diphtheria, pertussis and tetanus.

Dosage: 0.5 mL deep IM, anterolateral aspect of thigh. As a booster at 15-18 months and 5 years after the 3 primary doses of DTwP/DTaP given during infancy.

In children >7 years who have not received DTwP/DTaP, 2 doses of Tdap/Td, 4 weeks apart, with a booster dose 1 year later.

Contraindications: Severe reaction to previous dose, progressive neurological disease, seriously ill patients who need hospitalization, mild fever, febrile seizure, epilepsy, cerebral palsy with fits.

Special features: Vaccine should not be frozen. Stored in a refrigerator at 4-8°C.

Adverse effects: Fever, mild local reactions.

DTaP/DT, Td and Tdap

	Diphtheria	Tetanus
DTaP, DT	7–8 Lf units	5–12.5 Lf units
Td, Tdap (adult)	2–2.5 Lf units	5 Lf units

DTaP and pediatric DT used through age 7 years. Adult Td for persons 7 years and older. Tdap for persons 10-64 years.

Diphtheria Toxoid
- Formalin-inactivated diphtheria toxin
- *Schedule:* Three or four doses + booster
  Booster every 10 years
- *Efficacy:* Approximately 95%
- *Duration:* Approximately 10 years
- Should be administered with tetanus toxoid as DTaP, DT, Td, or Tdap.

DTaP, DT, Td and Tdap

	Diphtheria	Tetanus
DTaP, DT	7–8 Lf units	5–12.5 Lf units
Td, Tdap (adult)	2–2.5 Lf units	5 Lf units

DTaP and pediatric DT used through age 7 years. Adult Td for persons 7 years and older. Tdap for persons 7–64 years.

Pertussis Inactivated/Component Vaccine
- Formalin-inactivated diphtheria vaccine
- *Schedule:* Three or four doses + booster every 10 years
- *Efficacy:* Approximately 95%
- *Duration:* Approximately 10 years
- Should be administered with tetanus toxoid as DTaP, Tdap.

DTaP, DT, Td and Tdap

	Diphtheria	Tetanus
DTaP, DT	7–8 Lf units	5–12.5 Lf units
Td, Tdap (adult)	2–2.5 Lf units	5 Lf units

DTaP and pediatric DT used through age 7 years. Adult Td for person 7 years and older. Tdap for persons 7–64 years (Boostrix) or 10–64 years (Adacel).

Tetanus Toxoid
- Formalin-inactivated tetanus toxoid
- *Schedule:* Three or four doses +booster
  Booster every 10 years
- *Efficacy:* Approximately 100%
- *Duration:* Approximately 10 years
- Should be administered with diphtheria toxoid as DTaP, DT, Td, or Tdap.

Routine DTaP Primary Vaccination Schedule

Dose	Age	Interval
Primary 1	2 months	—
Primary 2	4 months	4 weeks
Primary 3	6 months	4 weeks
Primary 4	15–18 months	6 months

Children who receive DT

- The number of doses of DT needed to complete the series depends on the child's age at the first dose:
  - If first dose given at younger than 12 months of age, 4 doses are recommended.
  - If first dose given at 12 months or older, 3 doses complete the primary series.

Routine DTaP Schedule for Children Younger than 7 years of Age

Booster Doses
- 4 through 6 years of age, before entering school
- 11 or 12 years of age if 5 years since last dose (Tdap)
- Every 10 years thereafter (Td)

Routine Td Schedule for Unvaccinated Persons 7 Years of Age and Older

Dose*	Interval
Primary 1	—
Primary 2	4 weeks
Primary 3	6–12 months
Booster dose every 10 years	

*ACIP recommended that one of these doses (preferably the first) be administered as Tdap.

Diphtheria and Tetanus Toxoids

Contraindications and Precautions

- Severe allergic reaction to vaccine component or following a prior dose
- Moderate or severe acute illness.

Adverse Reactions

- Local reactions (erythema, induration)
- Fever and systemic symptoms not common

- Exaggerated local reactions (Arthus-type)
- Severe systemic reactions

DTwP/DTaP Vaccines

Current Concepts

- Both DTwP and DTaP vaccines have been registered in India.
- *Current recommendations for use of DTaP:*
  - For unimmunized children >7 years of age
  - For adolescents
  - For infants who were already immunized with DTaP
  - For booster doses routinely.
- DTwP-HB combination vaccine formulation is used as a diluent for dissolving the Hib component.
- DTwP-HB-Hib ready to use liquid formulation is now registered in India.

DTwP/DTaP/Tdap Vaccines

Current Concepts

- Tdap adult formulation has now been recommended as booster by WHO for adults.
- Tdap formulation is now recommended for adolescents by ACIP and AAP.
- Causal relationship to various complications attributed earlier to the use of DTwP have now been negated.
- *Absolute contraindications for DTwP:*
  - Anaphylaxis to previous dose
  - Progressive neurological disorder
  - Hypotensive hyporesponsive episodes.
- Adverse reactions following administration of DTwP/DTaP—almost comparable.

Haemophilus influenzae type b Vaccine

This is a solution of conjugate of oligosaccharides of the capsular antigen of *H. influenzae* type diphtheria protein or tetanus protein in saline. Its efficacy is about 90%.

Indications: For immunization of children against invasive diseases caused by *H. influenzae*.

Dosage: Both PRP-T and PRP-CRM conjugate Hib vaccines are available in India. A combination formulation which includes DTwP/DTaP along with Hib vaccine can also be used.

Contraindications: Children <6 weeks. Hypersensitivity to any of the components.

Special features: Avoid injection into a blood vessel.

Adverse effects: Local erythema, warmth or swelling, fever, rash, urticaria.
- DTwP or DTaP can be offered in primary series.

Haemophilus influenzae Type to Risk Factors for Invasive Disease
- *Exposure factors:*
    - Household crowding
    - Large household size
    - Childcare attendance
    - Low socioeconomic status
    - Low parental education
    - School-aged sibling.
- *Host factors:*
    - Race/ethnicity
    - Chronic disease.

Haemophilus influenzae type b polysaccharide vaccine
- Was available 1985–1988
- Not effective in children younger than 18 months of age
- Effectiveness in older children variable.

Polysaccharide vaccines
- Age-related immune response
- Not consistently immunogenic in children 2 years of age and younger
- No booster response
- Antibody with less functional activity.

Polysaccharide conjugate vaccines
- Stimulates T-dependent immunity
- Enhanced antibody production, especially in young children
- Repeat doses elicit booster response.

Haemophilus influenzae type b vaccines
- Recommended interval 8 weeks for primary series doses
- Minimum interval 4 weeks for primary series doses

- Vaccination at younger than 6 weeks of age may induce immunologic tolerance to Hib antigen.

Haemophilus Influenzae Type b Vaccine—Delayed vaccination schedule
- Children starting late may not need entire 3 or 4 dose series
- Number of doses the child requires depends on current age
- All children 15–59 months of age need at least 1 dose.

Haemophilus Influenzae type b Vaccine—Vaccination following invasive disease
- Children younger than 24 months may not develop protective antibody after invasive disease.
- Vaccinate during convalescence
- Complete series forage
- *Consider for high-risk persons:* Asplenia, immunodeficiency, HIV infection
- One pediatric dose of any conjugate vaccine.

Pentaxim Vaccines

- Contains lyophilized Hib (Act Hib) vaccine that is reconstituted with a liquid DTaP-IPV solution
- Approved for doses 1 through 4 among children 6 weeks through 4 years of age
- The DTaP-IPV solution should not be used separately (i.e. only use to reconstitute the Hib component).

Hexaxim Vaccines

- Contains liquid DTaP-IPV-HB-HIB solution
- Approved for doses 1 through 4 among children 6 weeks through 4 years of age

Haemophilus Influenzae Type b Vaccine

Contraindications and Precautions
- Severe allergic reaction to vaccine component or following a prior dose
- Moderate or severe acute illness
- Age younger than 6 weeks

Adverse Reactions
- Swelling, redness or pain in 5–30% of recipients

- Systemic reactions infrequent
- Serious adverse reactions

Hib vaccine—Current Status/How Many Doses?
- Hib vaccine now included in national immunization schedule in India
- Recommended as routine vaccine in IAP immunization timetable PRP-T/PRP_{CRM197} covalently bound to Hib conjugate antigen
- *Dose related to age:*
  <6 months—6, 10 and 14 weeks interval: 3 doses
  6 months: ≥2 doses at 4–8 weeks interval
  ≥12 months: 1 dose
  All three schedules should be followed by a single booster dose at 15–18 months.
- Early primary Hib immunization is mandatory at 6, 10 and 14 weeks since majority of invasive Hib disease (meningitis/pneumonia) occur in infants 6–11 months of age.
- No booster dose is required when given beyond 15 months and when aluminium salt adjuvanted vaccine formulation is used according to the manufacturer's recommendations.
  - *Hib vaccine is not indicated beyond 5 years:* Not to be considered as a panacea against brain fever of varying etiology
    - Monovalent, lyophilized/liquid combination formulations are available, e.g. DTwP-Hib/ DTwP-HB/DTaP-HB – Hib/DTaP-HB-Hib-IPV
  - Seroconversion of Hib component is well above the required protective titer when given in DTwP/DTaP combination formulation.
  - Hence, combination formulation of DTwP/DTaP can be used without fear of immunosuppression for the Hib component.

Pneumococcal Vaccines

Pneumococcal vaccine is used for active immunization against *Strep. pneumonia* which is the most common cause of bacterial pneumonia worldwide. It is prepared from purified pneumococcal capsular antigens and includes 10/13 serotypes which are responsible for at least 85% of pneumococcal infections and has greater than 90% coverage against serotypes that are penicillin resistant.

Indications: Prevention of pneumococcal infections, particularly those of respiratory origin in all subjects over the age of 2 years who are at risk of serious pneumococcal infections.

Dosage: SC or IM route: 10/13 valent preparation suitable for administration at 6, 10 and 14 weeks/2, 4, 6 months is now available which confers protection against pneumococcal types contained in the vaccine. Booster is advised at 16–18 months. *Revaccination:* Should not be carried before at least 5 years, unless the subject is particularly exposed.

Special precautions: Store between +2°C and +8°C. Do not freeze.

Contraindication: Safety during first trimester of pregnancy has not been established.

Side-effects: Possible reactions of hypersensitivity. Redness, slight pain and induration at the site of injection. Rarely fever may occur.

A 13-valent conjugate pneumococcal polysaccharide vaccine PCV13 is licensed in India.

Pneumococcal Vaccines
1977: 14-valent polysaccharide vaccine licensed
1983: 23-valent polysaccharide vaccine licensed (PPSV23)
2000: 7-valent polysaccharide conjugate vaccine licensed (PCV7)
2019: Pneumosil (PCV10) Indian vaccine pre-qualified by WHO.

Pneumococcal Polysaccharide Vaccine

- Purified capsular polysaccharide antigen from 23 sero-types of *Pneumococcus.*
- Account for 88% of bacteremic pneumococcal disease
- Cross-react with types causing additional 8% of disease protection.

Pneumococcal Conjugate Vaccine

- Pneumococcal polysaccharide conjugated to nontoxic diphtheria toxin (10/13 serotypes)
- Vaccine serotypes account for 86% of bacteremia and 83% of meningitis among children <6 years of age.

Pneumococcal Polysaccharide Vaccine

- Purified pneumococcal polysaccharide (23 types)
- Not effective in children <2 years
- 60–70% against invasive disease
- Less effective in preventing pneumococcal pneumonia

Pneumococcal Conjugate Vaccine

- Highly immunogenic in infants and young children, including those with high-risk medical conditions
- >90% effective against invasive disease
- Less effective against pneumonia and acute otitis media

Pneumococcal Polysaccharide Vaccine: Recommendations

- Adults 65 years of age or older
- Persons 2 years of age or older with:
  - Chronic illness
  - Anatomic or functional asplenia
  - Immunocompromised (disease, chemotherapy, steroids)—HIV infection
  - Environments or settings with increased risk
  - Cochlear implant

Pneumococcal Polysaccharide Vaccine: Revaccination

- Routine revaccination of immunocompetent persons is not recommended.
- Revaccination recommended for persons age ≥2 years at highest risk of serious pneumococcal infection
- Single revaccination dose ≥5 years after first dose

Pneumococcal Polysaccharide Vaccine

Candidates for revaccination:

- Persons ≥2 years of age with:
  - Functional or anatomic asplenia
  - Immunosuppression
  - Chronic renal failure
  - Nephrotic syndrome.
- Persons vaccinated at <65 years of age.

Contraindications and Precautions

- Severe allergic reaction to vaccine component or following prior dose of vaccine
- Moderate or severe acute illness.

Adverse Reactions

- *Local reactions:*
  - Polysaccharide   30–50%
  - Conjugate   10–20%
- *Fever, myalgia:*
  - Polysaccharide   <1%
  - Conjugate   15–24%
- *Severe adverse reactions:* Rare

Vaccines Recommended by IAP

Pneumococcal vaccine—For whom?

- *Conjugate 10/13 valent pneumococcal vaccine:* Each 0.5 mL contains a mixture of purified capsular polysaccharides containing 13 serotypes 1, 3, 4, 5, 6B, 7F, 9V, 14, 18C, 19A 19F and 23F: Dose—0.5 mL/IM (India- IBIS study, the prevalent serotypes were 1, 4, 5, 6, 7, 12, 19, 45). Serotypes 6 and 19 are omnipresent.
- Conjugate 10/13 valent pneumococcal vaccine (PCV10/13) since registered in India
- For routine use, the vaccine is recommended in prime boost schedule along with other EPI vaccines at 6, 10 and 14 weeks followed by a booster at 15–18 months.

Pneumococcal vaccine—increasing valance?

	7 valent	10 valent	13 valent
Invasive isolates			
IBIS <5 years	54.5%	72.3%	76.3%
IBIS >5 years	21.4%	56.9%	64.1%
Lakshmy <5 years	19.1%	45.2%	53%
Lakshmy >5 years	17.1%	60.3%	67.1%
Nasal Carriage isolates			
ANSORP <5 years	50.0%	52.5%	53.0%
Jabaraj <1 year	46.0%	-	-

IBIS: Invasive Bacterial Infection Surveillance Group; ANSORP: The Asian Network for Surveillance of Resistant Pathogens.

Vaccines, Immunoglobulins and Antisera

Pneumococcal Vaccine—For High-risk Group

IAP recommends administration of both the PCV13 and PPV 23 for the following high-risk groups of children <5 years and PPV for children above 2 years (including those who had received the 7 valent PCV < 2 years) if already received PCV, a gap of 2 months must be maintained between PCV 7 and subsequent PPV 23.

- Sickle cell disease
- Nephrotic syndrome on remission
- Congenital or acquired asplenia or splenic dysfunction
- HIV infection
- Chronic cardiac and pulmonary disease
- Immunodeficiency conditions
- Cerebrospinal fluid fistula, cochlear implants
- Diabetes mellitus
- Congenital immunodeficiency, HIV
- Immunosuppressive therapy, organ transplant recipient

Recommendations for Pneumococcal Immunization with PCV13 or PPV23 Vaccine for Children at High Risk

Age	Previous dose of any pneumococcal vaccine	Recommendations
23 months or younger	None	PCV7, as in Chapter 4
24 through 59 months	4 doses of PCV7	• 1 dose of PPV23 vaccine at 24 months of age, at least 8 weeks after last dose of PCV7 • 1 dose of PPV23, 5 years after the first dose of PPV23
24 through 59 months	1–3 previous doses of PCV7	• 1 dose of PCV7 • 1 dose of PPV23, 8 weeks after the last dose of PCV7 • 1 dose of PPV23, 5 years after the first dose of PPV23
24 through 59 months	1 dose of PPV23	• 2 doses of PCV7, 8 weeks apart, beginning at 6–8 weeks after last dose of PPV23 • 1 dose of PPV23 vaccine, 5 years after the last dose of PPV23 and at least 8 weeks after PCV7
24 through 59 months	No previous dose of PPV23 or PCV7	• 2 doses of PCV7, 8 weeks apart • 1 dose of PPV23 vaccine, 8 week after the last dose of PCV7 • 1 dose of PPV23 vaccine, 5 years • after the first dose of PPV23 vaccine

PCV7 heptavalent pneumococcal conjugate vaccine, PPV23 valent pneumococcal polysaccharide vaccine. A second dose of PPV23 5 years after the first dose is recommended only for children who are immunocompromised, have sickle cell disease, or have functional or anatomical splenia. All other children with underlying medical conditions should receive 1 dose of PPV23.

Inactivated Polio Vaccine (IPV) (SALK)

The inactivated polio vaccine (IPV) is the oldest of the 2 polio vaccines currently available. Developed by Dr Jonas Salk in 1954. IPV was improved with several fold potency and currently available enhanced potency inactivated polio vaccine (eIPV) was developed in 1987. The vaccine contains killed poliovirus type 1, 2 and 3 viz. Type 1 = 40UD*, Type 2 = 8 UD* and Type 3 = 32 UD*

Indications: In prophylaxis against poliomyelitis in immunodeficient patients and those undergoing corticosteroid or radiation therapy. It is now recommended for routine immunization in certain developed countries and also in India along with OPV to protect the individual child from vaccine associated paralytic polio (VAPP).

Dosage: First three doses at intervals of 1–2 months and fourth dose 6–12 months after the third dose.

Contraindications: During epidemics of poliomyelitis

Special features: Prevents paralysis but does not prevent reinfection by wild polio viruses. Does not require any stringent conditions of storage and transportation. It can be combined with DTP to form a quadruple vaccine. Simplifies the vaccination schedule. No risk of vaccine associated paralytic polio (VAPP).

Adverse effects: No serious adverse effects reported with currently used vaccines.

Inactivated Polio Vaccine
- Highly effective in producing immunity to poliovirus
- 90% or more immune after 2 doses
- At least 99% immune after 3 doses
- Duration of immunity not known with certainty.

[*Unidad antigen D] is administered in 3 primary doses preferably at 6, 10 and 14 weeks/2, 4 and 6 months followed by a single booster at one and half-year.

Polio Vaccination Schedule in the United States

Age	Vaccine	Minimum interval
2 months	IPV	—
4 months	IPV	4 weeks
6–18 months	IPV	4 weeks
4–6 years*	IPV	4 weeks

*The fourth dose of IPV may be given as early as 1½ years.

Schedules that Include Both IPV and OPV in the US
- Only IPV is available in the United States
- Schedule begun with OPV should be completed with IPV
- Any combination of 4 doses of IPV and OPV by 4–6 years of age constitute a complete series.

Polio Vaccine: Contraindications and Precautions

- Severe allergic reaction to a vaccine component or following a prior dose of vaccine
- Moderate or severe acute illness.

Rotavirus Vaccine

Currently 4 live-attenuated oral vaccines are registered in India, viz. monovalent (GSK) and Bharat Biotech and Tetravalent rotavirus vaccine (MSD) should be administered strictly by oral route for infants 6 weeks through 32 weeks in 2–3 doses at minimum interval of 4 weeks.

Types of Rotavirus Vaccines

- *RV5 (RotaTeq):*
  - Contains five reassorted rotavirus strains developed from human and bovine parent rotavirus strains
  - Vaccine viruses suspended in a buffer solution
  - Contains no preservatives or thimerosal.
- RV1 (Rotarix)
- *RV116E neonatal human strain (Rotavac, Indian):*
  - Contains one strain of live-attenuated human rotavirus (type G1P1A [8])
  - Provided as a lyophilized powder that is reconstituted before administration
  - Contains no preservatives or thimerosal.

- Rotasiil (Indian—thermostable) contains five reassorted rotavirus strains developed from human and bovine parent rotavirus strains.
  - *Rotavirus vaccine effectiveness:*
    - *Condition:* Effectiveness
    - *Any rotavirus gastroenteritis:* 74–87%
    - *Severe gastroenteritis:* 85–98%

All vaccines significantly reduced physician visits for diarrhea, and reduced rotavirus-related hospitalization.

Rotavirus Vaccine: Recommendations

- Routine vaccination of all infants without a contraindication
- 2 (RV1) or 3 (RV116E) or (RV5) oral doses beginning at 6 weeks or 2 months of age
- Subsequent doses in the series should be separated from the previous dose by 1–2 months.
- *For both rotavirus vaccines:*
  - Maximum age for first dose is 14 weeks 6 days
  - Minimum interval between doses is 4 weeks
  - Maximum age for any dose is 7 months and 6 days
- ACIP US did not define a maximum interval between doses.
- If the interval between doses is prolonged, then the infant can still receive the vaccine as long as the 2nd dose can be given on or before 8 months of age.
- It is not necessary to restart the series or add doses because of a prolonged interval between doses.

Rotavirus Vaccine
- IAP-ACVIP recommends that providers need not repeat the dose if the infant spits out or regurgitates the vaccine.
- Any remaining dose should be administered on schedule.
- Doses of rotavirus vaccine should be separated by at least 4 weeks.

Rotavirus Vaccine—conditions not considered to be precautions
- *Pre-existing chronic gastrointestinal conditions:*
  - No data available
  - IAP ACVIP considers the benefits of vaccination to outweigh the risk.
- *Recent receipt of an antibody-containing blood product:*
  - No data available

- IAP-ACVIP recommends that rotavirus vaccine may be administered at any time before, concurrent with, or after administration of any blood product.

Rotavirus Vaccine and Preterm Infants
- IAP-ACVIP supports vaccination of a preterm infant if:
  - Chronological age is at least 6 weeks
  - Clinically stable
  - Vaccine is administered at time of discharge or after discharge from neonatal intensive care unit or nursery.

Immunosuppressed Household Contacts of Rotavirus Vaccine Recipients
- Infants living in households with persons who have or are suspected of having an immunodeficiency disorder or impaired immune status can be vaccinated.
- Protection provided by vaccinating the infant outweighs the small risk of transmitting vaccine virus.

Pregnant Household Contacts of Rotavirus Vaccine Recipients
- Infants living in households with pregnant women should be vaccinated.
  - Majority of women of childbearing age have pre-existing immunity to rotavirus
  - Risk for infection by vaccine virus is very low.

Rotavirus Vaccine and Intussusception*
In the United States

	Number of infants	Vaccine recipients	Placebo recipients
RV1	63,225	7 cases	7 cases
RV5	69,625	6 cases	5 cases

* RV1—0–30 days after either dose, RV5—0.42 days after any dose

Rotavirus Vaccine: Adverse Reactions
- Vomiting — 15–18%
- Diarrhea — 9–24%
- Irritability — 13–62%
- Fever — 40–43%
- Serious adverse reactions — None

Rotavirus vaccine storage and handling
- Store at 35°–46°F (2–8°C) and protect from light

- Do not freeze vaccines
- Administer RV5 as soon as possible after being removed from refrigeration

Rotavirus Vaccine
- Currently, 4 vaccine formulations are available; RV1, RV5, 116E and RV4
- Monovalent rotavirus vaccines formulation contains live-attenuated human strain—RIX 4414 HRV (further purified from isolate 89—12 belonging to G1P (8) serotype) or human neonatal 116E strain.
- 1st dose to be given at 6-8 weeks of age followed by a 2nd dose at 4-8 weeks interval; should be completed before 32 weeks of age; lyophilized formulation to be reconstituted with recommended diluent and given orally.
- *Serological evidence of protection:* Serum anti-rotavirus IgA by ELISA
- Re-assorted pentavalent human-bovine vaccine (G1, G2, G3, G4, and P1a) is licensed in India. 3 oral doses at 2, 4, and 6 months should be completed before 32 weeks of age; Liquid formulation to be given orally.
- In case of Rotavirus vaccine, RV1 can be used in 6, 10 weeks schedule.

VACCINES ADMINISTERED AT 9 MONTHS

Measles Vaccine/MMR Vaccine

Measles Vaccine

The vaccine is presented as a freeze-dried preparation.

Schwartz: Lyophilized preparation of live-attenuated Schwartz strain of measles virus obtained from chick embryo tissue culture.

Edmonston Zagreb: This contains live-attenuated measles virus (Edmonston–Zagreb strain) cultivated on human diploid cells. Most used strain.

Indications: For routine immunization, contraindicated in acute illnesses, deficient cell-mediated immunity, while using steroids and other immunosuppressive drugs.

Special features: The reconstituted vaccine should be kept refrigerated (at 4–8°C) and used within 4 hours.

Provides immunity even in severely malnourished children. Immunity develops 11–12 days after vaccination.

Adverse effects: Mild 'measles' like illness (fever and rash) 5–10 days after immunization. Fever, few red spots over abdomen.

Measles Vaccines: History

1963	Killed and live-attenuated vaccines
1965	Live further attenuated vaccine
1967	Killed vaccine withdrawn
1968	Live further attenuated vaccine (Edmonston–Enders strain)
1971	Licensure of combined measles-mumps-rubella vaccine
1989	Two-dose schedule
2005	Licensure of combined measles-mumps-rubella-varicella vaccine

Measles Vaccines

- Composition: Live virus
- Efficacy: 95% (range 90–98%)
- Duration of immunity: Lifelong
- Schedule: 2 doses
- Should be administered with mumps and rubella as MMR or with mumps, rubella and varicella as MMRV.

Measles Vaccine: Newer Developments

- Intranasal (aerosol) administration has been tried with fewer side effects—May be available in India soon.
- Currently available measles vaccine is supplied as freeze-dried powder, (single dose/10 dose) in brown-colored vials to be reconstituted with the recommended diluents and used within 4 hours of reconstitution.
- Measles vaccine containing MMR vaccine is now recommended by IAP-ACVIP at 9 months followed by MMR vaccine at 15 months and 4–6 years. 3 doses of MMR vaccine are the current recommendation of IAP-ACVIP.
- However, for sustained protection when the vaccine is given for children above 1 year of age for the first time it is

preferable to give 2 doses in the form of MMR vaccine, as it has now been proved that even for measles protection 2 doses are mandatory.
- Good control with ≥95% coverage
- Efficacy and safety well established with very minimal breakthrough infection (modified measles).

Measles–Mumps–Rubella (MMR) Vaccine

Measles vaccine combined with other live-attenuated vaccines such as mumps and rubella (MMR). Single dose in a lyophilized preparation consists of at least 1000 TCID50 of live hyper-attenuated measles virus (strain Schwartz), at least 5000 TCID50 of live-attenuated mumps virus (UrabeAM-9), at least 1000 TCID50 of attenuated rubella (Wilstar RA27/3M).

Indications: In joint prevention of measles, mumps and rubella. Given in children of both sexes aged ≥15 months.

Dosage: 0.5 mL single dose given subcutaneously/any time after the age of 15 months.

Contraindications: Immunodeficiency—congenital or acquired. Anaphylactic reactions. Recent injection of immunoglobulins.

Special features: Immunity persists for at least 14–16 years probably lifelong.

Adverse effects: Hyperthermia, respiratory symptoms of short duration. Sometimes febrile convulsions. Lymphadenitis or parotitis.

Measles-Rubella (MR) Vaccination Campaign

India, along with 10 other WHO South East Asia Region member countries, have resolved to eliminate measles and control rubella/congenital rubella syndrome (CRS) by 2020. In this direction, Ministry of Health & Family Welfare has initiated measles-rubella (MR) vaccination campaign in the age group of 9 months to less than 15 years in a phased manner across the nation. The campaign aims to cover approximately 41 crore children. All children from 9 months to less than 15 years of age will be given a single shot of Measles-Rubella (MR) vaccination during the campaign. Following the campaign, MR vaccine will become a part of routine immunization and will replace measles vaccine, currently given at 9-12 months and 16-24 months of age of child.

For those children who have already received such vaccination, the campaign dose would provide additional boosting to them.

Measles (MMR) Vaccine: Indications in the United States

- All children 15 months of age and older
- Susceptible adolescents and adults, except pregnant women, without documented evidence of immunity.

Measles-Mumps-Rubella Vaccine
- 9 months is the recommended and minimum age, with 2 doses at 15-18 months
- 3rd dose at 4-6 years of age.

Second Dose of Measles Vaccine

- Intended to produce measles immunity in persons who failed to respond to the first dose (primary vaccine failure)
- May boost antibody titers in some persons
- First dose of MMR at 9 months
- Second dose of MMR at 15-18 months
- Third dose may be given any time 4 weeks after the first dose
- Third dose preferably at 4-6 years

MMR Vaccine: Failure
- Measles, mumps, or rubella disease (or lack of immunity) in a previously vaccinated person
- 2-5% of recipients do not respond to the first dose
- Caused by antibody, damaged vaccine, in correct records
- Most persons with vaccine failure will respond to second dose.

MMR Vaccine: Contraindications and Precautions
- Severe allergic reaction to vaccine component or following prior dose
- Pregnancy
- Immunosuppression
- Moderate or severe acute illness
- Recent blood product.

Measles and Mumps Vaccines and Egg Allergy

- Measles and mumps viruses grown in check embryo fibroblast culture.
- Studies have demonstrated safety or MMR in egg-allergic children
- Vaccinate without testing

Measles Vaccine and HIV Infection

- MMR recommended for persons with asymptomatic and mildly symptomatic HIV infection
- Not recommended for those with evidence of severe immunosuppression
- Pre-vaccination HIV testing not recommended

Tuberculin Skin Testing (TST)* and Measles Vaccine

- Apply TST at same visit as MMR
- Delay TST at least 4 weeks if MMR given first
- Apply TST first and administer MMR when skin test read (least favored option because receipt of MMR is delayed.

MMR Vaccine: The Old and New Controversies

- MMR vaccine is supplied as freeze-dried powder (single dose) in brown-colored vials, to be reconstituted with the recommended diluent and used within 4 hours of reconstitution
- Old controversy of causal association of MMR vaccine with occurrence of autism, Guillain–Barré syndrome, inflammatory bowel disease, etc. have been negated.
- New controversy about different strains of measles and mumps components is being debated: Aseptic meningitis has not emerged as a major problem in India following MMR vaccine; so also, postvaccination parotitis.
- *All strains are equally immunogenic:* Measles 98.7%, mumps 95.5%, Rubella 99.5% *Efficacious:* Inter-changeable
- *Ideal to start at 15 months:* If given during adolescents and for students going abroad 2 doses at 4–8 weeks interval.
- Second dose of MMR vaccine at 15 months and 3rd dose at 4–6 years is recommended by IAP-ACVIP due to demonstrable waning immunity for measles component.

- MMR-V combination vaccine is now registered in India. IAP-ACVIP recommends MMR-V vaccine *only* for 2nd dose to 4–6 years.

VACCINE ADMINISTERED AT 15 MONTHS

Varicella (Chickenpox Vaccine)

Live-attenuated varicella–zoster virus (Oka strain), obtained from human diploid cell culture.

Indications: For active immunization from age of 15 months onwards. *Dosage:* 0.5 mL subcutaneous.

For all ages: 2 doses—1st dose at 15 months and 2nd dose at 4–6 years.

Contraindications: Acute severe febrile illness. Lymphocytes <1200/mm^3.

Hypersensitivity to neomycin—special features: The vaccine should not be mixed with other vaccines in the same syringe.

Adverse effects: Mild, transient reaction at injection site.

Varicella in the United States

- Increasing proportion of cases as a result of breakthrough infection
- Outbreaks reported in schools with high varicella vaccination coverage
- Persons with breakthrough infection may transmit virus.

Herpes Zoster

- 5,00,000 to 1 million episodes occur annually in the United States
- Lifetime risk of zoster estimated to be 32%
- 50% of persons living until age 85 years will develop zoster.

Varicella-containing Vaccines

- Varicella vaccine (Varivax, Varilrix, OKA vac, Zuvicella, Nexipox)
  - Approved for persons 12 months and older.
- Measles-mumps-rubella-varicella vaccine (MMR TETRA) now registered in India
  - Approved for children 12 months through 12 years.

- Herpes zoster vaccine (Zostavax), not available in India now.
  - Approved for persons 60 years and older.

Varicella Vaccine Immunogenicity and Efficacy

- *Detectable antibody:*
  - 97% of children 12 months–12 years following 1 dose
  - 99% of persons 13 years and older after 2 doses.
- 70–90% effective against any varicella disease
- 95–100% effective against severe varicella disease.

Varicella Breakthrough Infection

- Immunity appears to be long-lasting for most recipients
- Breakthrough disease much milder than in unvaccinated persons
- No consistent evidence that risk of breakthrough infection increases with time since vaccination.
- Risk of breakthrough varicella 2–5 times higher if varicella vaccine administered less than 30 days following MMR.
- No increased risk if varicella vaccine given simultaneously or more than 30 days after MMR.

Varicella Vaccine Recommendations: Children

- Routine vaccination at 12–15 months of age
- Routine second dose at 4–6 years of age
- Minimum interval between doses of varicella vaccine for children younger than 13 years of age is 3 months

Varicella Vaccine Recommendations: Adolescents and Adults

- All persons 13 years of age and older without evidence of varicella immunity
- Two doses separated by at least 4 weeks
- Do not repeat first dose because of extended interval between doses.

Varicella Vaccine Recommendations: Healthcare Personnel

- Recommended for all susceptible heathcare personnel
- Pre-vaccination serologic screening probably cost-effective
- Post-vaccination testing not necessary or recommended

Herpes Zoster Vaccine

- ACIP recommends a single dose among persons 60 years and older
- May vaccinate regardless of prior history of herpes zoster (shingles)
- Persons with a chronic medical condition may be vaccinated unless a contraindication or precaution exists for the condition.

Herpes Zoster Vaccine: Efficacy

- Compared with placebo group vaccine group had:
  - 51% fewer episodes of zoster
  - Lower efficacy for older recipients
  - Less severe disease
  - 66% less postherpetic neuralgia

MMR-V Vaccine (Priorix Tetra)

Qualitative and Quantitative Composition

Each dose (0.5 mL) of the reconstituted vaccine contains:

- Live-attenuated measles virus 1 (Schwarz strain) not less than $10^{3.0} CCID_{50}^{3}$
- Live-attenuated mumps virus 1 (RIT4385 strain, derived from Jeryl Lynn strain) not less than $10^{4.4}$ $CCID_{50}^{3}$ live-attenuated rubella virus 2 (Wistar RA 27/3 strain) not less than $10^{3.0} CCID_{50}^{3}$
- Live-attenuated varicella virus 2 (OKA strain) not less than $10^{3.3} PFU^{4}$
- Water for injections IP 0.5 mL
- (i) Produced in chick embryo cells, (ii) Produced in human diploid (MRC-5) cells, (iii) cell culture infective dose 50% (iv) plaque-forming units
- This vaccine contains a trace amount of neomycin, 14 mg of sorbitol
- Before reconstitution, the powder is a white to slightly pink-colored cake and the solvent is a clear colorless liquid.
- PRIORIX-TETRA is indicated for active immunization in subjects from the age of 1 year to 12 years of age inclusive against measles, mumps, rubella and varicella.

- As it is associated with increased incidence of febrile seizures in children less than 4 years, IAP-ACVIP advocates its use only at 4–6 years.
- May be used for second doses of MMR and varicella vaccines at 4–6 years.

Varicella Vaccine Post-exposure Prophylaxis

- Varicella vaccine is recommended for use in persons without evidence of varicella immunity after exposure to varicella
  - 70–100% effective if given within 72 hours of exposure
- Not effective if administered more than 5 days after exposure but will produce immunity if not infected.

Zoster Vaccine

Contraindications and Precautions

- Severe allergic reaction to a vaccine component or following a prior dose
- Pregnancy or planned pregnancy within 4 weeks
- Immunosuppression from any cause.

Adverse Reactions

- Local reactions (pain, erythema)
  - 19% (children)
  - 24% (adolescents and adults)
- Generalized rash—4-6%
  - May be maculopapular rather than vesicular
  - Average lesions
- Systemic reactions not common
- Adverse reactions similar for MMRV.

Zoster Following Vaccination

- Most cases in children
- Not all cases caused by vaccine virus
- Risk from vaccine virus less than from wild-type virus
- Usually a mild illness without complications, such as post-herpetic neuralgia.

Varicella-containing Vaccines

Contraindications and Precautions

- Severe allergic reaction to vaccine component or following a prior dose

- Immunosuppression
- Pregnancy
- Moderate or severe acute illness
- Recent blood product (except herpes zoster vaccine)

Varicella Vaccine

Use in Immunocompromised Persons
- MMRV not approved for use in persons with HIV infection
- Do not administer zoster vaccine to immunosuppressed persons.

Varicella-containing Vaccine: Storage and Handling
- Store frozen at −15°C or lower at all times
- Store diluents at room temperature or refrigerate
- Discard if not used within 30 minutes of reconstitution

Varicella Vaccine

- Varicella vaccine is supplied as freeze-dried powder (single dose) in brown-colored vials, to be reconstituted with the recommended diluent and used within 4 hours of reconstitution.
- Varicella vaccine is now recommended ≥15 months of age in infant immunization.
- Now recommended for universal use by IAP-ACVIP.
- Varicella and MMR vaccines can be given on the same date at different sites: If not, they should be given at 4 weeks interval
- 2 doses at 15 months and 4–6 years is the current IAP-ACVIP recommendation for all children.
- 1st dose ≥15 months, for greater immunogenicity followed by 2nd dose at 4–6 years
- Breakthrough infection after 1st dose manifests as 'modified chickenpox.'

VACCINES ADMINISTERED AT 18 MONTHS (BOOSTER)

- DTwP/DTaP
- DTwP/DTaP-Hib
- DTwP/DTaP-Hib–IPV
- OPV/IPV
- Pneumococcal

VACCINES ADMINISTERED AT 12 MONTHS

Hepatitis A Vaccine (Inactivated)

This is a suspension-containing formaldehyde inactivated HM 175 strain hepatitis A virus. Aluminum hydroxide is used as the adsorbent. The pediatric dose ensures a viral antigen content of not less than 360/720 ELISA units in a dose volume.

Indications: Active immunization against hepatitis A virus infections.

Dosage: 0.5 mL/not less than 360 ELISA units given IM. The 1st dose is given on an elected date. Booster dose is recommended anytime between 6 and 12 months after initiation of the primary course.

Contraindications: Actuate severe febrile illness

Adverse effects: Nausea, loss of appetite, mild headache, malaise, fatigue, fever.

Hepatitis A Vaccines

- Inactivated whole virus vaccines
- Pediatric and adult formulations
  - Pediatric formulations approved for persons 12 months through 18 years
  - Adult formulations approved for persons 19 years and older

Hepatitis A Vaccine—Immunogenicity

Adults

- >95% seropositive after one dose
- 100% seropositive after two doses.

Children (>12 months) and Adolescents

- >97% seropositive after one dose
- 100% seropositive after two doses
- In India HAVRIX (GSK) AVAXIM (SANOFI) and HAVPUR (Virosome adjuvanted) (Novartis) Hep A vaccines are available. Hep A-Hep B combined vaccine should be given at 0, 1, 6 months schedule.

Recently, IAP ACVIP has endorsed use of live-attenuated HA vaccine (Biovac-A) which needs to be given SC in single dose at

1 year. No booster is needed. Seroconversion and sero-protection of both vaccines are comparable.

IAP-ACVIP Recommendations for Routine Hepatitis: A Vaccination of Children

- All children should receive hepatitis A vaccine at 12 months of age and booster as per vaccine used.
- Vaccination should be integrated into the routine childhood vaccination schedule.
- Children who are not vaccinated by 2 years of age can be vaccinated at subsequent visits.

VACCINES ADMINISTERED AT 2 YEARS OF AGE

Typhoid Vaccines

Polysaccharide Typhoid Vaccine

This is prepared from purified Vi capsular polysaccharides of *S. typhi* in endemic areas, protection offered: About 60–65%.

Indications: In prevention of typhoid fever in children >2 years old.

Dosage: 1 dose of 0.5 mL (subcutaneous or intramuscular). Booster every 3 years.

Contraindications: Hypersensitivity to any of the vaccine components.

Special features: No protection against *S. paratyphi* A or B Postpone the vaccination in cases of acute infections or fever.

Adverse effects: Local pain, rash, rise in temperature in few cases.

Conjugate Typhoid Vaccine

Typhoid Vi capsular polysaccharide tetanus toxoid conjugate vaccine (Typbar TCV and Pedatyph) stimulates specialized T cells in the human body, which the typhoid Vi capsular polysaccharide vaccine alone cannot do. Engagement of T-cells by Vi conjugate vaccine results in superior and longer lasting antibody response, which helps in the prevention of typhoid disease not only in adults but also in children and infants. Further, the typhoid Vi capsular polysaccharide tetanus toxoid conjugate vaccine is the only approved vaccine for children and infants less than 2 years of age. During the Phase III clinical study, a single dose of Typbar-TCV elicited 4-fold seroconversion rates of 98.05%, 99.17% and 92.13% in subjects between ≥6 months to 2 years, >2–15 years and >15–45 years, respectively.

1st dose can be given to babies 6 months and older and followed by a booster in 2nd year, which should confer lifelong immunity as per present studies.

- Vi antigen vaccine currently available in India is given in a prime boost schedule: Initially a single dose ≥2 years of age followed by booster doses every 3 years are mandatory for continuous protection.
- IAP-ACVIP recommends routine typhoid vaccination for children 9 months (minimum age 6 months) of age with TCV formulation currently available or at 2 years with typhoid Vi vaccine at 2 years
- Efficacy rated at 65–75%: Breakthrough infection is therefore a concern. Efficacy is better with TCV after completion of 2 dose schedule.
- Single dose of any of typhoid conjugate vaccine (TCV 25 mg) is recommended from 6 months onwards and can be administered with MMR also.
- Booster dose of Typhoid conjugate vaccine not recommended in subsequent years.
- Stress to be laid on personal hygiene and other universal precautions for prevention of water-borne infections in general.

VACCINES ADMINISTERED AT 5 YEARS

1. Diphtheria and Tetanus Vaccine (Pediatric Formulation)

This is a combination of diphtheria and tetanus toxoid adsorbed on aluminum phosphate and suspended in isotonic sodium chloride solution. Adsorption increases the immunological effectiveness. 2 doses provide more than 80% protection.

Indications: In primary immunization of school-going children 5 years and above against diphtheria and tetanus.

Dosage: 0.5 mL deep IM, lateral aspect of thigh. As a booster at 10 years, after the 3 primary doses of DPT given at infancy and booster doses (DPT) given at 15–18 months and 5 years.

In children >6 years who have not received DPT, 2 doses of DT, 4 weeks apart, with a booster dose 6 months–1 year later.

Contraindications: Seriously ill patients who need hospitalization.

Special features: Vaccine should not be frozen. Stored in a refrigerator at 4–8°C.

Adverse effects: Fever, mild local reactions

2. DTwP/DTaP booster: *Refer vaccines administered at 6, 10 and 14 weeks*

3. OPV booster

4. Typhoid booster: *Refer vaccines at 2 years*

5. MMR second dose: *Refer vaccines at 9 months and 15 months*

6. Varicella second dose

VACCINES ADMINISTERED AT 10 YEARS

TT/Td/Tdap Booster

Tetanus toxoid
This is a suspension of tetanus toxoid adsorbed on aluminum phosphate and suspended in isotonic saline.

Indications: To actively immunize all children from age 6 weeks onwards as DTP and as monovalent formulation from 10 years onwards against tetanus.

Dosage: 2 doses of 0.5 mL each at an interval of 4–6 weeks given intramuscularly. 1st booster does 1 year after the initial 2 doses.

Contraindications: Fever or other acute illness. *Special feature:* Stored at 4–8°C.

Adverse effects: Mild local reactions. Rarely neurological complications.

Td vaccine intended to maintain the diphtheria immunity is now recommended in place of TT for wound prophylaxis and against neonatal and maternal tetanus for pregnant women.

Tdap vaccine containing tetanus toxoid, acellular pertussis component and reduced quantity of diphtheria. Toxoid is also available which is indicated for boosters above 7 years of age, in adolescents and adults in regions endemic for pertussis. The vaccine is given only as a single booster whereas Td boosters are recommended very 10 years.

DTaP, DT, Td and Tdap

	Diphtheria	Tetanus
DTaP, DT	7–8 Lf units	5–12.5 Lf units
Td, Tdap (adult)	2–2.5 Lf units	5 Lf units

DTaP and pediatric DT used through age 6 years. Adult Td for persons 7 years and older. Tdap for persons 10–18 years (Boostrix) or 10–64 years (Adacel).

Tetanus Toxoid

- Formalin-inactivated tetanus toxin
- Schedule: Three or four doses + booster
  Booster every 10 years
- Efficacy: Approximately 100%
- Duration: Approximately 10 years
- Should be administered with diphtheria toxoid as DTaP, DT, Td, or Tdap.

Routine DTaP Primary Vaccination Schedule

Dose	Age	Interval
Primary 1	2 months	—
Primary 2	4 months	4 weeks
Primary 3	6 months	4 weeks
Primary 4	15–18 months	6 months

Children who receive DT
- The number of doses of DT needed to complete the series depends on the child's age at the first dose:
  - If first dose given at younger than 12 months of age, 4 doses are recommended.
  - If first dose given at 12 months or older, 3 doses complete the primary series.

Routine Tdap Schedule: Children Younger than 7 years of Age

Booster doses
- 4 through 6 years of age, before entering school

- 11 or 12 years of age if 5 years since last dose (Tdap)
- Every 10 years thereafter (Td).

Routine Td Schedule: Unvaccinated Persons 7 years of Age or Older

Dose*	Interval
Primary 1	....
Primary 2	4 weeks
Primary 3	6–12 months
Booster dose every 10 years	

*ACIP recommends that one of these doses (preferably the first) be administered as Tdap

Diphtheria and Tetanus Toxoids

Contraindications and Precautions
- Severe allergic reaction to vaccine component or following a prior dose
- Moderate or severe acute illness

Adverse Reactions
- Local reactions (erythema, induration)
- Fever and systemic symptoms not common
- Exaggerated local reactions (Arthus-type)
- Severe systemic reactions rare

DT/TT/Td/Tdap vaccines—For whom and when?
- DT is recommended for children at 5 years as booster in National Immunization Schedule
- IAP recommends a second booster of DTwP/DTaP at 5 years instead of DT
- After 7 doses of TT the adequately immunized pregnant woman needs only a single booster dose of Tdap/Td during each pregnancy.
- No need to repeat Td at less than 5 years interval for clean wound: For contaminated wound TIG may be administered.
- Tdap is now recommended by IAP-ACVIP instead of TT at 10 years because of re-emergence of adolescent pertussis in certain regions of India and Td every 10 years thereafter in view of re-emergence of diphtheria in adolescents.
- Td/Tdap vaccines since registered in India.

DT/TT/Td/Tdap Vaccines

- Repeated TT injections following trivial injuries may result in:
  - Reduced immunogenicity
  - Hypersensitivity
  - Hemolytic anemia
  - Amyloidosis
  - Increased risk of hemorrhagic disease of the newborn
  - 7 doses of TT injections, 5 doses as DTwP/DTaP at 6, 10 and 14 weeks followed by a booster at 5 years and 2 doses as Tdap/Td at 10 and 20 years, respectively.

HPV Vaccine

Human Papillomavirus

Human papillomaviruses are small, double-stranded DNA viruses that infect the epithelium. More than 100 HPV types have been identified; they are differentiated by the genetic sequence of the outer capsid protein L1. Most human papillomavirus (HPV) types infect the cutaneous epithelium and cause common skin warts. About 40 types infect the mucosal epithelium; these are categorized according to their epidemiologic association with cervical cancer. Infection with low-risk or non-oncogenic types, such as types 6 and 11, can cause benign or low-grade cervical cell abnormalities, genital warts and laryngeal papilloma. High-risk, or oncogenic, HPV types act as carcinogens in the development of cervical cancer and other anogenital cancers. High-risk types (currently including types 16, 18, 31, 33, 35, 39, 45, 51, 52, 56, 58, 59, 68, 69, 73, 82) can cause low-grade cervical cell abnormalities, high-grade cervical cell abnormalities that are precursors to cancer, and anogenital cancers. High-risk HPV types are detected in 99% of cervical cancer. Type 16 is the cause of approximately 50% of cervical cancers worldwide, and types 16 and 18 together account for about 70% of cervical cancers. Infection with a high-risk HPV type is considered necessary for the development of cervical cancer, but by itself it is not enough to cause cancer because most women with HPV infection do not develop cancer.

In addition to cervical cancer, HPV infection is also associated with anogenital cancers less commonly than cervical cancer, such as cancer of the vulva, vagina, penis and anus. The association of genital types of HPV with non-genital cancers is less well established, but studies support a role for these HPV types in a subset of oral cavity and pharyngeal cancers.

Human Papillomavirus (HPV): Features

- Small DNA virus
- More than 100 types identified based on the genetic sequence of the outer capsid protein L1
- 40 types infect the mucosa epithelium.

Human Papillomavirus: Types and Disease Association (Flowchart 5.1)

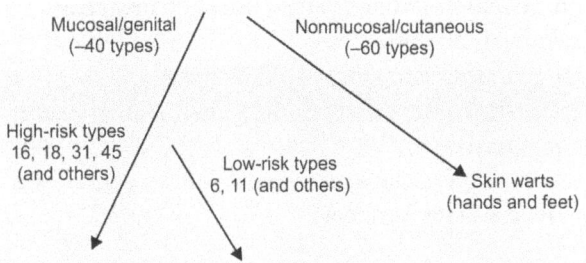

Flowchart 5.1: Types and disease association of HPV.

- Low-grade cervical abnormalities
- Cancer precursors
- Anogenital cancers
- Low-grade cervical abnormalities
- Genital warts
- Laryngeal papilloma

HPV-associated Disease

Type	Women	Men
16/18	• 70% of cervical cancers • 70% of anal/genital cancers	• 70% of anal cancers • Transmission to women
6/11	• 90% of genital warts • 90% of RRP* lesions	• 90% of genital warts • 90% of RRP lesions • Transmission to women

* RRP: recurrent respiratory papillomatosis

Natural History of HPV Infection (Flowchart 5.2)

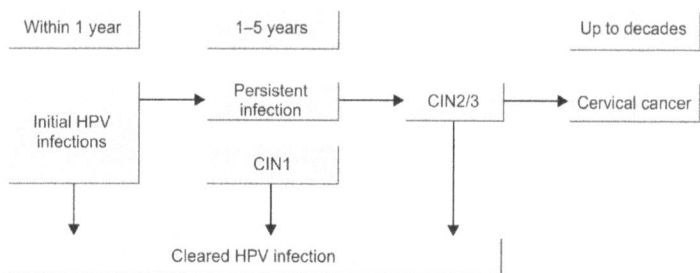

Flowchart 5.2: Natural history of HPV infection.

HPV: Clinical Features

- Most HPV infections are asymptomatic and result in no clinical disease.
- Clinical manifestations of HPV infection include:
  - Anogenital warts
  - Recurrent respiratory papillomatosis
  - Cervical cancer precursors (cervical intraepithelial neoplasia)
  - Cancer (cervical, anal, vaginal, vulvar, penile, and some head and neck cancer)

HPV: Epidemiology

- Reservoir: Human
- Transmission: Direct contact, usually sexual
- Temporal pattern: None
- Communicability: Presumed to be high

Cervical Cancer Screening

- Cervical cancer screening—no change
  - 30% of cervical cancers caused by HPV types not prevented by the quadrivalent HPV vaccine
  - Vaccinated females could subsequently be infected with non-vaccine HPV types
  - Sexually active female could have been infected prior to vaccination.
- Providers should educate women about the importance of cervical cancer screening.

Human Papillomavirus Vaccine

- HPV L1 major capsid protein of the virus is antigen used for immunization
- L1 protein expressed in yeast cells using recombinant technology
- L1 proteins self-assemble into virus-like particles (VLP)
- Non-infectious and non-oncogenic.

HPV Vaccine: Efficacy*

Endpoint	Efficacy
HPV 16/18-related CIN 2/3 or AIS	100
HPV 6/11/16/18-related CIN	95
HPV 6/11/16/18-related genital warts	99

*Among 16–26 years old females.
CIN: cervical intraepithelial neoplasia; AIS: adenocarcinoma *in situ*.

- High efficacy among females without evidence of infection with vaccine HPV types
- No evidence of efficacy against disease caused by vaccine types with which participants were infected at the time of vaccination
- Prior infection with one HPV type did not diminish efficacy of the vaccine against other vaccine HPV types.

Routine HPV Vaccination: Recommendations

- ACIP recommends routine vaccination of females 9 to 14 years of age
- The vaccination series should be started as young as 9 years of age at the clinician's discretion.
- Catch-up vaccination recommended to females 15 through 45 years of age.
- If HPV vaccine initiated between 9 and 14 years of age only 2 doses are sufficient to provide comparable protection with 3 dose schedules.

HPV Vaccination: Schedule (Tetravalent)

- Routine schedule is 0, 2, 6 months
- Third dose should follow the first dose by at least 24 weeks

- An accelerated schedule using minimum intervals is not recommended
- Series does not need to be restarted, if the schedule is interrupted.

HPV Vaccine: Special Situations

Vaccine can be administered:
- Equivocal or abnormal pap-test
- Positive HPV-DNA test
- Genital warts
- Immunosuppression
- Breastfeeding

HPV Vaccine: Contraindications and Precautions

- *Contraindication:*
  - Severe allergic reaction to a vaccine component or following a prior dose
- *Precaution:*
  - Moderate or severe acute illnesses (defer until symptoms improve)

HPV Vaccine: Adverse Reactions

• Local reactions (pain, swelling)	84%
• Fever	10%
• No serious adverse reactions reported*	

* Similar reports in placebo recipients (9%)

Vaccination during Pregnancy: Provisional Recommendation

- Initiation of the vaccine series should be delayed until after completion of pregnancy.
- If a woman is found to be pregnant after initiating the vaccination series, remaining doses should be delayed until after the pregnancy.
- If a vaccine dose has been administered during pregnancy, there is no indication for intervention.
- Women vaccinated during pregnancy should be reported to Merck registry (800,986,8999).

HPV Vaccine: Storage and Handling
- Store at 35–46°F (2–8°C)
- Protect from light
- Administer immediately after removing from refrigeration
- Do not expose to freezing temperature

Human Papillomavirus Vaccine
- 36.1% of Indian women per one lakh population suffer from cervical cancer. Serotype 16 and 18 account for 76.4% incidence. Serotype 45 and 31 responsible for a small percentage. Over 40 serotypes identified as oncogenic.
- HPV and cervical disease; disease progression; from HPV infection to cervical cancer is a process which may take 10–20 years. One of the first histological signs of HPV infection is the presence of koilocytosis; epithelial cell with distinctive large, clear vacuoles around the nucleus.
- When the immune system fails to clear an oncogenic HPV infection, a persistent infection develops.
- Persistent oncogenic HPV infection are more likely to progress towards invasive cervical cancer, if they are left untreated.
- Cervical intraepithelial neoplasia (CIN) precedes development of cervical cancer.
- There are three stages of cervical intraepithelial neoplasia: CIN1, CIN2, and CIN3
- CIN1 referred to as "*Low Grade*" is squamous intraepithelial lesions whereas CIN2 and CIN3 are referred to as "*High Grade*" intraepithelial lesions and are considered oncogenic.
- Every sexually active woman is at risk of oncogenic HPV infection. Of the estimated 50–80% of women who will accrue an HPV infection in their lifetime, 50% are infected with oncogenic HPV type.
- Young woman aged 16–25 years are at greatest risk of oncogenic HPV infection.
- Currently two vaccine formulations are licensed in India.
- HPV2; Bivalent HPV vaccine (Serotype 16 and 18); to be given to adolescent girls from 10 to 12 years of age and women with upper age limit of 45 years; dose 0.5 mL IM at deltoid at 0, 1 and 6 months.

- HPV4; Tetravalent HPV vaccine (serotypes 6, 11, 16 and 18) to be given to adolescent girls and women from 9 to 45 years of age; 3 doses at 0, 2, and 6 months. 0.5 mL IM at deltoid, HPV4 vaccine can be given during lactation period also.
- Both vaccines are to be given in lying down posture; no boosters are recommended.
- Immunogenicity; 100% seroconversion against HPV 16 and 18; (responsible for over 90% of cervical cancer); some evidence of protection against types 45 and 31.
- Routine HPV testing is not recommended. However, screening for cervical cancer subsequent to vaccination is mandatory.
- HPV vaccine is only a cervical cancer preventive vaccine and not to be promoted as a vaccine against STDs.
- The vaccine is to be administered preferably before sexual activity is established in naïve population; in young women and women of childbearing age vaccine can be administered regardless of sexual activity.

Rubella Vaccine

This is live-attenuated rubella virus (Wilstar RA 27/3M propagated on human diploid cells.

Indications: In immunization of unvaccinated girls from 12 years of age to puberty (before Pregnancy)

Dosage: 0.5 mL subcutaneously into upper arm

Contraindications: Febrile respiratory illness.

Special features: Seroconversion occurs in more than 91% of vaccinated persons.

Adverse effects: Local pain, erythema or induration at the site of injections.

Rubella vaccine is now given to adolescent girls from 10 years of age where campaign approach is preferred.

Dengue Vaccine

DENGVAXIA (Dengue Tetravalent Vaccine, Live) is a sterile suspension for subcutaneous injection. DENGVAXIA is supplied as a vial of lyophilized vaccine antigen, which must be reconstituted at the time of use with 0.6 mL from the accompanying vial of diluent (0.4% sodium chloride). After reconstitution, DENGVAXIA is a clear, colorless suspension (trace amounts of white to translucent proteinaceous particles may be present).

After reconstitution, each 0.5 mL dose of DENGVAXIA contains 4.5–6.0 $\log_{10}$ CCID50 of each of the chimeric yellow fever dengue (CYD) virus serotypes 3 ,2 ,1, and 4. Each 0.5 mL dose is formulated to contain 2 mg sodium chloride and the following ingredients as stabilizers: 0.56 mg essential amino acids (including L-phenylalanine), 0.2 mg non-essential amino acids, 2.5 mg L-arginine hydrochloride, 18.75 mg sucrose, 13.75 mg D-trehalose dihydrate, 9.38 mg D-sorbitol, 0.18 mg trometamol, and 0.63 mg urea.

Each of the four CYD viruses (CYD1-, CYD2-, CYD3-, and CYD4-) in DENGVAXIA was constructed using recombinant DNA technology by replacing the sequences encoding the pre-membrane (prM) and envelope (E) proteins in the yellow fever (YF) 17D204 vaccine virus genome with those encoding for the homologous sequences of dengue virus serotypes 1, 2, 3, and 4, respectively. Each CYD virus is cultured separately in Vero cells (African Green Monkey kidney) under serum-free conditions, harvested from the supernatant of the Vero cells and purified by membrane chromatography and ultrafiltration. The purified and concentrated harvest of each CYD virus is then diluted in a stabilizer solution to produce the four monovalent drug substances. The final bulk product is a mixture of the four monovalent drug substances diluted in the stabilizer solution. The final bulk product is sterilized by filtration at 0.22 μm, filled into vials and freeze-dried.

DENGVAXIA does not contain preservative.

The vial stoppers for the Lyophilized Vaccine Antigen and Diluent vials of DENGVAXIA are not made with natural rubber latex.

Indications

DENGVAXIA® (Dengue Tetravalent Vaccine, Live) is a vaccine indicated for the prevention of dengue disease caused by dengue virus serotypes 1, 2, 3 and 4. DENGVAXIA is approved for use in individuals 9 through 16 years of age with laboratory-confirmed previous dengue infection and living in endemic areas.

Limitations of Use

- DENGVAXIA is not approved for use in individuals not previously infected by any dengue virus serotype or for whom this information is unknown. Those not previously infected are at increased risk for severe dengue disease when vaccinated and subsequently infected with dengue virus. Previous dengue infection can be assessed through a medical record of a previous laboratory-confirmed dengue infection or through serological testing prior to vaccination.
- The safety and effectiveness of DENGVAXIA have not been established in individuals living in dengue non-endemic areas.

Dosage and Administration

For subcutaneous use only.

Dose

Three doses (0.5 mL each) 6 months apart (at month 0, 6, and 12).

Preparation

- The package contains a vial of lyophilized vaccine antigen and a vial of saline diluent (0.4% NaCl).
- After removing the "flip-off" caps, cleanse the lyophilized vaccine antigen and diluent vial stoppers with a suitable germicide. Do not remove the vial stoppers or metal seals holding them in place.
- To reconstitute DENGVAXIA, use a sterile needle and syringe to withdraw 0.6 mL from the diluent vial and inject it into the vial of the lyophilized vaccine antigen. Swirl the vial gently.
- Changing needles between withdrawing the vaccine from the vial and injecting it into a recipient is not necessary unless the needle has been damaged or contaminated.
- DENGVAXIA should be used immediately after reconstitution.
- After reconstitution, the suspension is colorless and may develop trace amounts of white to translucent endogenous proteinaceous particles.
- Parenteral drug products should be inspected visually for particulate matter and discoloration prior to administration,

whenever solution and container permit. Discard the vial if the solution is cloudy or contains particles other than trace amounts of white to translucent particles.
- Discard reconstituted vaccine if not used within 30 minutes.
- DENGVAXIA should not be mixed in the same syringe with other parenteral products.

Administration

After reconstitution, withdraw 0.5 mL of DENGVAXIA and administer subcutaneously immediately or store refrigerated at 2°C to 8°C (36°F to 46°F) and use within 30 minutes. Do not administer DENGVAXIA by intramuscular injection.

How Supplied:

- *Dosage forms and strengths:* DENGVAXIA is a suspension for injection (supplied as a lyophilized powder to be reconstituted with the supplied diluent, 0.4% NaCl). A single dose, after reconstitution, is 0.5 mL.
- An outer package of 1 dose (NDC 49281-605-01) contains 1 single dose vial of lyophilized vaccine antigen (NDC 49281-606-58) and 1 single dose vial of saline diluent (NDC 49281-546-68).
- The vial stoppers for the lyophilized vaccine antigen vials and the saline diluent vials of DENGVAXIA are not made with natural rubber latex.
  Storage and Handling
- Store Lyophilized Vaccine Antigen and Saline Diluent in a refrigerator at 2°C to 8°C (36–46°F). Do not freeze. Protect from light.
- Do not use after the expiration date shown on the vial labels of the Lyophilized Vaccine Antigen and Saline Diluent.
- After reconstitution, administer DENGVAXIA immediately or store refrigerated at 2°C to 8°C (36–46°F) and use within 30 minutes. Discard reconstituted vaccine, if not used within 30 minutes.

SEASONAL/TRAVEL-RELATED VACCINES

Flu Vaccines

Inactivated, purified split influenza vaccines containing 2A+ 1B/2B type antigens, is now available in India.

Composition

The antigen composition for the approaching influenza season (in view of frequent antigenic drift of the virus, more with type A) is determined by WHO. European community, US as well as Australian health officials as differences exist between northern and southern hemispheres. In India, only limited studies available regarding antigenic prevalence/drift. If antigenic shift occurs the result will be a pandemic.

Contents

0.5 mL of the vaccine contain 15 µg hemagglutinin of each of the recommended strains phosphate buffered saline, saccharide, thiomersal and traces of form—aldehyde (used for inactivation).

Indications

Routine
- Flu vaccine in routine immunization is not recommended in India.

High-risk groups: Who should receive the vaccine include:
- Asthma and other chronic pulmonary diseases, e.g. cystic fibrosis
- Hemodynamically severe cardiac disease
- Immunosuppressive disorder/therapy
- HIV infection
- Sickle cell anemia and other hemoglobinopathies
- Diseases requiring long-term aspirin therapy
- Chronic renal dysfunction
- Chronic metabolic diseases including diabetes mellitus
- Medical and health personnel
- Businessmen, travelers, military institutions, sports.

Dose and route: Infants from 6 months to 3 years: 0.25 mL 2 doses at 4–6 weeks interval (one dose of 0.25 mL will suffice, if vaccinated previously) 0.5 mL one dose for children over 9 years, adolescents and adults beyond 9 years a single dose will suffice at anterolateral thigh in infants and deltoid in adults.

Efficacy: Protection for 6 months to 1 year only.

Adverse effects:
- *Local*: Pain, redness, swelling will resolve spontaneously.

- Allergic reactions to vaccine components
- Anaphylaxis

Storage: +2°–8°C. No freezing. Shelf life 1 year.

Influenza Vaccine—For Whom?
- *Influenza vaccine:* Inactivated (split virion) vaccine contains 7.5–15 µg of the chosen strain: Dose—0.25 mL by IM route for 6–35 months old children in 2 doses 1 month apart from the first dose and 0.5 mL by IM route for children ≥3 years followed by one dose every year during the recommended season with the prevalent strain of the particular year, for routine immunization.
- *A new-generation influenza virus surface antigens (hemagglutinin neuraminidase) containing the following strains:* A/Brisbane/02/2018 (H1N1)-pdm 09-like strain (A/Brisbane/02/2018, IVR-190) 15 µg HA*; A/Kansas/14/2017(H3N2)—like strain (A/Kansas/14/2017 X-327) 15 µg HA*; B/Phuket/3073/2013—like strain (B/Phuket/3073/2013) 15 µg HA* and B Colorado/06/2017—like strain (B/ Maryland/15/2016 BX-69A) 15 µg HA* for 2019-20 Northern Hemisphere is available.
- Recently a new injectable pH1N1 influenza vaccine suitable for administration of individuals in the age group 16–60 years has been registered in India (Zydus Cadila). Single dose annually is the recommendation. An intranasal pH1N1 influenza vaccine suitable for administration in children above 3 years adolescents and adults has also been registered in India (S and I). Single annual dose is the current recommendation.

Dose of Inactivated Seasonal Flu Vaccine

Age 6 months to 3 years 0.25/0.5 mL booster after 4 weeks 0.25/0.5 mL.

Age 36 months to 9 years 0.5 mL booster after 4 weeks 0.5 mL. Age more than 9 years 0.5 mL; booster not required.

- IAP recommends the seasonal flu vaccine for the following high-risk groups of children
  - Asthma and other chronic pulmonary diseases, e.g. cystic fibrosis
  - Hemodynamically severe cardiac disease
  - Immunosuppressive disorder or therapy
  - HIV infection

- Sickle cell anemia and other hemoglobinopathies
- Diseases requiring long-term aspirin therapy
- Chronic renal dysfunction
- Chronic metabolic disease including diabetes mellitus
- Current available data on prevalence of influenza in children in India do not support recommendation for routine infant immunization.

Japanese B Encephalitis Vaccine

Japanese Encephalitis

Japanese encephalitis (JE) is the leading cause of viral encephalitis in Asia, but the disease is rare in travelers. Its incidence has been decreasing in China, Korea, and Japan but increasing in Bangladesh, India, Nepal, Pakistan, Northern Thailand, and Vietnam. It occurs in epidemics in late summer and early fall in temperate areas and sporadically throughout the year in tropical areas of Asia.

Immunization should generally be considered for those who will spend one month or more in endemic or epidemic areas during the transmission season, especially, if travel will include rural areas. In special circumstances, immunization should be considered for some people spending <1 month in endemic areas, e.g. travelers to areas where there is an epidemic, travelers making repeated short trips or people with extensive outdoor rural exposure. Under specific circumstances, vaccine should be considered for persons spending <30 days in endemic areas, e.g. travelers to areas experiencing epidemic transmission and persons whose activities, such as extensive outdoor activities in rural areas, place them at high risk for exposure.

In all instances, travelers should be advised to take personal precautions, e.g. to reduce exposure to mosquito bites. Laboratory workers at risk of exposure to JE virus should also be vaccinated.

Two types of JE vaccines are available. (see Chapter 4)
1. *Inactivated JE vaccine:* These were mouse brain/hamster kidney derived. Thus, because of their potential to cause serious anaphylactic reactions, they are no longer in use.
2. *Cell culture JE vaccine:* This is a live-attenuated vaccine produced from JE virus [SA-14-14-2]. The efficacy with single dose is almost 98%. The optimal time to give the vaccine is

at nine months of age with the measles vaccine. In China, the vaccine is routinely used at eight months. It is safe in infants as young as six months of age. Studies have already documented ongoing protection from a single dose for a minimum of five years in JE-endemic areas.

Dosage and route: The schedule is a single dose 0.5 mL given subcutaneously.

Side effect: Mild side effects such as fever, malaise may occur.

IAP-ACVIP has since fixed upper age limit for JE vaccine as 8 years. GOI has introduced JE vaccination in campaign mode at hyperendemic regions of the country ahead of anticipated epidemic.

Japanese B Encephalitis Vaccine

- Two brands of Japanese B encephalitis vaccine are now available in India.
- Vaccine indicated only in endemic areas during epidemic situations.
- Types of vaccines—mouse brain-derived inactivated vaccine given subcutaneously in doses of 0.5 mL for children below 3 years and 1.0 mL for children above 3 years.

Schedule: 3 doses SC on days 0, 7 and 30/0, 7 and 14 till 15 years of age

- To be given one month ahead of the anticipated epidemic in all the hyperendemic areas.
- A booster dose of 0.5 mL/1.0 mL should be given every year.
- IAP recommends JE vaccine for children 1–3 years in all hyperendemic regions: 3 doses at 0, 7 and 30 days with booster every 2 years till 10–15 years of age—not to be used as an '*outbreak response*' vaccine during epidemic.
- *Newer JE vaccine:* DNA multivalent single dose IM recombinant JE vaccine is under trial.
- A new live-attenuated vaccine, SA-14-14-2 (Chinese) has been successfully tried in JE hyperendemic areas as a single dose on a "campaign approach".

Japanese Encephalitis (Fig. 5.4)

- JE vaccination introduced by Golin 2006 with SA-14-14-2 live-attenuated vaccine.

- *Strategy:* Administered as a single dose vaccine in campaign mode (age 1–15 years)
- Campaigns followed by introduction in routine immunization at 18 months in the districts to cover the new cohort.

Year	States	Districts covered/ targeted	Reported coverage
2006–07	4	11	93, 08, 688 (88.4%)
2007–08	10	28	181, 95, 974 (87.4%)
2008–09	10	21	168, 81, 941 (84.2%)
2009–10	8	30	-
2010–11	4	14	-

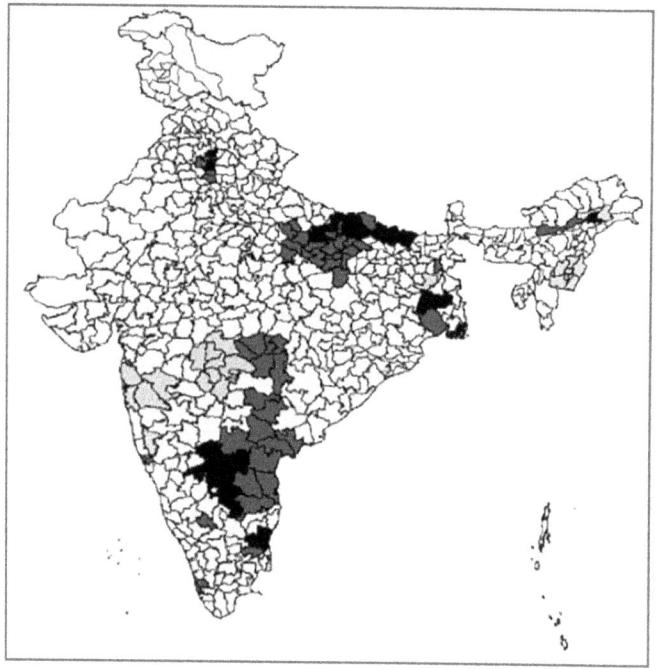

Fig. 5.4: India: Japanese encephalitis (JE) endemic regions where JE vaccinations in campaign mode was done.

Meningococcal Vaccine

This vaccine prepared from meningococcal polysaccharides (One dose lyophilizate containing 50 µg purified polysaccharide of *Neisseria meningitids* group A and C lactose/excipients diluent buffered isotonic 0.5 mL).

Indications: For prophylaxis against cerebrospinal meningitis due to meningococci of A and C groups.

Dosage: 0.5 mL subcutaneous or intramuscular.

Contraindications: Acute infectious disease. Children <2 years.

Adverse effects: Low-grade fever. Pain at injection site.

Meningococcal Polysaccharide Vaccine (MPSV4)

- Menomune (Sanofi Pasteur)
- Quadrivalent polysaccharide vaccine (A, C, Y, W-135)
- Administered by subcutaneous injection
- 10-dose vial contains thimerosal as preservative.

Meningococcal Endemic Areas 2004

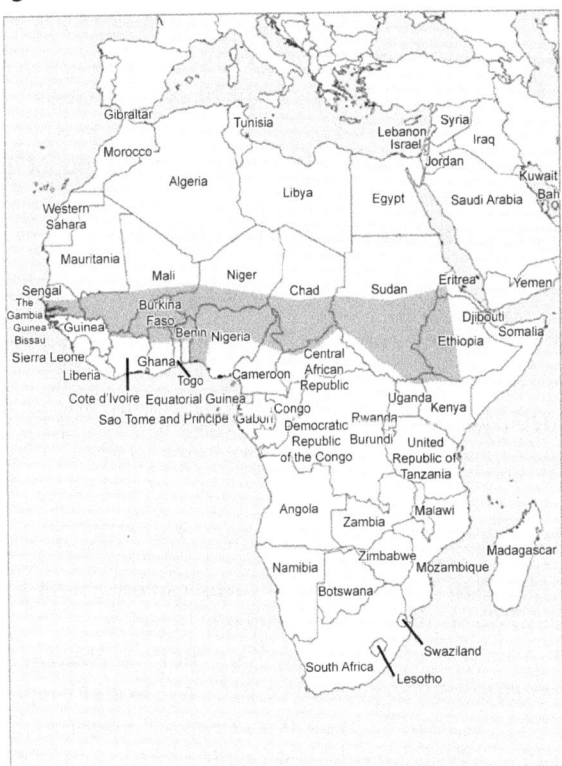

Meningococcal Conjugate Vaccine (MCV4)

- Menactra (Sanofi Pasteur)
- Quadrivalent polysaccharide vaccine (A, C, Y, W-135) conjugated to diphtheria toxoid
- Administered by intramuscular injection
- Single-dose vials do not contain a preservative.

Meningococcal Vaccine

- *Recommended for persons at increased risk of meningococcal disease:*
  - Microbiologists who are routinely exposed to isolates of *Neisseria meningitidis.*
  - Military recruits
  - Persons who travel to and US citizens who reside in countries in which *N. meningitidis* is hyperendemic or epidemic
  - Terminal complement component deficiency
  - Functional or anatomic asplenia
- Both MCV4 and MPSV4 recommended for control of outbreaks caused by vaccine preventable serogroups
- *Outbreak definition:*
  - 3 or more confirmed or probable primary cases
  - Period for 3 months
  - Primary attack rate ≥ 10 cases per 100,000 population.

Meningococcal Vaccines: Adverse Reactions

	MCV4	MPSV4
Local reactions for 1–2 days	4–48%	11–59%
Fever ≥100°F	3%	5%
Systemic reactions (headache, malaise, fatigue)	3–60%	4–62%

Meningococcal Vaccine—for whom?

- Two types of meningococcal vaccines containing A and C and ACWY strains are now available in India.
- The vaccine contains purified polysaccharide of *N. meningitidis* serogroups of A and C, W-135 and Y types.
- *Meningo A and C:* Each 0.5 mL dose contains purified capsular polysaccharide of *N. meningitidis* serogroups A and C.
- *Meningo ACWY:* Each dose of 0.5 mL contains purified capsular polysaccharide of *N. meningitidis* serogroups A, C, W-135 and Y types—0.5 mL/SC.

- A single dose of 0.5 mL SC is recommended for children in endemic areas: Not recommended routinely
- Suitable for children ≥2 years, adolescents and adults
- Useful for students going abroad for higher studies/Travelers on Hajj pilgrimage.

Cholera Vaccine

This is a saline suspension of approximately 6,000 million each of killed classical Ogawa and Inaba serotypes of *V. cholerae*.

This is preserved by addition of 0.5% phenol. Protection is for a period of 36 months.

Dosage: 1-2 years: 0.2 mL/dose; *2-10 years:* 0.3 mL/dose

>10 years: 0.5 mL/dose 2 doses subcutaneously, at an interval of 4-6 weeks. Boosters are recommended every 6 months.

Contraindications: Previous history of sensitivity

Special features: Not very helpful in control and prevention of cholera. Used only as an adjuvant to other preventive measures.

Adverse effects: Generally, local tenderness, mild-to-moderate elevation of temperature.

CHOLERA VACCINE

Cholera vaccine has not been required for border crossing under International Health Regulations since 1973. Cholera vaccine is a vaccine recommended for travelers and at-risk individuals like healthcare professionals, help/aid workers in endemic areas. Cholera vaccine has not been required for border crossing under International Health Regulations since 1973.

The vaccine is available in two forms:

1. Oral Cholera Vaccine

The vaccine provides 60–90% protection against severe disease for 6 months. All individuals must complete the immunization course at least 1 week prior to potential exposure.

Dosage: Adults and children over 2 years of age are given two doses on day 0 and 14, 1.5 mL orally.

Children: It can be given to children over 2 years age. Age 2–6 years. Two doses of vaccine are necessary on day 0 and 14.

If there is a time gap of more than 6 weeks between any doses, the primary immunization course must be restarted.

Booster: A single booster may be given after 6 months in <6 years and after 2 years in >6 years age.

Side effects: Include nausea, abdominal cramps or diarrhea.

2. Combination Vaccine (Chol-Ecol-O)

This provides short-term protection against diarrhea caused by enterotoxigenic *Escherichia coli*. No cholera vaccine currently available has been shown to be protective against the O139 Bengal strain that emerged in south Asia starting in 1992.

Meningococcal Vaccine (For details see Chapter 4)

As a condition of entry, Saudi Arabia requires proof of meningococcal immunization for pilgrims to Mecca during the Hajj. Quadrivalent polysaccharide vaccine is recommended. The serotype of bacteria involved were serogroups A and W-135 in 2000 and 2001.

Two vaccines are available, both quadrivalent:
1. The meningococcal conjugate vaccine (MCV4) approved for use in persons 2–55 years of age.
2. Meningococcal polysaccharide vaccine (MPSV4).

Revaccination: For children vaccinated at <4 years of age, revaccination in 2–3 years should be considered if they remain at high-risk for infection. For children vaccinated at 4 years of age, revaccination should be considered in 5 years if they remain at high-risk.

3. Yellow Fever Vaccine

Yellow fever vaccine is the only vaccine required as a condition of entry under the World Health Organization's International Health Regulations. The yellow fever vaccine has been in use since the 1930s. A valid International Certificate of Vaccination, issued within the previous 10 years, is mandatory for entry into certain countries in Africa and South America. Other countries have requirements for proof of immunization from travelers who have passed through yellow fever endemic zones.

The decision to immunize against yellow fever will depend on the itinerary of the individual traveler and the specific requirements of the country to be visited (including stopovers).

As well as being necessary for entry into certain countries, immunization against yellow fever is recommended for all travelers who are visiting or living in countries in Africa and South America where yellow fever infection is officially reported. It is also recommended for travel outside of urban areas in countries that do not officially report yellow fever but lay in the yellow fever endemic zones. One should refer to the yellow fever maps for more information.

The period of validity of the International Vaccination Certificate for yellow fever is 10 years, beginning 10 days after primary vaccination and immediately after revaccination.

Children: Yellow fever vaccine should never be given to infants younger than 6 months of age. Infants 6–8 months of age should be vaccinated only if they must travel to areas of ongoing epidemic yellow fever and a high level of protection against mosquito bites is not possible.

Travelers with infants younger than 9 months of age should be strongly advised against traveling to areas within the yellow fever endemic zone. The vaccine provides almost 100% protection.

Yellow fever vaccine is an attenuated, live-virus preparation of the 17D strain of yellow fever virus grown in leukosis-free chick embryos.

In India, one has to take the old preparation which is available in certain Government hospitals. Only these centers can give the certificate that is accepted by the passport and visa authorities.

Dose and route: 0.5 mL given subcutaneously

Side effects: It may cause transient side effects rarely, encephalitis in the very young; hepatic failure.

Contraindications: To the vaccine include egg allergy, immune-suppressed state from medication or disease, symptomatic HIV infection, hypersensitivity to previous dose and pregnancy.

Recommended Immunization for Travelers to Developing Countries

Immunizations	Length of travel		
	Brief, <2 weeks	Intermediate, 2 weeks through 3 months	Long-term residential, >3 months
Review and complete age-appropriate childhood schedule (see Chapter 4 for details)	+	+	+
• DTaP, poliovirus, pneumococcal, and *Haemophilus influenzae* type b vaccines may be given at 4-week intervals if necessary, to complete the recommended schedule before departure			
• *Measles:* 2 additional doses given if younger than 12 months of age at first dose			
• Varicella[a]			
• Hepatitis B[b]			
Yellow fever[c]	+	+	+
Hepatitis A[d]	+	+	+
Typhoid fever[e]	±	+	+
Meningococcal disease[f]	±	±	±
Rabies[g]	±	+	+
Japanese encephalitis[h]	±	±	+

DTaP indicates diphtheria and tetanus toxoids and acellular pertussis: +, recommended; ±, consider.

[a] See disease-specific in section Chapters 4 for details. For further sources of information, see text.
[b] If insufficient time to complete 6-month primary series, accelerated series can be given (Chapter 4 for details).
[c] For regions with endemic infection (see *Health Information for International Travel*, chapter 5).
[d] Indicated for travelers to areas with intermediate or high endemic rates of HAV infection.
[e] Indicated for travelers who will consume food and liquids in areas of poor sanitation.
[f] Recommended for regions of Africa with endemic infection and during local epidemics and required for travel to Saudi Arabia for the Hajj.
[g] Indicated for people with high animal exposure (especially to dogs) and for travelers to countries with endemic infection.
[h] For regions with endemic infection (see *Health Information for International Travel*, chapter 5). For high-risk activities in areas experiencing outbreaks vaccine is recommended even for brief travel.

Source: RED Book. AAP Publication. 2009:101.

Post-exposure Prophylaxis Vaccines

Rabies Vaccine (Cell Culture)
(See Chapter 12 WHO Position Paper on Rabies for Latest Guidelines)
Inactivated 2nd generation tissue culture vaccine, derived from Wilstar rabies PM/WI 38-1-503-30 strain.

Indications: In pre-exposure and post-exposure immunization against rabies.

Pre-exposure prophylaxis (Pre-EP) is recommended in following two situations:
1. Children exposed to pets in home.
2. Children identified to have a higher risk of being bitten by dogs.

WHO recommends a "1-site vaccine administration on days 0 and 7 for intramuscular administration".

For post-exposure prophylaxis, recently the WHO has recommended a new 4-dose schedule of either of the following:
   (i) 1-site intramuscular administration of vaccine on days 0, 3, 7 and between day 14-28, or (ii) 2-sites intramuscular administration on days 0 and 1-site on days 7, 21 (intramuscular).
   Not given in the gluteal region.

Special features: 3-4 injections produce good antibody levels.

Adverse effects: No serious side effects. Rarely, local redness, pain, headache and fever.

WHO Recommendations for Management of Animal Bites

Step I: Liberal washing of the wound thoroughly with soap and water for 10 minutes. This step invariably reduces the virus load of the wound physically (running water) and inactivating the remaining particles of virus chemically (soap or detergent).

Step II: Application of 70% alcohol, tincture iodine, povidone iodine, or any other suitable disinfectant after removing all traces of soap—Alcohol and other disinfectant lead to further inactivation of remaining virus by chemical disruption.

The animal bite wound(s) is (are) better not to be covered. If suturing is unavoidable for the purpose of hemostasis, it must be ensured that immunoglobulin has been administered in the wound prior to suturing with only minimal loose sutures. Tight suturing will shorten incubation period.

Step III: Proper infiltration of the wound(s) with rabies immunoglobulins of human (hRIC) or equine (eRIC) origin—as much as anatomically feasible the RIG should be infiltrated into, and around the wounds.

The remaining portion of the calculated amount of the RIG (40 units per kg of bodyweight in case of eRIG or 20 units per kg of body weight in case of hRIG) if any is to be injected in the deltoid region away from the site of vaccine administration to prevent on site neutralization of vaccine antigen. RIGs are specific rabies virus neutralizing antibodies that immediately neutralize rabies virus on contact. RIG gives a coating to the virus so that it cannot enter the nerve ending resulting in reduction or total obliteration of inoculated virus.

Step IV: Immunization with rabies modern tissue culture vaccine. (Earlier Schedules)

Post-exposure Prophylaxis

Regimes of rabies vaccine worldwide as accepted by WHO

Reference	Dose	Day	Site
Standard WHO IM regimen (ESSEN)	One IM dose (0.5 or 1.0 mL)	0, 3, 7, 14, 28	1-1-1-1 Deltoid
2-1-1 intramuscular regimen (Zagreb)	One IM dose (0.5 or 1.0 mL)	0, 7, 21	2-1 Deltoid
2-site intradermal regimen (TRC-ID)	One-fifth of IM dose (0.1 or 0.2 mL)	0, 3, 7, 28, 90	2-2-2-1 Deltoid
8-site intradermal regimen (Oxford-ID)	One-fifth of IM dose (0.1 or 0.2 mL)	0, 7, 28, 90	8-4-1-1-1 Deltoid, Pectoralis-major, over the scapular region, anterolateral thighs
Modified TRC	(0.1 or 0.2 mL)	0, 3, 7, 28	2-2-2-0-2-0

Note:
1. In case of re-exposure for persons who have received pre-exposure or at least 3 doses of any post-exposure regimen, only the first 2 doses on day 0 and 3 are needed.
2. For category III bites, RIG is also mandatory along with first dose(s) of ARV.
3. Modified TRC (0.1 or 0.2 mL) 0, 3, 7, 28 2-2-2-0-2-0

Adverse Reactions

- Reactions are less serious and less common than with previously available vaccines.
- A few vaccines may experience local redness, pain, headache and fever.
- An immune complex like reaction has been reported among approximately 6% of persons who received booster doses, 2-21 days after administration of the booster doses.

Recommended post-exposure prophylaxis

Category	Type of contract with a suspect or confirmed rabid domestic or wild animal, or animal unavailable for testing	Type of exposure	Recommended post-exposure prophylaxis
I	Touching or feeding of animals licks on intact skin	None	None, if reliable case history is available
II	Nibbling of uncovered skin minor scratches or abrasions without bleeding	Minor	Administer vaccine immediately. Stop treatment if animal remains healthy throughout an observation period of 10 days or if animal is proven to be negative for rabies by a reliable laboratory using appropriate diagnostic techniques
III	Single or multiple transdermal bites or scratches, licks on broken skin. Contamination of mucous membrane with saliva (i.e. licks). Exposure to bats	Severe	Administer rabies immunoglobulin and vaccine immediately. Stop treatment if animal remains throughout an observation period of 10 days or if animal is found to be negative for rabies by a reliable laboratory using appropriate diagnostic technique.

Source: WHO (1992), Tech Rep Ser No 824.
Note: The observation period of 10 days applies only for domestic dogs and cats.

Post-exposure Prophylaxis

(See Chapter 12 WHO Position Paper on Rabies for Latest Guidelines)

Five doses on day 0, 3, 7, 14, 28. Day '0' is the date of 1st vaccination and not the day of animal bite. Revaccination whenever the antibodies fall below 0.5 IU/mL as recommended. For re-exposure, irrespective of the interval between past-exposure prophylaxis and present bite administer 2 more doses on day 0 and 7.

2. Hepatitis B Vaccine

Refer chapters 4 and 5.

Combination Vaccines

DTwP/DTaP, DTwP/DTaP–HB, DTwP/DTaP-Hib, DTaP-IPV–Hib, DTwP–HB–Hib

Spectacular advances made in vaccine production especially in the field of molecular biology and genetic engineering, are revolutionizing the concept of childhood immunization. The successful combination of 2 or more antigens in a single vaccine formulation way back in 1940s has since culminated in combining as many as 6 antigens with excellent compatibility and high immunogenicity. The future naked DNA gene vaccines will perhaps be available in more combination formulations.

Advances in technology have enabled the development of a whole range of new and improved vaccines. Currently, new vaccines are being developed against more than 20 different diseases which until recently, appeared to be a distant dream. These include vaccines against major killer diseases-diarrheal diseases, acute respiratory infections and malaria. As of date, of the 25–30 vaccines available world over, nearly 20 of them are available in India, either in monovalent of combination formulation.

Attempts had been made in the past to reduce the number of injections by combining diphtheria, tetanus, pertussis antigens into a single DTP vaccine in 1945 and further in the year 1971 by combining measles, mumps and rubella vaccine as MMR vaccine. But for these developments, an infant would have had to receive 10 injections during first three months of life and coverage of the immunization program would not have reached the level of ≥85% that it has today. Benefits of combination vaccines are given in **Table 5.1**.

Table 5.1: Benefits of combination vaccines.

To the end-user	To the health planner
Reduced number of pricks	Reduced storage
Reduced parental anxiety	Reduced burden on cold chain
Reduced pain to the child	Improved logistics, distribution, lesser paperwork.
Reduced number of visits	
Increased compliance	

The successful combination of diphtheria, tetanus and pertussis as DTP has laid the foundation that opened up exciting prospects for present and future combination vaccine development. In fact, the tetravalent and pentavalent combination that exist today are essentially built by integrating the antigens around DTP combination vaccines.

Combination vaccines: The issues concerning combination vaccines can be related to manufacturing, developmental or related to researchers and pediatricians.

Manufacturing Issues

- Antigenic compatibility with other antigens
- Immunological interference with live virus vaccine
- Volume of the vaccine that can be given
- Use of adjuvant in the combination

Developmental Issues

- Each component antigen to be indicated at the same time in the immunization schedule.
- Each antigen should produce good immunogenic response.
- Product should be stable for at least 18–24 months.

Researcher's Point of View

- Potential to reduced antigenic response
- Antigenic competition
- Epitopic suppression
- Increased antigenic/adjuvant ratio
- Competition for B-cells.

Pediatrician's Point of View

- Apprehension of cumulative side effects
- Difficulty in assessing the severe reactions
- Some components can be given too often.

Combination Vaccines Available

A summary of the combination vaccines that are presently available or are under development are listed here under:

DTaP/IPV

This was the first tetravalent vaccine in use since early 1990s. In developed countries where IPV is preferred to OPV, this tetravalent vaccine is recommended for routine immunization.

DTwP/Hib, DTaP/Hib

This vaccine represents a new generation of vaccines that simultaneously prevent Hib disease and 3 major childhood diseases (diphtheria, pertussis and tetanus). It has an excellent immunogenicity and response to Hib (PRP-T) which is not affected by the combination process when given in the primary series as DTP alone. This vaccine is in use since early 1990s in the developed countries.

DTaP–IPV–Hib

It is a penta-valent reconstituted vaccine. Hib (PRP-T) and DTP-IPV are mixed extemporaneously prior to administration. The response to each antigen is excellent not affected by the combination. This combination vaccine induces, diphtheria and anti-tetanus titers >0.01 IU/mL in 99–100% of infants, anti-PRP titers >0.5 mg/mL in more than 94%, polio neutralizing titers >5 in more than 98%, pertussis agglutinin titers >80 in more than 78% of infants. It has also been found that the combination does not increase the frequency and severity of side effects. It is given at 6, 10, 14 weeks as a primary schedule and a booster dose at 18 months of age. This vaccine is currently in use in over 21 countries.

This combination vaccine formulation had been in use in western countries since 1996. DTwP-HB-Hib combination vaccine is now available in India. A single 0.5 mL dose of the combined vaccine formulations contains 10 µg of hepatitis B surface antigen, not less than 30 IU of absorbed D-toxoid, not less than 60 IU of T-toxoid and not less than 4 IU of Pw, Pertussis whole cell component and PRP (T). When given in either of the schedule given below the vaccine offer at least 95% protection against hepatitis B with titers of >10 mIU/ mL along with over 98% sero-protection against tetanus.

Vaccines, Immunoglobulins and Antisera

Table 5.2: WHO recommendation on HB and Hib immunization.

Age	Schedule I	Schedule II	Schedule III
Birth	–	Hep B$_1$*	Hep B*
6 weeks	Hep B$_1$**+ Hib$_1$	Hep B$_2$**	Hep B# + Hib1#
10 weeks	Hep B$_2$**+ Hib$_2$	+ Hib	Hep B# +Hib2 #
14 weeks	Hep B$_3$**Hib$_3$	Hep B$_3$**	Hep B# Hib3 #

Note: *Monovalent vaccine, **Monovalent or combination vaccine, # Combination vaccine

Table 5.2 illustrates the latest WHO recommendation on the use of this combine formulation.

Hep A–Hep B

A combined vaccine against hepatitis B 20 µg and hepatitis A 1440 units adsorbed on aluminum hydroxide has produced good immunogenicity and tolerance results in the study trials according to a 0, 6 months schedule with 100% seroconversion results for both the components. The improved immunogenicity against both the antigens could be explained on the basis of increased local production of cytokines and consequent enhancement of the macrophage activity. The vaccine is also available in pediatric formulation with 10 µg of hepatitis B and 720 ELU of hepatitis A, suitable for older children and adolescents up to 15 years at 0, 6 months schedule. This vaccine has been licensed in India.

Combination Vaccines Recently Developed DTaP–Hib, DTaP Hib–eIPV, MMR-V

One of the consequences of remarkable technical advance, that in the future will greatly influence the art of immunization, is the development of the acellular pertussis vaccine. Five immunogenic components of *Bordetella pertussis* have been identified, that in various combination have been found to confer immunogenic protection. The acellular pertussis vaccine development has redefined the tolerance profile of pertussis prophylactic intervention. These vaccines are comparable to the traditional whole cell pertussis vaccine with regards to efficacy and in the future will be more often used in combination vaccine development. Today 13 acellular pertussis vaccines are under evaluation by different manufactures and will be the building blocks of future combination vaccines. A combination vaccine of Hib and DTaP has shown adequate antibody response to Hib at 2, 3, 4 months and has replaced the whole cell pertussis-based vaccine in a few developed countries.

The pentavalent DTaP–eIPV–Hib is now available in India and has been recommended for use in private practice by the Indian Academy of Pediatrics (IAP).

MMR–Varicella Vaccine

A combination of measles, mumps rubella and varicella vaccines has been developed and registered in European countries and found to be safe and immunogenic in children. Seroconversion responses produced so far are 100%. Thus, the combined MMR-V vaccine could be administered as a second dose for both the vaccines at 4 to 6 years as per current Global recommendation.

DTaP–Hib–IPV Hep B

A combination formulation incorporating 6 components is also now developed. Preliminary data have indicated that immune response to the combination antigens including diphtheria, acellular pertussis and hepatitis B inactivated polio viruses are comparable with those seen when vaccines are administered separately. Some studies of combination vaccines that includes Hib antigen show a diminished antibody response whereas some studies have indicated the same immunogenic response as whole cell pertussis-based combination with significantly better safety profile. Combination vaccines development current status is given in **Table 5.3**.

New Thinking and Rethinking

There is no doubt that the coming era in vaccinology belongs to the new and wonderful concept of combination vaccines. However, various issues other than pharmaceutical and developmental aspects are to be considered and examined.

- Different countries follow different immunization schedules, either for social and administrative or epidemiological reasons. Combination vaccines can only in corporate those antigens which can be given at the same time or can be given relatively at an early starting age and to be effective over a range of immunization schedules. Different countries may

Table 5.3: Status of combination vaccines.

Vaccine	Developed	Under development
DTwP–eIPV	+	
DTwP–Hib	+	
DTwP–HepB	+	
DTwP–eIPV–Hib	+	
HepA–HepB	+	
DTaP–Hib	+	
DTaP–eIPV	+	
DTaP–Hib–IPV	+	
DTaP–HB	+	
DTaP–HB–eIPV	+	
MMR-V	+	
DTaP–Hib–eIPV–HepB	+	

prefer a different vaccine combination in their vaccination schedules.
- Since, epidemiological situations and immunization schedules vary from country to country, the cost benefit of a combined vaccine will also vary. The cost benefit estimates should therefore precede the development effort and will be important in ensuring acceptance of these vaccines in the immunization schedules of the countries.
- Since, these vaccines seek to combine many more antigens from multiple different pathogens, it makes them difficult to study in controlled double blind, randomized trials because of the increased number of the study arms required for complete evaluation. Also, the determination of the serological response to different antigens should be evaluated in relation to protective immunological responses to the lowest antibody protection level rather than equivalent mean titer of antibodies towards individual components.

TO SUMMARIZE

Combination Vaccines

'Lyophilized/liquid' combinations. What we need to know?

Is immunogenicity disturbed?	**No**
Are they safe?	**Yes**
Have they been tested in Indian infants?	**Yes**
Can we use them even for booster series?	**Yes**

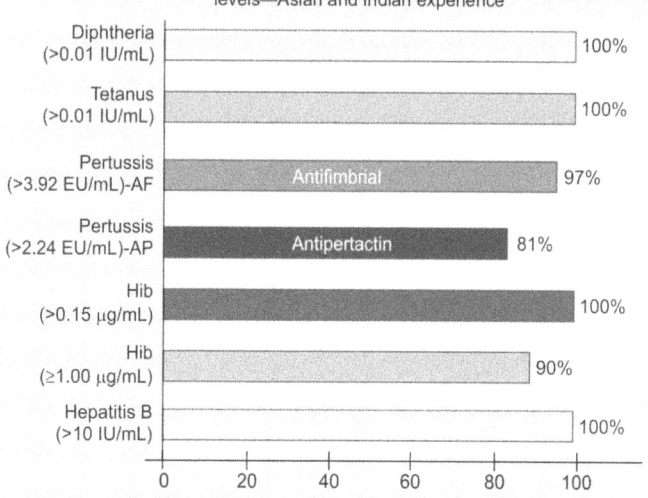

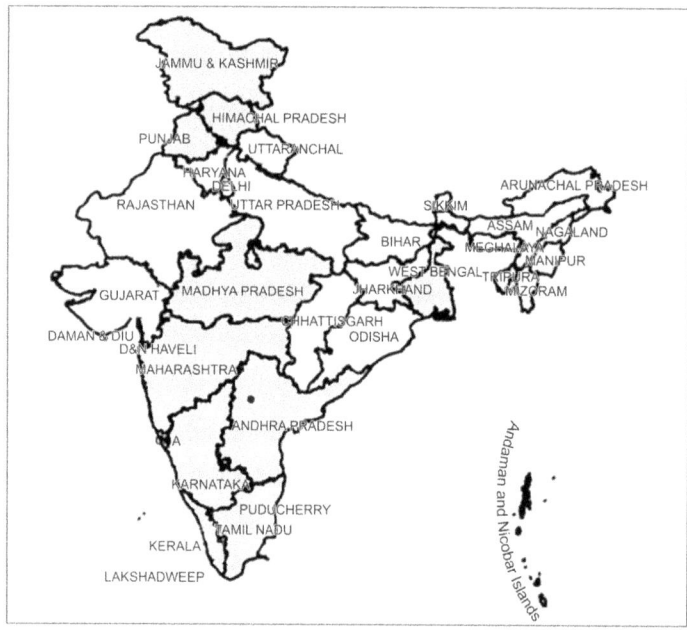

Map showing all states have started using gray (DTwP-HB-HIB) now 'Lyophilized/liquid' combinations. Percentage of infants having post-immunization antibody titres above minimum protective levels—Asian and Indian experience have combined their antigenicity.

Triple "I" Strategy

Integrated Infant Immunization Strategy

- 4-4-9 concept
- 4 vaccine formulations
- Before the infant attains 4 months of age
- To prevent 9 vaccine preventable diseases
- DTwP-HB-Hib pentavalent vaccine to prevent 5 VPDs + BCG to prevent TB and bOPV/eIPV to prevent polio.

IMMUNOGLOBULINS

These are preparations containing antibodies against infectious microorganisms and are usually prepared from human plasma or serum. Normal immunoglobulins are prepared from material from blood donors and contain several antibodies against infectious diseases prevalent in the general population. Specific immunoglobulins contain minimum specified levels of one antibody.

Anti-D immunoglobulins are given to prevent the formation of rhesus antibodies in rhesus negative (Rh-ve) persons on exposure to rhesus positive red blood cells.

Special precautions: A live vaccine should be given after an interval of 3 months of immunoglobulin administration.

Hepatitis B Immunoglobulin

Hepatitis B Immunoglobulin (HBIg) provides immediate passive immunity for those individuals with acute exposure to HBsAg positive blood/blood derivatives. Clinical trials have demonstrated reduction in attack rate of clinical hepatitis B following its use. After administration of the usual recommended dose of the HBIg, there is a detectable level of circulating anti-HBsAg antibody which will persist for 3 months. No case of transmission of hepatitis B has been associated with the use of this product anywhere in the world.

HBIg does not interfere with generation of antibody response to hepatitis B vaccine. Ideally, persons known to be exposed to blood which is known to contain hepatitis B virus should be given combined passive-active immunization.

Adverse effects: Transient, mild pain at the site of injection, itching are the common side effects in a small proportion of recipients.

Contraindication: No specific contraindications.

Route of administration: Intramuscular

Special precautions: More as a precautionary measure, some experts recommend caution when administering HBIg to humans with history of previous systemic allergy subsequent to administration of immunoglobulin preparations.

Hepatitis B Immunoglobulin: Preparations

Hepatitis B immunoglobulin can be given by IM route as per manufacture's recommendation. The needle should not be in a blood vessel and this should be ascertained by drawing back the plunger of the syringe.

Indications: For prophylaxis of hepatitis B after exposure to HBsAg, e.g. by accidental "needle-stick", contact by accidental splash or oral ingestion (pipetting accident) involving HBsAg positive materials such as blood, plasma or serum. For prophylaxis of hepatitis B in neonates born to HBsAg positive mothers.

Dosage: Following exposure to HBsAg: *Adults:* 1,000–2,000 IU, IM.

Children: 32–48 IU/kg body weight. This should be administered within 7 days (preferably within 48 hours) after exposure to HBsAg.

Neonates: Initial dose is 100–200 IU; should be administered within 12–24 hours after birth.

Tetanus Immunoglobulin

Tetanus Immunoglobulin (TIg) is a liquid freeze-dried preparation containing immunoglobulins, mainly IgG obtained from plasma or serum- containing specific antibodies against the toxin of *Clostridium tetanus.*

Adverse effects: Local pain, fever flushing, headache and chills may occur.

Indications: Subjects already sensitized with serums of animal origin, existence of prior or present allergic manifestations (asthma, eczema, etc.). Burns, injuries, open and compound fractures. Unimmunized or inadequately immunized smothers.

Dosage

Prophylaxes: 250–500 IU intramuscular.

Therapeutic: Tetanus neonatorum 500–1000 IU intramuscular or 250 IU intrathecal. In adults and children, 500–10,000 IU intramuscular and/or 250–500 IU intrathecally.

Rabies Immunoglobulin

It is a liquid or freeze-dried preparation containing immunoglobulins mainly IgG obtained from plasma or serum of donors immunized against rabies and contains specific antibodies that neutralize that rabies virus. It is prepared from plasma or serum of not fewer than 1,000 donors. It contains not less than 150 units/mL.

It provides passive protections when given immediately to individuals exposed to rabies virus. This provides maximum circulating antibody with minimum interference of active immunization with human diploid-cell vaccine. Rabies Human Monoclonal Antibody (RHMAB) Access to Rabies immunoglobulin (RIg) is limited resulting in high rabies mortality. RHMAB is a completely human IgG1 monoclonal antibody that binds to the ectodomain of the G-glycoprotein produced by recombinant technology. It has been demonstrated to neutralize 25 different isolates of wild-type or street isolates of rabies virus. A recent study found that it is not inferior to human rabies immunoglobulin (HRIg) in producing rabies virus neutralizing antibody in 200 subjects with WHO category III suspected rabies exposures. The study subjects received either RMHAB or HRIg (1:1 ratio) in wounds, and intramuscularly wherever necessary, on day 0. All these patients also received five doses of rabies vaccine intramuscularly on 0, 3, 7, 14 and 28 days. This newly introduced monoclonal antibody has emerged as a safe and potent alternative to rabies immunoglobulin. The WHO position paper on rabies in 2018 has also suggested encouragement of use of this product, if available, instead of RIG.

The comparative advantages include easy availability, standardized production quality, possibly greater effectiveness, no requirement of animals in its production, and less adverse events. In view of the irregular availability and high cost of Rabies immunoglobin (RIG), ACVIP endorses the use of RHMAB as an alternative to RIG—human or equine—along with rabies vaccines in all category-III bites. RHMAB is licensed in India (as Rabisheild, Serum Institute of India; 40 IU/mL) since 2017. The recommended dose is 3.33 IU/kg body weight, preferably at the time of the first vaccine dose. However, this may also be administered up to the 7th day after the first dose of vaccine is given. If the calculated dose is insufficient (to infiltrate all the wounds), it should be diluted in sterile normal saline to get a volume that is enough to be infiltrated around all the wounds.

Adverse effects: Local tenderness, muscle soreness or stiffness at the injection site, low-grade fever sensitization to repeated injections of human globulin in immunoglobulin deficient patients.

Contraindications: Do not administer repeated doses once vaccine treatment has been initiated.

Indications: Category III bites of suspected rabies animals.

Gamma-globulin

Intravenous gamma-globulin preparations are available for replacement therapy for patients with congenital agammaglobulinemia and hypogammaglobulinemia, idiopathic thrombocytopenic purpura and Kawasaki syndrome. It is also used for prophylaxis of infection following bone marrow transplantation.

Human Normal Immunoglobulin

It is sterile solution of globulins that contain many antibodies normally present in human adult blood. It is prepared from plasma or serum or from normal placentas frozen immediately after collection from not fewer than 1,000 donors. It has a protein concentration of approximately 16%.

Adverse effects: Rarely flushing with chills, nausea and headache.

Contraindications: Selective IgA deficiencies, hypersensitivity.

Special precautions: Signs of anaphylactoid reactions.

Indications: Prophylaxis of infectious diseases, immunotherapy.

Dosage

Therapy: 10%: 0.6 mL/kg body weight of 16.5%: 0.4 mL/kg body weight.

Prophylaxis: 10%: 0.4mL/kg body weight or 16.5% : 0.25 mL/kg bodyweight.

Human Anti-D Immunoglobulin

It is sterile solution containing IgG anti-D for use in preventing Rh-immunization. A single dose of human anti-D immunoglobulin contains sufficient anti-D to suppress the immune response to 2.5 mL or less of Rh-positive red blood cells.

Adverse effects: Discomfort at the site of injection; a slight elevation in temperature has also been reported.

Contraindications: Rh-o (D) positive 2 or D-u positive. Rh-o (D) negative or D-u negative patient previously sensitized to Rh-o (D) positive infant.

Special precautions: Patients with IgA antibodies or a history of reaction to blood or blood products. Concomitant administration of live vaccines. Warm to body temperature before injecting. Store between 2–8°C.

Indications: Prevention of development of anti-D antibodies in Rh-negative mothers after childbirth, abortion beyond 13 weeks gestation, antepartum prophylaxis at 26–28 weeks gestation.

Dosage

Adults: Prophylaxis after delivery, abortion, and amniocentesis: 300 µg IM within 72 hours. Massive transplacental hemorrhage: 25 µg/mL of fetal erythrocytes.

Children: Not applicable.

ANTISERA

Antisnake Venom

The venom of snake is a complex mixture of protein which have enzymatic activity and may also provoke local inflammatory reaction. The venom may have effect with sensory, motor and respiratory involvement. Management of snake bite involves general supportive care and monitoring of vital functions but in a systemic snake bite poisoning, specific antivenom is the most effective therapy. It is highly recommended to wait for clear clinical evidence of systemic poisoning before giving antivenom. Monospecific anti-venoms are more effective and are less likely to cause side effects than polyvalent anti-venoms. Manufacturer's guidelines should be followed

VACCINES LICENSED IN INDIA

Parents may be aware through the media or information from non-authoritative Internet Websites of controversial issues above vaccines their child is scheduled to receive. Many issues about childhood vaccines communicated by these means are presented inaccurately. When a parent initiates discussion about a vaccine controversy, the healthcare professional should discuss the specific concerns and provide factual information, using language appropriate or parents. Through direct dialogue with parents and the use of available resources, healthcare professionals can help prevent acceptance of media reports and information from non-authoritative Internet Websites on scientific facts. So much so the practices of today has to be well versed with the vaccines licensed in the country/their schedule **(Tables 5.4 and 5.5)**.

LEARNING POINTS

- Vaccines, Antisera and Immunoglobulins are lifesaving; Use them judiciously following Guidelines issued by the Manufacturer, WHO, Local Governments and Professional Bodies.
- Recommended routes of administration must be scrupulously followed for optimal immunogenic responses.
- The recommended needle size should be followed for different routes of administration such as ID, SC, IM and IV routes.
- Always be 'Needle Smart' by using auto disabled/disposable syringes by following 'Safe Injection Practices' guidelines.
- After use destroy the needle using a 'needle cutter' and dispose the used needles and syringes in a separate bag and dispose it at the appropriate disposal bag.

Table 5.4: Vaccines licensed in India and their routes of administration.

Vaccine*	Type	Route
BCG	Live bacteria	ID
Diphtheria-tetanus (DT)	Toxoids	IM
DTwP	Toxoids and inactivated bacteria	IM
DTaP	Toxoids and inactivated bacterial components	IM
Hepatitis A	Inactivated viral antigen	IM
Hepatitis B	Inactivated viral subunit	IM
Hib conjugate CRM197	Polysaccharide-protein conjugate-Diphtheria Toxin CRM197	IM
Hib conjugate PRPT	Polysaccharide-protein conjugate-Tetanus toxoid	IM
PRP-T Hib conjugate reconstituted with DTP-HB	Polysaccharide-protein conjugate-killed bacteria, diphtheria toxoid, tetanus toxoid, subunits	
Hepatitis B	Subunit	IM
Hepatitis B+ DTwP	Subunit, toxoid and inactivated bacteria	IM
Japanese encephalitis	Inactivated virus	IM
Measles	Live virus	SC
Meningococcal	Polysaccharide	SC
MMR	Live viruses	SC
Measles rubella	Live viruses	SC
Mumps	Live virus	SC
Pneumococcal	Polysaccharide	IM or SC
Poliovirus • OPV • IPV	Live virus inactivated virus	Oral IM
Rabies	Inactivated virus	IM or ID
Rubella	Live virus	SC
Tetanus	Toxoid	IM
Typhoid • Parenteral • Parenteral • Oral	Inactivated bacteria Capsular polysaccharide Live bacteria	SC SC (boosters may) Oral
Varicella	Live virus	SC
HPV	Virus like particles	IM

*BCG, Bacillus Calmette–Guérin; DTP, diphtheria and tetanus toxoids and pertussis, absorbed; DTaP, diphtheria and tetanus toxoids and acellular pertussis, absorbed; Hib, *Haemophilus influenza* type b; MMR, live measles-mumps-rubella viruses; OPV, oral poliovirus; IPV, inactivated poliovirus; dT, diphtheria and tetanus toxoids (for children 7 years of age or older and adults); and DT, diphtheria and tetanus toxoids (for children older than 5 years of age.); SC, subcutaneous; ID, intradermal; IM, intramuscular.

Table 5.5: A ready reckoner for vaccines is given below for quick reference.

Vaccine	Age	Route/Dose	Remarks	Adverse reactions	Prevention and management
BCG	Birth	0.1 mL intradermal over left deltoid region	• Use reconstituted vaccine in 4 hours • Uses sterile water to wipe • The skin; if alcohol is used, allow it to evaporate before giving the vaccine	• Regional adenitis (1–10%) • Usual reaction is a papule or nodule after 2-3 weeks with ulceration, and scar at 4–6 weeks	• Adenitis <1.5 cm increasing size or fluctuation, give 3–6 months INH or aspirate cold abscess • Avoid in immunodeficient individuals
OPV	Birth 6,10,14 weeks; 15–18 months, 5 years	• 2 drops orally • Avoid repeated thawing the total thaw times should not exceed 23 hours	• Store in freezer	None	
Hepatitis B	Birth 6 weeks, 14 weeks	0.5 mL IM over right deltoid/ anterolateral aspect of mid- thigh (in newborns and young infants)	• Avoid gluteal region • First does preferably within 12 hours of birth	• Soreness at the site of injection • Mild fever • Rarely anaphylaxis	• Paracetamol for fever

Contd...

Contd...

Vaccine	Age	Route/Dose	Remarks	Adverse reactions	Prevention and management
DTwP/DTaP	6, 10, 14 weeks; 15–18 months 5 years	0.5 mL IM anterolateral aspect of mid-thigh/ over right deltoid to previous dose and	DT is used if DPT is contraindicated in progressive neurological conditions or severe reaction prolonged cry syndrome	• Pain, fever • High pitched cry • Hypotonic, hypersensitive episode of reactions • Convulsion (Primarily febrile convulsion) • Acute encephalopathy (very rare)	• Paracetamol for pain and fever • Symptomatic treatment
MMR	9 and 15 months and 4–6 years	0.5 mL subcutaneous over right deltoid	Once reconstituted should be used within 4 hours	Fever, transient rashes in few vaccines 5–7 days after immunization	Paracetamol
TT/Td	10, 20 years	0.5 mL intramuscular	–	–	–
H. Influenzae b conjugate vaccine		0.5 mL IM/SC	Upper limit age upto 5 years only antero-lateral thigh 2–6 months 3 doses 15–18 months	Local reaction; After 15 months, only one does no booster	Paracetamol for fever

Contd...

Contd...

Vaccine	Age	Route/Dose	Remarks	Adverse reactions	Prevention and management
Typhoid:					
(a) Killed TA vaccine		0.25 mL SC, deltoid 2 doses, 4 weeks apart from 6–9 months of age: Booster every 3 years	Inexpensive and highly effective with Vi antigenicity	Severe local pain, high fever and other systemic symptoms the previous dose	Avoid if there is a severe reaction to
(b) Typhoid Vi Polysaccharide antigen vaccine		0.5 mL SC/IM, single dose, anterolateral thigh or deltoid Booster every 3 years	From 2 years of age 'Expensive	Ever <3%, local reaction 7% forever	Paracetamol
(c) Oral Ty 21a attenuated vaccine		One capsule on alternate days for 3 days. Booster every 3 years	'From 5 years of age 'Avoid antibiotics effective against *S. typhi* 5–7 days prior to and after vaccine administration. Strict cold chain mandatory	Minor gastrointestinal side effects	–
Varicella vaccine		0.5 mL SC	>1 year of age	Mild fever, local pain	Paracetamol
Hepatitis A vaccine		0.5 mL IM over deltoid 2 doses at 1 month interval. Third 6–12 months later	>2 years	Mild fever and local pain	Paracetamol for fever

Contd...

Vaccines, Immunoglobulins and Antisera

Contd...

Vaccine	Age	Route/Dose	Remarks	Adverse reactions	Prevention and management
Pneumococcal vaccine		0.5 mL SC/IM anterolateral thigh, single dose. Booster every 5 years	2 years and above-indicated in asplenia and immunocompromised children	None	–
DTP-HB/DTP-Hib DTP-HB-Hib		6, 10, 14 days IM anterolateral thigh 3 doses	Substitute for monovalent formulations where indicated	Pain, local induration, fever	Paracetamol for fever
Rotavirus vaccine,		2 doses orally 1st dose 6 weeks 2nd dose 28–32 weeks	Note indicated >32 weeks of age 10–45 years of age preferably, gives before the adolescents is sexually active. To be given in lying down posture		
Bivalent Tetravalent HPV vaccine		Bivalent; 3 doses 0, 1, 6 months tetravalent 3 doses 2, 4, 6 months preferably adolescents for 10 years of age			

Source: Bhave SY, Yadav S. Future vaccines. In: a ready-reckoner for vaccinations adult, adolescent and pediatric. Jaypee Brothers Medical Publishers: New Delhi; 2009.

- Administer the full course of vaccines in Primary and Booster schedules to obtain maximum protection.
- Remember the twin objectives of any Immunization are: a) to protect the individual vaccinee and b) to control, eliminate and eradicate the targeted VPD from the community.
- Store vaccines, antisera and immunoglobulins at the recommended temperature and cold chain equipment.
- Check the color of the VVM and ensure that the vaccine administered is within the expiry date.
- At least once go through the product leaflet supplied by the manufacture about the vaccine, antisera and immunoglobulins.

BIBLIOGRAPHY

1. ACVIP-IAP Guidelines; 2016.
2. Ambrosch F, Wiederman G, et al. Clinical and Immunological investigation of the new combined Hepatitis A and Hepatitis B vaccine. J Med Virol.1994;44:452-6.
3. American Academy of Pediatrics Varicella-infection, Recommendations for Immunization In: Pickering LK (Ed). 2000 Red Book. Report of the Committee in Infections Diseases. 25th edition. Elk Grove Village II: American Academy of Radiations.2000;634-8.
4. American Academy of Pediatrics. In: Pickering LK (Ed). Active immunization, recommendation for care of children in special circumstances, Summaries of Infectious Diseases. 2009 RedBook: Report of the Committee on Infectious Diseases, 28th edition. Elk Grove, IL: American Academy Pediatrics.2009;29:30, 65, 101, 329-6.
5. Bhave SY, Yadav S. Future vaccines. In: a ready reckoner for vaccinations adult, adolescent and pediatric. Jaypee Brothers Medical Publishers: New Delhi;2009.
6. Centers for Disease Control and Prevention. In: Atkinson W, Wolfe S, Hamborsky J, McIntyre L (Eds). Epidemiology and Prevention of Vaccine: preventable diseases. 11th edition. Washington DC: Public Health Foundation; 2009.
7. Centers for Disease Control and Prevention. Pertussis Vaccination Use of Acellular Pertussis Vaccines Among Infants and Young Children. Recommendations of the Advisory Committee on Immunization Practices. (ACIP). MMWR. 1997;46(RR-7):1-25.
8. Cherian T, Thomas N, Raghupathy P, et al. Safety and Immunogenicity of *Haemophilus influenzae* type B vaccine given in combination with DTwP at 6, 10 and 14 weeks of Age. Indian Pediatr. 2002;39(5):427-36.
9. Chutivongse S, Wilde H, Supich C, Baer G. Postexposure prophylaxis for rabies with antiserum and intradermal vaccination. Lancet. 1990;335:896-8.
10. Dutta AK, Agrawal A. Newer Vaccines. In: Parthasarathy A, Manon PS, Nair MKC (Eds). IAP Textbook of Pediatrics. Jaypee Brothers Medical Publishers: New Delhi; 2009.

Vaccines, Immunoglobulins and Antisera

11. Dutta AK, Kanwal SK. The past, present and future of combined vaccines. Ind J Pract Ped. 1999;7(1):43-4.
12. Edwards KM, Decker MD. Combination vaccines consisting of the acellular pertussis vaccines. Paediatr Infect Dis. 1997;16(4):97-102.
13. Goswami A. Safety and tolerance of equine rabies immunoglobulin in the Indian population. J Assoc Prev Control Rabies India.2000;1:30-4.
14. Invasive Bacterial Infections Surveillance (IBIS) Group of the International Clinical Epidemiology Network. Are *Haemophilus influenzae* infection a significant problem in India? A Prospective Study and Review. Clin Infec Dis. 2002;34:949-57.
15. Lambert PH, Siegrist CA. Vaccines and vaccination. Br Med J. 1998;14(3):71-5
16. Lang J, Duong Q Hoa, Nguyen VG. Randomized feasibility trial of pre-exposure rabies vaccination with DPT–IPV in Infants. Lancet. 1997;349:1663-5.
17. Levine OS, Wenger JD. Defining the Burden of HIB Disease in India. Indian Pediatr. 2002;39:5-1.
18. Parthasarathy A. Combination vaccines. The Choice Ahead. In: Kumar A, Mohan M, Heena M (Eds). Pediatric Index. Vol1 No.3. Meditch Publications and Distributor, New Delhi. 2001:13-8.
19. Pichicharo ME, Passador S. Administration of combined diphtheria and tetanus toxoids and pertussis vaccine, hepatitis B vaccine and *Haemophillus influenzae* type B vaccine to the infants and response to a booster dose of HIB conjugate vaccine. Clin Infect Dis.1997;25(6);1378-84.
20. Biswas S, Reddy GS, Srinivasan VA, Rangarajan PN. Preexposure efficacy of a novel combination DNA and inactivated rabies virus vaccine. Hum Gene Ther. 2001;12:1917-22.
21. Recommendation of First National Conference of the Association of the Prevention and Control of Rabies in India (APCRI) held at Rotary Sadan, kolkata; 1999.
22. Pharmaceutical, Regulatory and Policy-Making Aspects. Second European Conference on Vaccinology: Combined Vaccines for Europe. In: Vaccine. Brussels: 1994 Butterworth-Heinemann Ltd; p. 1482-3.
23. WHO State of the World's Vaccines and Immunization. Geneva, World Health Organization, 1996 (http://www.who.ch/programmes/gpv/gpv_home.htm; accessed 11 November 2019).
24. Steven P. Tartagila J, Paoletti E. Pox virus based vectors as vaccine candidates. Biologicals. 1995;23:159-64.
25. Sudarshan MK, Mahendra BJ, Ashwathnarayan DH, Gangaboriah. Clinical trials on newer antirabies vaccines: results and some experiences. J Assoc Prev Control Rabies India. 2000;1:21-5.
26. The Centers for Disease Control and Prevention. General recommendations on immunization: Recommendations of the Advisory Committee on Immunization Practices (ACIP) and then American Academy of Family Physicians (AAFP). MMWR. 2002;51:1-82.
27. The Centers for Disease Control and Prevention. Measles, Mumps, and Rubella: Vaccine Use and Strategies for Elimination of Measles,

Rubella, and Congenital Rubella Syndrome and Control of Mumps: Recommendations of the Advisory Committee on Immunization Practices (ACIP). MMWR. 1998;47:1-57.
28. Tripathi KK, Madhusudana SN. Safety of Equine Rabies Immunoglobulin. Vaccine. 1989;7:372-3.
29. Weibel RE, Villarejos VM, Klein EB, Buynak EB, McLean AA, Hilleman MR. Clinical and laboratory studies of live attenuated RA27/3 and HPV 77-DE rubella virus vaccines. *Proc Soc Exp Biol Med.* 1980;165:44-9.
30. Warell MJ, Nicholson KG, Sitharasami P, Udomaskadi D. Economical multiple site intradermal immunization with human diploid cell strain vaccine is effective for postexposure rabies prophylaxis. Lancet. 1985;1:1059-62.
31. Widle H, Chomchey P, Prakongsri S, Punyaratha Bandhu P. Safety of equine rabies Immunoglobulin. Lancet.1987;2:1285.
32. WHO Rabies vaccines: WHO Position Paper. Geneva, World Health Organization, 2018. (Weekly epidemiological record, 93) (Available at http://www.who.int/immunization/position_papers/position_paper_process.pdf: accessed 05 November 2019).
33. Indian Academy of Pediatrics (IAP) Advisory Committee on Vaccines and Immunization Practices (ACVIP). Recommended Immunization Schedule (2018–19) and Update on Immunization for Children Aged 0 Through 18 Years. S Balasubramaniyum, et al. Indian Paediatrics. 2018;55:1066-74.
34. WHO Dengue and Severe Dengue. Geneva, World Health Organization, 2019. (https://www.who.int/news-room/fact-sheets/detail/dengue-and-severe-dengue; accessed 05 November 2019).

Immunization in Special Clinical Circumstances

Alok Gupta

Certain immunizations are mandatory in special clinical circumstances. The following resume gives an account of the same.

IMMUNIZATIONS REQUIRED OR RECOMMENDED BECAUSE OF RISK OF DISEASES

Preterm Infants Born to Mothers not Tested During Pregnancy for HBsAg

The maternal hepatitis B virus surface antigen (HBsAg) status should be determined as soon as possible, and the infant should receive hepatitis B vaccine, as recommended for term infants in this category. For preterm infants who weigh less than 2 kg at birth, hepatitis B immunoglobulin (HBIg, 0.5 mL) should be given if the mother's HBsAg status cannot be determined within the initial 12 hours of birth because of the poor immunogenicity of vaccine in these infants. The initial vaccine dose should not be counted in the required three doses to complete the immunization series. The subsequent three doses (or a total of four doses) are given in accordance with the recommendations for the immunization of preterm infants with birth weights less than 2 kg born to HBsAg-negative women.

RECOMMENDED SCHEDULE OF HEPATITIS B IMMUNOPROPHYLAXIS TO PREVENT PERINATAL TRANSMISSION (TABLE 6.1)

Table 6.1: Hepatitis vaccination schedule.

Hep B vaccine and HBIg dose	Age
Infant born to mother known to be HBsAg positive	
First dose of Hep B vaccine	Birth (within 12 hours)
HBIg	Birth (within 12 hours)

Contd...

Contd...

Hep B vaccine and HBIg dose	Age
Second dose of Hep B vaccine	6 weeks
Third dose of Hep B vaccine	14 weeks/24 weeks
Final dose of Hep B vaccine (3rd or 4th)	24 weeks (6 months)
Infant born to mothers not screened for HBsAg	
First dose of Hep B vaccine	Birth (within 12 hours)
HBIg	If mother is HBsAg-positive, give 0.5 mL, as soon as possible, not later than 1-week after birth
Second dose of Hep B vaccine	6 weeks
Third dose of Hep B vaccine	14 weeks/24 weeks
Final dose of Hep B vaccine (3rd or 4th)	24 weeks (6 months)

(HBsAg: hepatitis B surface antigen; HBIg: hepatitis B immunoglobulin)

HBIg (0.5 mL) given intramuscularly at a site different from that used for vaccine.

Breastfeeding

Breastfeeding of the infant by an HBsAg positive mother poses no additional risk for acquisition of HBV infection by the infants by human milk.

Household Contacts of Persons with Acute Hepatitis B Virus (HBV) Infection

Infants (i.e. younger than 12 months of age) who have close contact with primary caregivers with acute infection and who have begun the immunization series should complete the series on schedule. If immunization has not been initiated, the infant should receive HBIg (0.5 mL), and hepatitis vaccine should be given in accordance with the routinely recommended 3-doses schedule (see Pre-exposure Universal Immunization).

RECOMMENDATIONS FOR POSTEXPOSURE IMMUNE PROPHYLAXIS OF HEPATITIS A INFECTION (TABLE 6.2)

Table 6.2: Postexposure Immune prophylaxis of hepatitis A infection.

Time since exposure, week	Future exposure likely, or immunization	Age of patients	Recommended prophylaxis
≤2 weeks	No Yes	Younger than 12 months 12 months through 40 years 41 years or older People of any age who are immunocompromised or have chronic liver disease	IgIM (0.02 mL/kg)* Ig (0.02 mL/kg)* and hepatitis A vaccine IgIM 0.02 mL/kg* HEPA vaccine^ can be used if IgIM unavailable*
>2 weeks	No Yes	Younger than 12 months 12 months or older	No prophylaxis Hepatitis A vaccine No prophylaxis but hepatitis A vaccine may be indicated for ongoing exposure^

*IgIM should be administered deep into a large muscle mass. Ordinarily no more than 5 mL should be administered in one site in an adult or large child; lesser amounts (maximum, 3 mL) should be given to small children and infants
^Dosage and schedule of hepatitis A vaccine as recommended as per age.
(IgIM: immunoglobulin intramuscular)
Source: Kimberlin DW, Brady MT, Jackson MA, et al. (Eds). Red Book. 2015 Report of the Committee on Infectious Diseases, 30th edition. American Academy of Pediatrics; 2015. pp. 386-8.

RECOMMENDED IMMUNIZATION SCHEDULES FOR CHILDREN NOT IMMUNIZED IN THE FIRST YEAR OF LIFE (TABLE 6.3)

Table 6.3: Immunization schedules for children not immunized in the first year of life.

Recommended time/age	Immunization	Comments
1. Younger than 5 years—First Visit	BCG, IPV1/OPV1, DPT1, HB1, Hib1	If indicated, tuberculin testing may be done at same visit. If child is 5 years of age or older, Hib is not indicated in most circumstances

Contd...

Contd...

Recommended time/age	Immunization Comments
Second visit (after 4 weeks' of above)	DTP2, IPV2/OPV2, HB2, Hib2, MMR1
Third visit (after 4 weeks of above)	DTP3, IPV3/OPV3, HB3, Hib3, MMR2
2. Age 5 years and above (at or before school entry)	Hepatitis B—three doses at 0, 1, and 6 months, Td—three doses at 4 weeks' interval, Varicella—two doses preferably at 3 months' interval MMR—two doses at minimum 4 weeks' interval
3. Age 10 years and above	Hepatitis A (inactivated)—two doses at 0 and 6 months Varicella—two doses preferably at 3 months' interval
4. Age 16 years and above	Hepatitis B—three doses at 0, 1, and 6 months Tdap—single dose Hepatitis A—two doses at 0 and 6 months Varicella—two doses at 4 weeks' interval MMR—two doses at minimum 4 weeks' interval

Note:
1. **Table 6.3** is not completely consistent with all package inserts. For products used, also consult manufacturer's package insert for instruction on storage, handling, dosage, and administration. Biologicals prepared by different manufacturers may vary and package inserts of the same manufacturer may change. Therefore, the physician should be aware of the contents of the current package insert. Vaccine abbreviations: HB indicates hepatitis B virus; Var, varicella; DTP, diphtheria and tetanus toxoids and whole cell pertussis; Hib, Haemophilus influenzae type b conjugate; IPV, inactivated polio vaccine, OPV, live poliovirus, MMR, live measles-mumps-rubella; Td, adult tetanus toxoid (full dose) with reduced dose of diphtheria toxoid.
2. If all needed vaccines cannot be administered simultaneously, priority should be given to protecting the child against the diseases that pose the greatest immediate risk. In the United States, these diseases for children younger than 2 years usually are measles and Hemophilus influenza type infection, for children older than 7 years, they are measles, mumps, and rubella. Before 13 years of age, immunity against hepatitis B and varicella should been ensured. DTaP, HBV, Hib, MMR, and varicella can be given simultaneously at separate sites if failure of the patient to return for future immunizations is a concern.
3. Varicella vaccine can be administered to susceptible children anytime after 15 months of age. Unimmunized children who lack a reliable history of varicella should be immunized before their 13th birthday.
4. Minimal interval between two doses of MMR is 1 month (4 weeks).
5. HBV may be given in a 3-dose schedule with minimum 4 weeks interval, ideal being 0-1-6-month schedule.

SIMULTANEOUS ADMINISTRATION OF MULTIPLE VACCINES

Most vaccines can be safely and effectively administered simultaneously. No contraindication is known to the simultaneous administration of multiple vaccines routinely recommended for infants and children. Immune responses to one vaccine generally do not interfere with those to other vaccines; concerns include interference among the three oral poliovirus serotypes in trivalent OPV vaccine and concurrent administration of measles and MMR (measles, mumps, and rubella) vaccines. Simultaneous administration of oral poliovirus vaccine (OPV), MMR, varicella, or diptheria, tetanus toxoids and pertussis (DTP) vaccines has resulted in similar rates of seroconversion and of side effects such as those observed when thevaccines are administered at separate times. Because simultaneous administration of common vaccines is not known to affect the efficacy or safety of any of the routinely recommended childhood vaccines, simultaneous administration of all vaccines (DTP, OPV, MMR, varicella, Hep B, and Hib vaccines) appropriate for the age and previous immunization status of the recipient is recommended. Simultaneous administration of multiple vaccines can raise immunization rates significantly.

For persons preparing for foreign travel, multiple vaccines generally can be given concurrently. An exception is the simultaneous administration of yellow fever and cholera vaccines. Antibody responses to both cholera and yellow fever vaccines are decreased if given simultaneously or within a short time of each other. If possible, these vaccines should be separated by at least 3 weeks; alternatively, cholera vaccine could be omitted since its effectiveness is limited and few indications for its use exist.

If both vaccines are necessary and time constraints exist, these vaccines can be given simultaneously or within a 3-week period with the understanding that antibody responses may not be optimal.

When vaccines commonly associated with substantial local or systemic reactions, e.g. cholera, parenteral typhoid vaccines, and plague are given simultaneously, the reactions can be accentuated. Thus, in most circumstances, if feasible, these vaccines should be given on separate occasions.

Measles, mumps, and rubella vaccine and typhoid conjugate vaccine (TCV) should be separated by an interval of 4 weeks pending studies of concurrent administration.

LAPSED IMMUNIZATIONS

A lapse in the immunization schedule does not require re-instituting of the entire series. If a dose of DTP, OPV, Haemophilus influenzae type b (Hib), or Hep B vaccine is missed, immunizations should be given at the next visit as if the usual interval had elapsed. The medical charts of children in whom immunizations have been missed or postponed should be flagged to remind healthcare professionals to complete immunization schedules at the next available opportunity. If status is unknown, consider them as unimmunized and administer age-appropriate vaccine at recommended schedule.

UNKNOWN OR UNCERTAIN IMMUNIZATION STATUS

A physician may encounter some children with an uncertain immunization status. Many young adults and some children do not have adequate documentation of immunizations and recollection by the parent or guardian may be of questionable validity. In general, these persons should be considered disease susceptible and age-appropriate immunizations should be administered. No evidence indicates that administration of MMR, varicella, Hib, Hep B, or poliovirus vaccine to already immune recipients is harmful.

ACTIVE IMMUNIZATION OF PERSONS WHO RECENTLY RECEIVED IMMUNOGLOBULIN

Live-virus vaccine given parenterally can have diminished immunogenicity when given shortly before or during a period of several months after receipt of immunoglobulins. High doses of immunoglobulin have been demonstrated to inhibit the response to measles vaccine for a prolonged period. The duration of inhibition varies directly with the dose of immunoglobulin administered. Inhibition of immune response to rubella, while of shorter duration than measles, also has been demonstrated. The appropriate suggested interval between immunoglobulin administration and measles immunization will vary with the indication for immunoglobulin (which determines the dose) and specific product, e.g. immune globulin vs immunoglobulin intravenous. If immunoglobulin must be given within 14 days after administrations of measles or measles-containing vaccines, these live-virus vaccines should be administered again after the period specified unless serologic testing at an appropriate interval after immunoglobulin administration indicates that adequate serum antibodies were produced.

The effect of administration of immunoglobulin on the antibody response to varicella vaccine is not known. Because of potential inhibition of the response, varicella vaccine should not be administered after receipt of an immunoglobulin preparation or a blood product (except washed red blood cells), as recommended for measles vaccine. In addition, immune globulin preparations, if possible, should not be administered for 14 days after immunization. If an immune globulin preparation is given in this interval, the vaccine recipient should be reimmunized after the period or tested for varicella immunity at that time and reimmunized if seronegative.

In contrast with live-virus vaccines given parenterally, administration of immune globulin preparations has not been demonstrated to cause significant inhibition of the immune responses to inactivated vaccines and toxoids. For example, concurrent administration of recommended doses of hepatitis B immunoglobulin, tetanus immunoglobulin, or rabies immunoglobulin (RIG) and the corresponding inactivated vaccine or toxoid indicate long-term immunity, i.e. active and passive immune prophylaxis. Standard doses of the corresponding vaccines are recommended. Increase in the vaccine dose volume or number of immunizations are not indicated. Vaccines should be administered at sites different from that of intramuscularly administered immunoglobulin.

Administration of hepatitis A vaccine together with immunoglobulin has been recommended for situations in which immediate and prolonged protection against hepatitis A virus (HAV) infection is desired. Although this combined active-passive immunization has been demonstrated to result in significantly lower serum antibody concentrations than those induced by vaccine administration only, these concentrations are still many times higher than those considered protective and seroconversion rates are not affected. The reduced immunogenicity, therefore, is to be considered clinically significant.

On the other hand, MMR and varicella vaccines, as previously discussed, these recipients should be immunized as per the recommended schedule for routine childhood immunization.

Administration of immune globulin preparations does not interfere with antibody responses to yellow fever or OPV vaccines. Hence, OPV and yellow fever vaccines can be administered simultaneously with or at any time before or after immunoglobulin, such as to travelers whose departure is imminent.

PREGNANCY

TT/Td/Tdap and inactivated influenza can safely be given. Live-virus vaccines are contraindicated in general. Hep A, Hep B, and pneumococcal vaccines can also be given. All vaccines except yellow fever vaccine are safe in lactating women. Rabies vaccination for postexposure prophylaxis is not contraindicated.

CHILDREN ON STEROIDS

- *Topical therapy or local injections of corticosteroids:* Administration of topical corticosteroids, either on the skin or in the respiratory tract (i.e. by aerosol) or eyes, and intra-articular, bursal, or tendon injections of corticosteroids usually do not result in immunosuppression that would contraindicate administration if clinical or laboratory evidence of systemic immunosuppression results after prolonged application until corticosteroid therapy has been discontinued for at least 1 month.
- *Physiologic maintenance doses of corticosteroids:* Children who are receiving only maintenance physiologic doses of corticosteroids can receive live-virus vaccines during corticosteroid treatment.
- *Low or moderate doses of systemic corticosteroids given daily or on alternate days:* Children receiving less than 2 mg/kg/day of prednisone or its equivalent, or less than 20 mg/day if they weigh more than 10 kg can receive live-virus vaccines during corticosteroid treatment.
- *High doses of systemic corticosteroids given daily or on alternate days for fewer than 14 days:* Children receiving 2 mg/kg/day

or more of prednisone or its equivalent, or 20 mg or more daily if they weigh more than 10 kg, can receive live-virus vaccines immediately after discontinuation of treatment. Some experts; however, would delay immunization until 2 weeks after corticosteroid therapy, if possible (i.e. provided the patient's condition allows temporary cessation).

- *High doses of systemic corticosteroids given daily or on alternate days for fewer than 14 days or more:* Children receiving 2 mg/kg/day or more of prednisone or its equivalent, or 20 mg or more daily if they weigh more than 10 kg, should not receive live-virus vaccines until corticosteroid therapy has been discontinued for at least 1 month.
- *Children with a disease that is considered to suppress the immune response and who are receiving systemic or locally administered corticosteroids:* These children should not be given live-virus vaccines except in special circumstances.

HODGKIN'S DISEASE

Children suffering from Hodgkin's disease should receive pneumococcal and Hib vaccines as per recommendations.

ASPLENIC CHILDREN (CONGENITAL ASPLENIA, SICKLE CELL DISEASE, AND SPLENECTOMY)

Children with congenital asplenia or after splenectomy (functional asplenia) or sickle-cell disease should receive Hib as well as pneumococcal and meningococcal vaccines.

CHILDREN WITH HIV-AIDS

In India, children with HIV-AIDS should receive immunization as per the **Table 6.4**.

Table 6.4: Immunization of Indian children to prevent HIV-AIDS.

Vaccines	Known symptomatic HIV infection	Symptomatic HIV infection
BCG	Yes	Yes*
Hepatitis B	Yes	Yes
DTP	Yes	Yes
OPV	Yes	Yes

Contd...

Contd...

Vaccines	Known symptomatic HIV infection	Symptomatic HIV infection
MMR	Yes	Yes**
Hib	Yes	Yes
Pneumococcal	Yes	Yes
Influenzae	Yes	Yes
Hepatitis A	Consider	Consider
Varicella	Consider	Consider

*Yes, in India where TB is highly endemic
**Severely immunocompromised HIV infected children should receive MMR.

IMMUNIZATION IN BLEEDING DISORDERS

Subcutaneous route preferred unless contraindicated. Aluminium salt adjuvanted vaccines can be given IM with caution by applying deep pressure after vaccination at the injectionsite. It is ideal to immunize after factor replacement therapy. Facilities for immediate blood transfusion should be available if uncontrolled bleeding occurs at injection site. Always immunize these children in a hospital setup.

IMMUNIZATION IN CHILDREN WITH HISTORY OF ALLERGY

If previous history of hypersensitivity/anaphylaxis is to any vaccine is present, do not use the same vaccine again. If history of egg allergy is present, only influenza and yellow fever vaccines are contraindicated. Measles and MMR vaccines can be given as they are propagated in chick embryo cells only. If history of any hypersensitivity present, JE vaccination should be done cautiously, facilities for cardiopulmonary resuscitation (CPR) is mandatory.

ORGAN TRANSPLANT INDIVIDUALS

All inactivated/subunit vaccines may be given safely to all transplant patients. In planned transplant, the donor may be given the required vaccines. However, in bone marrow transplant patients, the entire age appropriate series should be restarted in view of marrow ablation.

VACCINATION OF THE INDIVIDUAL WITH CANCER/CHEMOTHERAPY

General Principles

- Avoid administration of all live vaccines to patients on chemotherapy and within 6 months following completion of chemotherapy.
- Avoid administration of live vaccines, except MMR, VZV (varicella zoster virus), LAIV (live-attenuated influenza vaccine) and rotavirus vaccines, to siblings of patients on chemotherapy (or within 6 months following completion of chemotherapy).
- Inactivated influenza vaccine (IIV) is recommended annually for all patients on chemotherapy or within 6 months of its completion.
- Catch up DTwP/DTaP, Hep B, pneumococcal, varicella and MMR vaccines should be given before initiation of chemotherapy or 3–6 months after chemotherapy.
- All live vaccines should be avoided at least 3 months after chemotherapy or radiotherapy.

IMMUNIZATION IN RELATION TO ANTIBODY CONTAINING PRODUCTS

Inactivated vaccines are safe. Live vaccines viz. MMR, varicella, etc. should be avoided for 3 months. Antibody containing products should be avoided at least for 2 weeks after these vaccinations. Oral typhoid vaccine, LAIV, OPV, and yellow fever vaccines may be given at any time indicated as for age. Rotavirus vaccines should be avoided for 6 weeks.

IMMUNIZATION FOR TRAVELERS

Travelers to India should receive typhoid, HAV, HBV, varicella, rabies vaccines and JE vaccine if traveling to JE endemic areas during JE session. Travelers from India if traveling to South Africa, sub-Saharan should receive yellow fever vaccine. If on Hajj pilgrimage, polio and meningococcal vaccines are indicated. Travelers to Africa should receive meningococcal vaccine in addition to yellow fever vaccine.

LEARNING POINTS

- Specific vaccines recommended by professional bodies should be administered to children and adolescents at appropriate ages and situations.
- Each country specifies travel-related vaccines to be taken for those visiting the country and for students proceeding abroad for higher studies.
- For Hajj pilgrims, meningococcal vaccination is mandatory.

BIBLIOGRAPHY

1. American Academy of Pediatrics. Immunization in special clinical circumstances. In: Kimberlin DW, Brady MT, Jackson MA, et al. (Eds). Red Book: 2015 Report of the Committee on Infectious Diseases. 30th edition. American Academy of Pediatrics; 2015. pp. 68-107.
2. Bonanni P, Grazzini M, Niccolai G, et al. Recommended vaccinations for asplenic and hyposplenic adult patients. Hum Vaccin Immunother. 2017;13(2):359-368. doi:10.1080/21645515.2017.1264797.
3. https:/www.england.nhs.uk 2019.
4. Immunization in special situations. In: Vashishtha VM, Choudhury P, Bansal CP, Yewale YN, Agrawal R (Eds). IAP Guide Book on Immunization 2013-14. Indian Academy of Pediatrics; 2014. pp. 363-82.
5. Vaccination in special situations, Course material Advanced Science of Vaccinology workshop. Indian Academy of Pediatrics; 2009.

Adverse Events Following Immunization

Mohit Vohra

Several scientific, ethical and statutory obligations are fulfilled by manufacturers; elaborate field trials regarding safety and protection offered by individual vaccines are established before it is recommended for routine use. Being product of biological nature certain adverse reactions and mishaps may rarely occur following vaccination.

Complications following administration of vaccination may be broadly categorized into different categories depending on the reactions and their severity. All these are grouped under adverse effects following immunization (AEFI). An anticipated reaction to the vaccination is one which is expected but not severe enough to cause discomfort beyond short duration of time, e.g. pain/fever/discomfort after DTP vaccination, erythema at the site of vaccination, whereas severe complications following vaccine administration may be in the form of unexpected anaphylactic shock, induction of active disease, or complications such as toxic shock syndrome following measles vaccination.

Therefore, it is mandatory for the person administering vaccine to have sufficient knowledge regarding vaccines and expected side effects and to inform parents thoroughly regarding such adverse effects which may; however, occur very rarely. It is also essential to be prepared and to always have a "Kit" with life-saving drugs and equipment at each place of vaccination.

VACCINE SAFETY: A UNIVERSAL CONCERN

A steering committee on immunization safety has been formed since 1999, including the members nominated by the Director of World Health Organization (WHO), Department of Vaccines and Biologicals:
- To review critically the priorities and targets for the immunization projects.
- To assess the functioning of the programs and immunization safety.

- To provide guidance for improvement, modifications and efficacious implementation of the programs.

This Global Advisory Committee on Vaccine Safety particularly assesses the issues of vaccine safety and adverse events. The facts and challenges outlined are as follows:

- Up to one-third vaccine injections are not carried out in a way that guarantees sterility.
- Safe technologies are not available in many places or are not accessible.
- Adverse events are poorly understood, recorded, and investigated.
- Awareness of risk associated with vaccines is gaining importance and immunization programs are at risk of persistent rumors related to the damages of immunization.
- In 1998, only 78% countries producing vaccines and 30% countries procuring vaccines had monitoring systems for Vaccine Adverse Event Reporting System (VAERS).

The Immunization Safety Project includes WHO, UNICEF (United Nations Children's Fund), UNAIDS (United Nations Joint Programme on HIV/AIDS), World Bank, PATH, Bill and Melinda Gates Children's Vaccine Program, Industry and National/International Professional Organizations. The CIDA (Canadian International Development Agency), JICA (Japan International Cooperation Agency), USAID (US Agency for International Development), and CDC (Centers for Disease Control and Prevention) are partners and financial supporters.

The priority project has important sets of advocacy messages:
- Ensuring vaccine safety
- Securing safety of injections, auto disable syringes by 2003, adhere to sterilization procedures, no recapping syringes to prevent needle stick injuries.
- Controlling safety of disposal, include immunization safety and waste management in national immunization and ensure accountability for waste disposal.
- Use vaccines of good quality, safety and efficacy, strengthen national regulatory authorities and ensure commitment to child safety.

The organizations have four main areas of focus:
1. Vaccine safety
2. Research and development of safe, thermostable vaccine

3. Access to safe vaccine delivery systems, safe sharp disposal by 2002 and safe injection
4. Identification and management of risks related to immunization; develop resource material, training of all EPI managers in the surveillance and management of adverse events following immunization.

WHO RECOMMENDATIONS TO MINIMIZE AEFI

The adverse events can be completely preventable if the necessary guidelines for the proper storage and the handling of vaccines as per WHO are followed. These are:

- Measles and Bacillus Calmette-Guérin (BCG) vaccines must be reconstituted only with the diluents supplied by the manufacturer.
- Reconstituted vaccines must be discarded at the end of each immunization session and not to be retained for use in any further session.
- No other drugs and substances should be kept inside the refrigerator being used for vaccine storage.
- Training and supervision of workers to ensure the proper procedures.
- Careful epidemiological investigations must be carried out in the event of AEFI.

Prevention of Acute Vaccine Reactions

This depends on the adequate knowledge of possible side effects and due diligence in recording the history of any vaccination reaction in child or in family before vaccinations. It is prudent to read the manufacturers product labeling and the package insert. A contraindication indicates that a vaccine should not be administered, whereas a precaution specifies a situation in which the vaccine may be indicated if after careful assessment the benefits outweigh the risks. Minor illness with/without fever does not contraindicate immunization. A child with moderate or severe febrile illness should be recalled as soon as symptoms alleviate or resolve.

CAUSES AND ERRORS LEADING TO AEFI

The causes and errors leading to AEFI could be:
- Inherent to vaccine components/preservatives/small quantity of antibiotics (vaccine related).

- Improper cold chain maintenance/administration of the vaccine using unsterile syringes and needles/improper sterilization (programmatic errors).

The increasing success of childhood vaccines in the control and prevention of vaccine preventable diseases has made both the health professionals and the public aware and focused on the risks associated with the immunization. Vaccines continue to be given to the millions of persons every year, as the benefits of vaccine far outweigh the small risks associated with them. The vaccine recommendations are based on the characteristic of the immunobiological product, disease burden as well as its epidemiology in target population and the vaccine safety profile.

Vaccination risks range from common, minor, and local adverse effects to rare, severe, and life-threatening conditions. Thus, recommendations for immunization practices balance scientific evidence of benefits for each person and to the society, against the potential costs and risks of vaccination programs. Vaccines are intended to produce active immunity to specific antigens. An adverse reaction is an untoward effect that occurs after a vaccination, i.e. extraneous to the vaccine's primary purpose of producing immunity. Vaccination reactions to individual immunization agents have been discussed in the relevant chapters of this book. The present chapter primarily deals with general aspects related to adverse events following immunization.

All vaccines might cause adverse reactions. However, it is often difficult to prove a definite cause-effect relationship between the act of vaccination and a subsequent complication. Only some of these reactions have established correlation with a particular vaccine.

VACCINES AND CONTRAINDICATIONS

- *Avoid:*
  - *Live vaccine:*
    - Immunodeficient individuals
    - Immunosuppressant therapy
    - Chronic debilitating illness
  - *DPT (1st dose):*
    - Progressive neurologic disease
    - Uncontrolled seizure disorder

- Rubella vaccine during pregnancy
- Antibiotics effective against *Salmonella typhi*: Avoid week prior/later of TY21 vaccination.
- *Delay:*
  - Measles/MMR for 6 weeks following immunoglobulin therapy
  - Severe febrile illness
- *Discontinue:* DTPw/DTPa in case of severe postvaccination reactions
- *Do not stop vaccination in:*
  - Malnutrition
  - Mild fever
  - Upper respiratory tract infections
  - Mild diarrhea
  - Any benign ailment.

ANAPHYLAXIS AND DRUGS

Epinephrine in the Treatment of Anaphylaxis

Subcutaneous or Intramuscular Administration

Epinephrine* 1:1000 (aqueous): 0.01 mL/kg per dose repeated every 10–20 minutes[+]. Usual dose—dose may be repeated every 10–20 minutes. A continuous infusion should be started if repeated doses are required. One milliliter (1 mL) of 1:1000 dilution of epinephrine added to 250 mL of 5% dextrose in water, resulting in a concentration of 4 µg/mL, is infused initially at a rate of 0.1 µg/kg per minute and increased gradually to 1.5 µg/kg per minute to maintain blood pressure.

Patients should be observed even after remission of immediate symptoms; however, a specific period of observation has not been established. A period of observation of 4 hours would be reasonable for mild episodes and 24 hours for severe episodes.

Anaphylaxis occurring in persons already taking (3-adrenergic blocking agents presents a unique situation.

---

*In addition to epinephrine, maintenance of the airway and administration of oxygen are critical.

[+]If agent causing anaphylactic reaction was given by injection, epinephrine can be injected into the same site to slow absorption.

[+]If intravenous access cannot be obtained, IM dose can be injected into posterior one-third of sublingual region of the tongue.

In such persons, the manifestations are likely to be more profound and significantly less responsive to epinephrine and other adrenergic agonist drugs. More aggressive therapy with epinephrine may be adequate to override the receptor blockade in some patients. The use of IV glucagon for cardiovascular manifestations and inhaled atropine for management of bradycardia or bronchospasm also has been recommended in this situation.

Dosages of Commonly Used Secondary Drugs in the Treatment of Anaphylaxis

Drug	Dose*
H_1–blocking agents (antihistamines) Diphenhydramine	Oral, IM, IV: 1–2mg/kg, every 4–6 hours (100 mg, maximum—single dose)
Hydroxyzine	Oral, IM: 0.5–1 mg/kg, every 4–6 hours (100 mg, maximum—single dose)
H_2-blocking agents (also antihistamines) Cimetidine	IV: 5 mg/kg, slowly during 15 minutes, every 6–8 (300 mg, maximum single dose)
Ranitidine	IV: 5 mg/kg, slowly during 15 minutes, every 6–8 hour (50 mg, maximum single dose)
Corticosteroids Hydrocortisone	IV: 100–200 mg/kg, every 4–6 hours
Methylprednisolone	IV: 1.5–2 mg/kg, every 4–6 hours (60 mg, maximum—single dose) use corticosteroids as long as needed
β_2-agonist Albuterol	Nebulizer solution: 0.5% (5 mg/mL) 0.05–0.15 mg/kg per dose in 2–3 mL isotonic sodium chloride, maximum of 5.0 mg/kg per dose every 20 minutes for 1–2 hours or 0.5 mg/kg per hour by continuous nebulization (15 mg/hr, maximum dose)
Other dopamine	IV: 5–20 µg/kg per unit. Mixing 150 mg of dopamine with 250 mL of saline or 5% dextrose in water will produce a solution that, if infused at the rate of 1 mL/kg per hour, will deliver 10 mg/kg per minute The solution must be free bicarbonate, which may inactivate dopamine
Aminophylline	IV: 4–6 mg/kg in 20 mL saline by rapid drip every 6 hours or 0.9–1.1 mg/kg per hour continuous infusion

Source: Pickering LK, Baker CJ, Kimberlin DW, Long SS (Eds). Red Book: 2009 Report of the Committee on Infectious Diseases, 28th edition. American Academy of Pediatrics; 2009.

THREATS TO IMMUNIZATION: SAFETY CONCERNS

While the entire world is jubilant about the eradication of smallpox, effective control of poliomyelitis, reduction in mortality due to diphtheria, pertussis, tetanus and measles, it is unfortunate that an anti-vaccination lobby has emerged questioning the ethical aspects of immunization. To quote John Clements and Peter J Lachmann, "No valid ethical distinction exists between harm arising from a medical intervention and the harm arising from its omission", this is self-explanatory. Hence, the slogan "*Vaccines for all children of the World*" has been given by the Global Alliance for Vaccines and Immunization (GAVI).

Let us briefly analyze the "scares, cams and sickness" concerning vaccines (**Table 7.1**) and ascertain the scientific facts, as they have been proved to be baseless.

Table 7.1: Vaccination scares.

Vaccine	Supposed Link
Hepatitis B	Multiple sclerosis, lupus, diabetes
Whole-cell pertussis	Encephalopathy, epilepsy, learning disorders
Diphtheria, tetanus, and pertussis	Cot death/sudden infant death syndrome (SIDS)
Inactivated polio vaccine	HIV infection
Influenza	Diabetes mellitus
Haemophilus influenzae type b	Diabetes mellitus
Measles, mumps, and rubella	Autistic spectrum disorder, inflammatory bowel disease, childhood arthropathy
Rubella	Ethical concerns because grown in cells from an aborted fetus
Thimerosal-containing vaccines, aluminum-containing vaccines	Neurodevelopmental disorders, autism, muscular fibrosclerosis
Various vaccines	Diseases of unknown, or only partially understood etiology, e.g. asthma, autism, inflammatory bowel disease. Cot death, chronic fatigue syndrome. Immune deficiency, leukemia, autoimmune diseases, learning disorders, increase in violent crime

The AEFI are termed "Causal Relationship" or "Causal Link" scientific research and surveillance have identified proven causative links which includes the real, albeit very small, risk that rotavirus vaccine will cause intussusception and the higher risk of aseptic meningitis associated with mumps vaccines containing the Urabe strain rather than the Jerry Lynn strain, vaccine-associated paralytic polio (VAPP) which varies from region-to-region need extensive surveillance to link their real occurrence with the theoretical possibility. Fortunately, VAPP has not emerged as a concern in India both in National Immunization Program and Office Practice.

However, overwhelming scientific evidence for the overall safety of all the childhood vaccines recommended for universal immunization have negated most of these scares, scams, and sickness attributable to vaccines.

The reputable medical world had declared dead the hypothesis that MMR vaccines cause autism. Similarly, the risk complications from natural measles infection compared with known risks of vaccination with a live-attenuated virus, which is given below is self-explanatory **(Table 7.2)**.

Table 7.2: Risk of complications from natural measles infection compared with known risks of vaccination with a live-attenuated virus in immune competent individuals.

Complication	Risk after natural disease (%)[a]	Risk after vaccination (%)[b]
Postinfectious enchephalomyelitis	0.05–0.1	1 per million
Otitis media	7–9	0
Pneumonia	1–6	0
Diarrhea	6	0
SSPE	0.001	0
Anaphylaxis	0	1 per million to 1 per 100,000
Death	0.01–0.1 (industrialized countries) Up to 15 (developing countries)	0
		0

[a]Risks after natural measles are calculated in terms of events per number of cases.
[b]Risks after vaccination are calculated in terms of events per number of doses.
(PE: postinfectious encephalomyelitis; SSPE: subacute sclerosing panencephalitis)

To prove that the vaccines today are safe, similar scientific evidence is also available in respect of Hep B, whole-cell pertussis, DTP, inactivated polio, influenza, Hib vaccines.

The safety concern of vaccines containing thiomersal as preservative (the American Obsession) and aluminum salt adjuvant vaccines has also been negated. The ethyl alcohol in thiomersal never causes a neurological or neurodevelopmental disorder as compared to methyl alcohol, which is known to be neurotoxic. A recent study by Michael E Pichichero et al., concludes "Administration of Vaccines containing thimerosal does not seem to raise blood concentrations of mercury above safe values in infants". Ethyl mercury seems to be eliminated from blood rapidly via the stools. Similarly, the causal link between aluminum salts and muscular fibrosclerosis have also been negated.

Considering the above scientific facts, WHO advocates universal immunization with BCG, HB, DTP (whole-cell or acellular), OPV or IPV, measles, MMR, etc. and GAVI is working out strategies to make available all these vaccines at affordable cost to all world's children. Let us therefore dwell more on the benefits that vaccines have provided for the world's children rather than getting scared about stray and rare complications. However, it is imperative that every practitioner has access to cardiopulmonary resuscitation in case of an anaphylactic reaction and declares himself "needle smart" by using auto-destruct/disable syringes and needles.

ADVERSE EVENTS FOLLOWING IMMUNIZATION: PRACTICAL GUIDELINES

- *Definition:* An event following an immunization procedure attributable to the causal relationship between the vaccine/components in the vaccine formulation and the adverse event.
- *Types:* Local, systemic or anaphylaxis
  - *Local:* Swelling, redness and pain at the site of vaccination.
  - *Systemic:* Hypotensive, hyporesponsive episode attributable to DTP vaccine formulations, toxic shock syndrome (TSS) following administration of measles vaccine contaminated with *Staphylococcus aureus*, when used beyond there commended 4 hours after the constitution.

Cause-specific type of AEFI	Definition
Vaccine product-related reaction	An AEFI that is caused or precipitated by a vaccine due to one or more of the inherent properties of the vaccine product
Vaccine quality defect-related reaction (both 1 and 2 were earlier categorized in vaccine reaction)	An AEFI that is caused or precipitated by a vaccine that is due to one or more quality defects of the vaccine product, including its administration device as provided by the manufacturer
Immunization error-related reaction (formerly "program error")	An AEFI that is caused by inappropriate vaccine handling, prescribing or administration and thus by its nature is preventable
Immunization anxiety-related reaction (formerly "injection reaction")	An AEFI arising from anxiety about the immunization
Coincidental event	An AEFI that is caused by something other than the vaccine product, immunization error or immunization anxiety

Precautions

- Shake test for aluminum adjuvant vaccine formulations to prevent sterile abscess.
- Noticing color change in reconstituted measles/MMR vaccine vials from amber yellow to pink color.
- Use of recommended diluents of the same manufacturer.
- Not mixing up diluents with other injectable liquid preparations such as muscle relaxant, etc.
- Carrying emergency kit containing adrenaline, dopamine, IV fluids, oxygen mask with Ambu bag.
- Observing the child/person vaccinated at least for 30 minutes after an immunization procedure for any possible immediate adverse event.

DCGI (DRUGS CONTROLLER GENERAL OF INDIA) SUGGESTED SURVEILLANCE: ADVERSE EVENT REPORTING

In a modern developed democracy, no child should suffer from a vaccine-preventable disease. The immunization coverage in India is gradually increasing, and new vaccines are being added up in the national immunization program AEFI surveillance is a crucial program initiated long back to prevent the AEFI and to ensure safety. There is a need to improve the awareness about reporting among the medical professionals working in public as well as the private sectors to report all suspected adverse events (AEs) associated with immunization so that proper steps can be taken to prevent such incidents in future. The vibrant AEFI program will go a long way in winning the faith of people toward immunization.

Information related to AEs, if received, will go a long way in continuous efforts to update safety database and this will in turn help in our efforts to ensure patient safety. To facilitate safety reporting, most vaccine personnel are trained on reporting AEs, if received. Moreover, all promotional materials provided to the doctors have a mention of the email address for reporting AEs. The AE reporting process is well integrated and it has been been requested by Indian regulatory authorities to conduct an additional activity in the space of AE reporting so as to to carry out active surveillance for vaccines products.

COMMON ADVERSE EVENTS TO VACCINES

BCG Vaccine

Approximately 90–95% develop local reaction followed by healing and scar formation in 3 months.

DTwP/DTaP Vaccine

- Local reactions include erythema and indurations, with/without tenderness, which are usually self-limited and require no treatment.
- Systemic reactions, e.g. drowsiness, anorexia, vomiting, crying, and slight to moderate fever, are common. They subside spontaneously without sequelae.
- Severe systemic reactions include—(1) Severe allergic reactions, (2) seizures, (3) hypotensive, hyporesponsive episode/collapse or shock-like state, (4) temperature of >40.5°C, and (5) prolonged crying.

Hib Conjugate Vaccine

- Local reactions include swelling, redness, and pain, are reported in about 5–30% of the cases, and usually resolve in 24 hours.
- Systemic reactions, e.g. low-grade fever and irritability are infrequent.

Hepatitis A Vaccine

- Local reactions include pain, erythema, and swelling are reported in about 20% of recipients. These symptoms are mild- and self-limited.
- Systemic reactions—mild, e.g. low-grade fever and irritability are infrequent.

Hepatitis B Vaccine

- Local reactions include pain, erythema, and swelling reported in about 20% of recipients. These symptoms are mild- and self-limited.
- Systemic reactions—mild, e.g. low-grade fever and malaise, are reported (<10%). No serious adverse reactions have been reported.

Human Papillomavirus Vaccine

Human papillomavirus (HPV) vaccine was found to be safe and well-tolerated, with no serious adverse reactions to vaccination. The most common vaccine-related adverse event reported was local discomfort at the injection site.

Haemophilus Influenzae Type b Vaccines (Livestock Inactivated)

- Local reactions include transient soreness and erythema (10–20%). Generally lasting 1–2 days.
- Local reactions include fever and myalgia (<1%).
- Immediate hypersensitivity reaction is very rare, possibly related to egg protein allergy.

Japanese B Encephalitis Vaccines (Livestock Inactivated)

- Local tenderness, redness or swelling at injection, site occurs in 20% of recipients immunized with inactivated mouse brain-derived vaccines.
- Mild systemic symptoms, chiefly headaches, low-grade fever myalgia, malaise and gastrointestinal symptoms, are reported by 10–30% of vaccines
- Neurological manifestations and severe hypersensitivity reactions temporally associated with JE vaccines are rare.

Measles, Mumps, and Rubella Vaccine

- Fever (5-15%) occurs between 6 and 12 days after vaccination
- Transient rashes (5%)—appearing 7-10 days after vaccination
- Transient thrombocytopenia (1 : 30000)—within 2 months after vaccination
- Transient arthritis (10%)—7-21days after immunization
- Parotitis and orchitis have been reported rarely
- Aseptic meningitis after Urabe strain of live-attenuated mumps virus has been reported, with an incidence of 1:933-1:18868 doses in Japan.

Meningococcal Vaccine

- Rare and mild adverse reactions occur, the most common of which are localized and erythema for 1-2 days.
- There have been five case reports of Guillain-Barré syndrome following the use of conjugate Vaccines (A/C/Y/W135).

Pneumococcal Vaccine (PCV and PPSV)

The most common are local reactions, including pain, swelling, and erythema at the injection site in about 10-20% of vaccines recipients, systemic reactions, e.g. fever and myalgia, have being reported in 15-24% of recipients. Severe adverse reactions are very rare.

Polio Vaccines (OPV and IPV)

- Minor local reaction, i.e. pain and redness, may occur following IPV. Because IPV contains trace amounts of streptomycin, polymyxin B, and neomycin allergic reaction may occur in persons sensitive to these antibiotics.
- Vaccine-associated paralytic poliomyelitis (VAPP) is a rare adverse event following OPV. VAPP is more likely to occur in persons ≥18 years of ages than in children, and is much more likely to occur in immunodeficient children than in those who are immunocompetent usually following the first dose.
- The risk of VAPP is 7-21 times higher for the first dose than for any other dose in the OPV series. The overall ratio of VAPP was 1 case per 2.4 million doses.
- The risk for all other doses was 1 per 27.2 million doses.

Rabies Vaccine

- The adverse events of cell-culture derived vaccines were less and milder than those of nerve tissue vaccines.
- Most of the local reactions (15–25%) include pain and itching, especially in intradermal (ID) administration. Systemic reactions (2–8%), e.g. headache, nausea, and myalgia, may occur, especially with the first three doses of primary vaccination or in the booster dose. However, most of the reactions were mild and self-limited.
- Serum sickness-like reactions may be found (6–10%) 2–21days after receiving the booster vaccine. Anaphylaxis and Guillain-Barré syndrome were reported in some cases.

Rabies Immunoglobulin (RIg)

- Early local injection-site reactions consisting of erythema and itching are not uncommon with both human rabies immunoglobulin (hRIg) and purified equine rabies immunoglobulin (eRIg).
- Published data indicates that immunoglobulins can be safely injected into already infected animal bite wounds following proper wound cleansing and the administration of appropriate antibiotics.
- Because of the price and unavailability of hRIg and RIg is commonly used.
- To determine whether to use eRIg, a skin test needs to be done on the patient, as the risk of side effects which has now been reduced following purification process during manufacture.
- Most eRIgs that are presently manufactured are highly purified, and the occurrence of adverse effect has been significantly reduced to <1–2%.
- Serious adverse reactions, including anaphylaxis, may occur despite a negative skin test.

Rotavirus (RV) Vaccine

- The incidence of gastroenteritis, fever, and other adverse events was not different in the vaccine group when compared to the control group receiving the placebo group.
- Following administration of a previously licensed live RV, an increased risk of intussusceptions was observed.

- In large scale clinical trials, they did not show an increased risk of intussusceptions for both licensed vaccines when compared to placebo.
- In currently available bivalent-tetravalent rotavirus vaccine formulations the risk of intussusceptions is very rare. However, stray cases have been reported in India also, and hence follow-up of immunized child is mandatory.

Typhoid Vaccine

- Oral Ty21a vaccine produces minimal adverse reactions. Reported adverse effects have included abdominal discomfort, nausea, vomiting, fever, headache, and rash (urticaria).
- Reported adverse events from inactivated Vi CPS vaccine are also minimal and include fever, headache, and local reactions of erythema or indurations of 1 cm.

Varicella Zoster Vaccine

- Systemic reaction are uncommon complaints include pain, swelling, varicella-like rash, and maculopapular rash at the injection site.
- These local adverse events are generally mild and self-limited.

LEARNING POINTS

- Beware of adverse events following immunization.
- Follow the manufacturer's recommendations scrupulously.
- Administer vaccines by the recommended right technique, e.g. route, needle size, site of vaccination, etc.
- Two separate needles—one needle for loading and another needle for administration can be used in private practice with single dose vials.
- Gently roll between palms, the reconstituted lyophilized vaccine vials to get uniform solution; do not shake the reconstituted vaccine vial which may result in virus clumping.
- In case of reconstituted measles/MMR vaccine vials observe whether the amber yellow color changes to pink. If color change occurs possibility of contamination with *S. aureus* to be alerted to prevent toxic shock syndrome (TSS).
- Always be equipped with emergency kit for '0' hour management.

- Observe the child/person vaccinated at least for 15 minutes following any vaccination procedure.
- Report any adverse event to the local health authority.

BIBLIOGRAPHY

1. American Academy of Pediatrics. Passive immunization treatment of anaphylactic Reactions. In: Kimberlin DW, Brady MT, Jackson MA, et al. (Eds). Red Book: 2015 Report of the Committee on Infectious Diseases, 30th edition. American Academy Pediatrics; 2015. pp. 42-51.
2. Aston R. Scares, scams and sickness: countering the anti-vaccination lobby. Vaccines: Children and Practice. 2002;5(2):31.
3. Clements J, Lachmann PJ. Ethics and vaccination: irrelevant of imperative? Vaccines: Children and Practice. 2002;5(2):27-8.
4. Dubey AP, Banerjee S. Measles, mumps, rubella (MMR) vaccine: Indian J Pediatr. 2003;(7):579-84.
5. https://mohfw.gov.in/sites/default/files/Unit6Adverseevents followingimmunization.
6. India.pharmacovigilance@gsk.com.
7. Kher A, Shah N, Desai A. Adverse events following immunization. In: Shendurnikar N, Agarwal M (Eds). Immunization for Children. Palar Publishing, Hyderabad-Bangalore; 2002. pp. 191-4.
8. Mittal SK, Mathew JL. Vaccine associated paralytic poliomyelitis. Indian J Pediatr. 2003;7:573-7.
9. Pichichero ME, Cernichari E, Loprelato J, Treanor J. Mercury concentration and metabolism in infants receiving vaccines containing thiomersal: a descriptive studies. Lancet. 2002;360:737-41.
10. Rao IS. Vaccination complications, their management and contraindications: In: Lokeshwar MR, Shah N (Eds). Recent Concepts in vaccinology. Pediatric Clinics of India. 2001;36(1):30-5.
11. World Health Organization. Global Alliance for Vaccines and Immunization (GAVI). WHO Fact Sheet No. 169 March 2001 (cited 11 April 2002). [online] Available from: URL:http://www.who.int/inf-fs/en/fact169. html
12. World Health Organization. Vaccine safety—Vaccine safety Advisory Committee. Wkly Epidemiol Rec. 1999;74:37-8.
13. www.ijp-online.com.

CHAPTER 8

The Cold Chain for Vaccines

A Parthasarathy

COLD CHAIN

Cold chain is the vital link in immunization. However, potent the vaccine may be, if cold chain is not maintained properly the vaccine efficacy will be lost. From the manufacturing unit to the site of vaccine administration, stringent measures should be followed as per recommendation to avoid breaks in cold chain **(Fig. 8.1)**. It is always ideal to measure the temperature with a Dial thermometer twice daily to check any equipment fault and the consequences of breaks in the cold chain. Such vaccines not only lose their potency but also pose a serious setback to the credibility of immunization programs.

COLD CHAIN EQUIPMENT

The cold chain consists of two aspects that are complementary to each other: *"the set chain"* which includes walk in coolers, deep freezers, ice-lined refrigerators and *"the mobile chain"* which consists of vaccine carriers (VC), mobile storage device (MSD), vaccine vial monitor (VVM), etc.

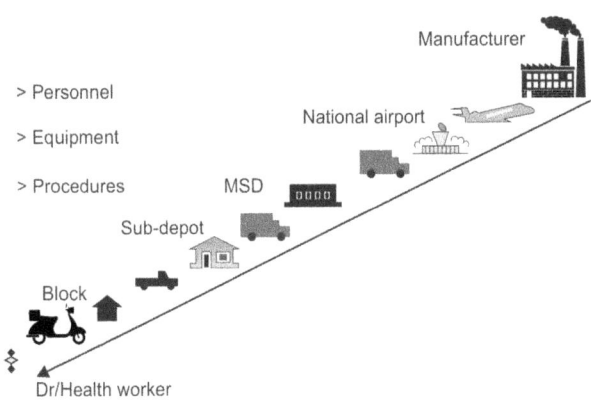

Fig. 8.1: Cold chain.

REFRIGERATORS

These are of two types: (1) Absorption type (powered by kerosene, bottled gas, or electricity) and (2) compression type (powered by electricity).

Domestic refrigerators are also commonly used for vaccine storage. Certain guidelines given below would help to improve the functioning of the equipment and thus, ensure proper storage of vaccines **(Fig. 8.2)**.

- Refrigerator should be protected from direct sunlight and should be at least 10 cm away from the wall to allow adequate air circulation and heat dispersal. Clear space above the refrigerator should be about 40 cm.
- It should be kept locked and opened only when necessary.
- It should be equipped with the ice packs in the freezer compartment and several bottles of chilled water in the shelves that are not being used for storage of vaccines. This will help keep the temperature down in case of power failure.
- It is always advisable to keep some empty spaces in between for proper air circulation.
- Refrigerators should be defrosted periodically (when the layer of ice in freezer exceeds >5 mm).
- Always follow the principle of First in, First out (FIFO), First expired, First out (FEFO).

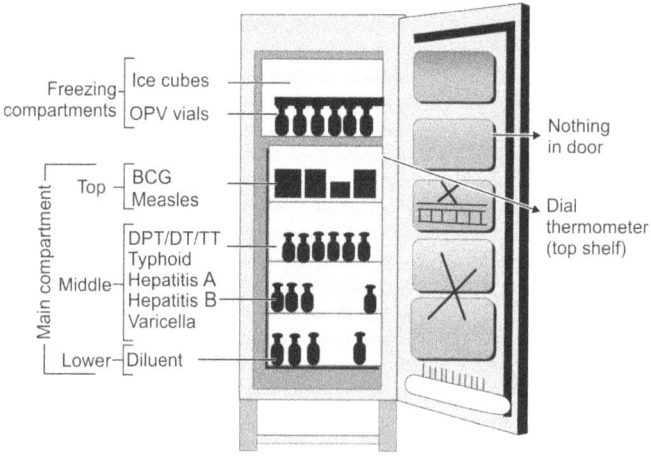

Fig. 8.2: Domestic refrigerator showing vaccine storage.
Source: Government of India, CSSM training module.

TECHNICAL SPECIFICATIONS OF COLD CHAIN EQUIPMENT (TABLE 8.1)

Table 8.1: Technical specifications of cold chain equipment.

Equipment	Temperature	Storage capacity	Holdover time
Deep freezer (large)	−15°C to −25°C	Ice packs or OPV stock for 3 months (275–300 L)	At 43°C for 2 hours 30 min (minimum)
ILR (large)	+2°C to +8°C	BCG, OPV, IPV, RVV, DPT, TT, measles/MR, Hep B, Penta, vaccine stock for 3 months (135–160 L)	At 43°C for 20 hours (minimum)
Deep freezer (small)	−15°C to −25°C	Ice packs (105–125 L)	At 43°C for 2 hours 30 min (minimum)
ILR (small)	+2°C to +8°C	BCG, OPV, IPV, RVV, DPT, TT, measles/MR, Hep B vaccine stocks for 1 month (90–105 L)	At 43°C for 20 hours (minimum)
Cold box (large)	+2°C to +8°C	All vaccines stored for transport or in case of power failure (20–25 L)	At 43°C for 96 hours (minimum)
Cold box (small)	+2°C to +8°C	All vaccines stored for transport or in case of power failure (5–8 L)	At 43°C for 48 hours (minimum)
Vaccine carrier (1.7 L)	+2°C to +8°C	All vaccines carried for 12 hours (4 conditioned ice packs and 16–20 vials)	At 43°C for 36 hours (minimum)

(ILR: ice-lined refrigerator; OPV: oral polio vaccine; RVV: rotavirus vaccine; DPT: diphtheria, pertussis, and tetanus; BCG: Bacillus Calmette–Guérin; TT: tetanus toxoid; IPV: Inactivated polio vaccine)

VACCINE VIAL MONITORS

Vaccine vial monitors (VVMs) are time and temperature-sensitive labels attached to the vials of the vaccine at the time of manufacture. Through a gradual and irreversible color change they warn the health workers, in case the vaccines have been degraded by an unacceptable exposure to heat. This facilitates decision-making at the worker level regarding the appropriateness of the vaccines for use in the community. VVMs

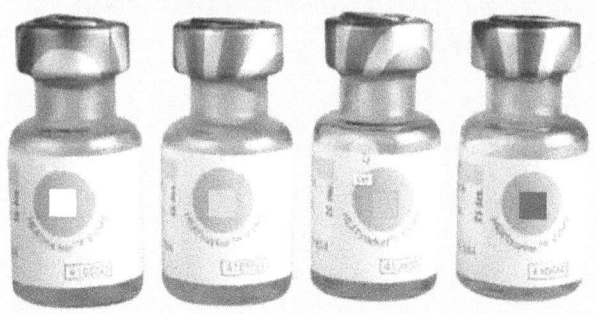

Fig. 8.3: Vaccine vial monitors.
Source: Government of India, CSSM Training Module.

are designed to meet the vaccines heat stability curve allowing a margin of safety. Thus, VVMs indicate problems in the cold chain, prevent delivery and use of heat-damaged vaccines, and serve as a tool for management of vaccine stocks.

Since the beginning of 1996 all the vials of OPV procured through the UNICEF come with a VVM. The VVM is a small square made up of heat sensitive material and placed on an outer colored circle printed on the label of OPV vial. Combined effects of time and temperature cause the VVM to change the color gradually from light at the starting point to dark with the exposure to the heat **(Fig. 8.3)**. The outer colored circle is used as a reference to compare the color of VVM.

STORAGE OF VACCINES IN DOMESTIC REFRIGERATOR

- A VVM is a label containing a heat-sensitive material which is placed on a vaccine vial to register cumulative heat exposure over time **(Figs. 8.4 and 8.5)**.
- The inner square (2 mm) is the indication, which is light at starting point than the outer circle (7 mm) and becomes darker with exposure to heat.

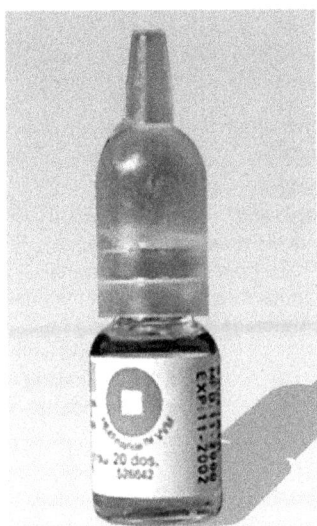

Fig. 8.4: OPV vial with VVM.
Source: Government of India, CSSM training module.

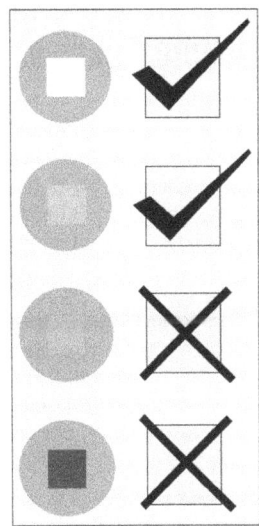

Fig. 8.5: Interpretation of color change of square in the circle on VVM.

The use of VVM in our country is increasing with the introduction of NIDs for polio eradication. A recent study conducted on a National Immunization Day observed lack of staff awareness regarding the interpretation of VVM. The study also recommended training of staff before the next PPI rounds for an effective cold-chain maintenance.

The VVM can be seen as a catalyst for much needed changes in the strategies for vaccines distribution via the cold chain. It should eventually allow immunization programs to exploit the stability of each vaccine to the greatest possible extent, minimize distribution costs and increase flexibility in the handling of vaccines in the field.

VVM is not a direct measure of the vaccine potency, but only provides information about the heat exposure of the vial over a period. VVM does not provide any information about other factors that could also affect the potency of a vaccine, such as exposure to sunlight, expiry date, etc.

RECOMMENDED STORAGE OF COMMONLY USED VACCINES

Vaccine	Recommended temperature	Duration of stability	Normal appearance
Diphtheria and little as 24 hours and acellular pertussis vaccine adsorbed (DTaP)	2–8°C (35°F), do not freeze. As not more than 18 months at <2°C (<35°F) or >25°C (>77°F) may cause antigens to fall from suspension and be difficult to resuspended	Markedly turbid and from the time of issue from manufacturer's cold storage	Tetanus toxoids whitish suspension. If product contains clumps of material that cannot be resuspended with vigorous shaking it should not be used.
Diphtheria and tetanus toxoids whole-cell pertussis vaccine adsorbed and *Haemophilus influenzae type b* vaccine	2–8°C, do not freeze. As little as 24 hours at <2°C or >25°C may cause antigens to fall from suspension and be difficult to resuspended	Not more than 2 years from the time of issue from manufacturer's cold storage	Markedly turbid white suspension. If product contains clumps of material that cannot be re-suspended with vigorous shaking, it should not be used.
(DTP-HbOC) Diphtheria toxoid adsorbed	2–8°C, do not freeze	Not more than 2 years from the time of issue from manufacturer's cold storage	Turbid and white, slightly pink suspension
H. influenzae type b conjugate vaccine HbOC (diphtheria toxoid conjugate)	2–8°C, do not freeze	Not more than 2 years from date of issue from storage	Clear, colorless liquid Manufacturer's cold storage
H. influenzae type b conjugate vaccine: PRP-T (tetanus toxoid conjugate)	*Lyophilized formulation:* 2–8°C. do not freeze Formulation or diluents	Not more than 2 years from date of issue from manufacturer's cold storage	Clear, colorless liquid
	Reconstituted formulation: 2–8°C, do not freeze	Vaccine should be used immediately when reconstituted.	*Reconstituted:* Clear and colorless

Contd...

Contd...

Vaccine	Recommended temperature	Duration of stability	Normal appearance
Hepatitis A virus vaccine, inactivated	2–8°C, do not freeze. Do not use if product has been frozen	2 years, if kept refrigerated	Opaque, white suspension
Hepatitis B virus vaccine, inactivated (recombinant)	2–8°C. Storage outside This temperature range may reduce potency. Freezing substantially reduces potency	2 years from date of issue from manufacturer's cold storage	After thorough agitation, a slightly opaque, white suspension
Influenza virus vaccine (subversion)	2–8°C. Freezing destroys potency	Use of vaccine is recommended only during the year for which it is manufactured antigenic composition differs annually	Clear, colorless liquid
Measles, mumps, and rubella (MMR) virus vaccine, live-attenuated	May be frozen. Protect from light, which may inactivate virus *Diluent:* Store at room temperature or refrigerated Do not freeze reconstituted formulation 2–8°C protect from light, which may inactivate virus	*Lyophilized formulation:* 2°C Discard reconstituted vials if not used within 8 hours	–8°C *Reconstituted:* Clear, yellow solution
Measles virus vaccine, live mumps virus vaccine, live Rubella virus vaccine, live	See MMR	See MMR	See MMR
Pneumococcal vaccine, polyvalent	2–8°C. Freezing destroys potency	See expiration date on vial	Clear, colorless, or slightly opalescent liquid

Contd...

Contd...

Vaccine	Recommended temperature	Duration of stability	Normal appearance
Poliovirus vaccines, live oral (OPV)	Must be stored at <0°C (<32°F). Because of sorbitol in the vaccine, it will remain fluid at temperatures above −14°C (7°F). Refreezing the thawed product is acceptable (maximum of 1° thaw-freeze cycles) if the temperature never exceeds 8°C and the cumulative thawing time is <24 hours	Not more than 1 year from date of issue from manufacturer's cold storage	Clear solution, usually red or pink, from the phenol red (pH) indicator, it contains; may be yellow if shipment was packed with dry ice. Color changes that occur during storage or thawing are unimportant, provided the solution remains clear.
Tetanus and diphtheria toxoids adsorbed (DT and dT)	2–8°C, do not freeze	Not more than 2 years from the time of issue from manufacturer's cold storage	Markedly turbid and white suspension. If product contains clumps of material that cannot be resuspended with vigorous shaking, it should not be used.
Varicella virus vaccine+	*Lyophilized formulation:* keep frozen, temperature of −15°C (5°F) or colder, protect from light. *Diluent:* Store at room temperature or refrigerated. Reconstituted formulation; use immediately; do not store. For temporary storage, reconstituted, vaccine may be stored at 2–8°C for a maximum of 72 hours	*Lyophilized formulation:* 18 months. Discard reconstituted vials if not used within 30 minutes. Discard reconstituted vaccine if not used within 72 hours (do not refreeze)	*Lyophilized formulation:* Whitish powder. Reconstituted formulation; clear, colorless to pale yellow liquid

Source: Red Book: 2009 Report of the Committee on Infectious Diseases. Pickering LK, Baker CJ, Kimberlin DW (Eds). 28th edition: American Academy of Pediatric; 2009.

The Cold Chain for Vaccines

For recently licensed combination vaccines, see package inserts; instructions may be different from those for products listed in Annexure IV. Also, any changes in the formulation of currently available immunizing agents may alter their appearance, stability, and storage requirements. Questions about the stability of biological subjected to potentially harmful environmental conditions should be addressed to the manufacturer of the product in question.

POWER FAILURE

Continue to keep all the vaccines in the refrigerator and ensure that door is kept closed. If power failure occurs too often or exceeds 6 hours shift vaccines in an Igloo box filled with icepacks. A closed refrigerator can retain +2°C to +8°C refrigerated state for 4–6 hour of power failure. IPV, liquid Hib formulation, hepatitis B and DTwP/DTaP, combination formulations of DTwP/ DTaP, DT, TT/Td are most cold sensitive in that order. Hence, they should be packed in plastic bags and direct contact with ice packs.

LEARNING POINTS

- Use continuous temperature monitoring devices (data loggers) to monitor vaccines that will be administered to children in the Vaccines for Children (VFC) program. This applies to:
  - Routine onsite storage of vaccine
  - Transport of vaccine
  - Mass vaccination clinic.
- Maintain primary and back-up thermometers that meet the CDC data logger requirements, which include having:
  - A temperature probe—a buffered probe is recommended and represents the vaccine temperature better than measuring the air temperature
  - An active temperature display that can be easily read from the outside of the unit
  - The capacity for continuous temperature monitoring and recording where the data can be downloaded routinely.
- Assess and record minimum and maximum temperatures at the start of each clinic day.

- Refrigerator temperature should measure between 2°C and 8°C. Freezer temperature should measure –15°C to –50°C.
- Do not freeze T series of vaccines of DTwP/DTaP, DT, TT, Td, Tdap, Typhoid and Aluminium salt adjuvanted vaccine such as hepatitis B and hepatitis B combination vaccine for fear of sterile abscess following desiccation of aluminium salts if frozen. Once frozen these vaccines should be discarded.
- Do not expose to sunlight most heat-sensitive vaccine such as OPV, measles, MMR, BCG, hepatitis B, DT, IPV, and Hib formulations.
- Always perform shake test before using aluminum salt adjuvanted vaccines to ensure homogeneous fluidity. If flocculation occurs after shake test discard.
- Reconstituted freeze-dried vaccines vials such as measles, MMR should be gently shaken after injecting the diluent. Vigorous shaking may result in clumping and reduce immunogenicity of the vaccine component.
- Always follow the rules of "*First in, First out*" while distributing or administering a vaccine. Notice the expiry date before administering any vaccine.

BIBLIOGRAPHY

1. American Academy of Pediatrics. Active immunization, vaccine handling and storage. In: Pickering LK, Baker CJ, Kimberlin DW (Eds). Red Book: 2009 Report of the committee on Infectious Diseases, 28th edition. American Academy of Pediatrics; 2009. pp. 13-7.
2. Cold Chain. Parthasarathy A, Dutta AK, Bhave S (Eds). IAP Guide Book on Immunization; Indian Academy of Pediatrics; 2001.
3. Cold Chain Maintenance. Child Survival and Safe Motherhood (CSSM) Module 1992. Government of India.
4. Cold Chain for vaccine. In: Parthasarathy A, Menon PSN, Nair MKC, Gupta P (Eds). IAP Textbook of Pediatrics. Jaypee Brothers Medical Publishers, New Delhi; 2015.
5. Unit 4: Cold chain and logistics management. Immunization handbook for Medical Officers. [online] Available from: https://mohfw.gov.in.
6. Immunizations and practice management, American Academy of Pediatrics. [online] Available from: https://www.aap.org.

CHAPTER 9

Vaccine Development

Srinivas G Kasi

Immunizations are one of the greatest success stories of public health. Every vaccine goes through a well-defined developmental process to ensure the development of safe and efficacious vaccines.

VACCINE DEVELOPMENT PROCESS

The clinical evaluation of a vaccine typically comprises three phases. The entire process takes 10–15 years and by present day standards, requires a budget of about 1 billion US Dollars[1] **(Table 9.1)**.

Vaccine development is highly pyramidal process, for every success, there are many failures. Most failures occur in the preclinical stage and in the Phase 1 clinical trial. Vaccines that reach the Phase 2 and 3 trials have an increased likelihood of reaching successful licensing and usage.[1,2]

The general stages of the development cycle of a vaccine are:
- Exploratory stage
- Preclinical stage

Table 9.1: Vaccine development process.

Identification and product characterization	Nonclinical (animal) testing	Clinical trials (Phase 1–3)	Licensing	Surveillance
Time taken for each stage				
2–5 years	1–2 years	4–8 years	1–2 years	>2 years
Cost of each stage				
10–20 M USD	50–100 M USD	500–1000 M USD	20+ M USD	
8–17 years and 560–1120 M USD				Commercial production

(M USD: Million US Dollar)

- Clinical development
- Regulatory review and approval
- Manufacturing
- Quality control.

Exploratory Stage

This is the first step and may last 2–4 years. In this stage, the antigens are identified, chemically characterized and the immunology studied to enable the selection of one or more candidate vaccines to continue the development process.

Preclinical Stage

This is the second step and lasts between 1 and 2 years. In this stage, the antigens are assessed in animals and the best candidate vaccine is selected for human testing. The formulation, pharmacokinetics, mechanism of actions and bioavailability are assessed. Initial manufacturing processes are setup in order to prepare the first clinical batches.

Clinical Development

This is the phase in which the candidate vaccine is tested in healthy human beings who volunteer for trials. Their safety is fundamental. This phase may last between 6 and 8 years. Trials in humans pass through four phases.

- In *Phase 1 studies*, which are done in humans, the primary endpoints studied are safety and tolerability, both the local and systemic levels. Additionally, dose-ranging studies and preliminary information on immunogenicity and efficacy may be collected. Phase 1 studies are usually randomized, double-blind, placebo-controlled, single-center studies. This stage is limited to short-term studies in a few patients or normal healthy volunteers (generally 20–80).
- In *Phase 2 studies*, the parameters assessed are primarily the immunogenicity and safety of the candidate vaccine within the target population, the optimal dose and the initial schedule. The number of subjects in this phase is still relatively limited (100–200). Phase 2 studies are often subdivided into phase 2A and phase 2B. The parameters assessed in Phase 2A studies include, dose-response studies, studies to determine vaccination schedules, route of administration,

and need for boosters. Phase 2B studies include small-scale pilot efficacy trials and larger confirmatory immunogenicity and tolerance studies in target populations.
- In *Phase 3 studies*, which are the final step in the clinical evaluation before the product is licensed for clinical usage, assessment of the vaccine's immunogenicity, efficacy and safety is studied, in a significantly larger group of subjects (several hundreds to several thousands). It may be conducted at different sites, and in different countries. The endpoint may be clinical endpoints or comparative (noninferiority or superiority) immunogenicity trials when an established reference vaccine is available. Serological data are usually collected from at least a subset of the immunized population at predefined intervals. Additional studies performed in Phase 3 studies include co-administration or interchangeability with other vaccines, minor extension of the age target, immunogenicity in special risk groups and validation of a different immunization schedule.
- *Phase 4 studies* are designed to collect additional safety data in large numbers of vaccine recipients or for seeking additional indications for product use.

Regulatory Processes in India

The Central Drugs Standard Control Organization (CDSCO), which functions under the Directorate General of Health Services, Ministry of Health and Family Welfare,

Government of India is India's National Regulatory Authority (NRA) and is responsible for regulating the production and import of biological product in India. It undertakes evaluation of safety, effectiveness, and quality of all prescription drugs and biologicals in the country. The Drug Controller General of India (DCGI) heads CDSCO. The DCGI is often referred to as the Central Licensing Authority. The CDSCO along with state regulators, deals with license of manufacturing for examination, tests and analysis, conduct of clinical trials, permission and license for manufacturing and marketing.[3]

The Department of Biotechnology in India is the department that governs the preclinical studies of all biologicals. The Review Committee on Genetic Manipulation (RCGM) and the Genetic Engineering Approval Committee (GEAC) are involved in the approval of any research involving genetic manipulation.

Following completion of all clinical studies, a dossier containing all the information is submitted to the DCGI at New Delhi. Following inspection, the Compliance report is submitted to both FDCA and CDSCO. If found satisfactory, State FDCA forward the recommendation to DCGI which issues the Permission for Market Authorization approval. The next step is to acquire the Manufacturing License from the State FDCA.[4]

Following release of the vaccine in the market for clinical usage, it is mandatory for the manufacturer to conduct post-marketing surveillance for adverse drug reactions for a variable period. Every lot released into the market must undergo rigorous quality control testing at Central Drug Laboratory, Kasauli, before release into the market.[4]

REFERENCES

1. Seunghoon Han. Clinical vaccine Development. Clin Exp Vaccine Res. 2015;4:46-53.
2. https://www.who.int/biologicals/expert_committee/WHO_TRS_1004_web_Annex_9.pdf?ua=1.
3. https://cdsco.gov.in/opencms/export/sites/CDSCO_WEB/Pdf-documents/biologicals/1CDSCOGuidanceForIndustry.pdf.
4. Maurya SK, Shukla V, Kaushik P, Yamini Kanti SP, Bansal A. Regulatory aspects for Biologic product Licensing in India. International Journal of Drug Regulatory Affairs. 2019;7(1):1-5. [online] Available from: http://ijdra.com/index.php/journal/article/view/287.

CHAPTER 10

Future Vaccines

Srinivas G Kasi

INTRODUCTION

Vaccination is a highly effective preventive strategy, and some vaccines are true success stories. These include vaccines against smallpox, diphtheria, poliomyelitis, measles, mumps, and rubella (MMR). Existing vaccines can be used more effectively for preventing influenza, hepatitis A, hepatitis B, meningococcal disease, pneumococcal infection, and varicella (including zoster). Of great promise are vaccines now in the development "pipeline". These include vaccines against anthrax, cytomegalovirus (CMV) infection, group B streptococcal disease, HIV disease, hepatitis C, genital herpes, dengue, tuberculosis (New), malaria, meningococcal disease caused by serotype B organisms, and infection with multidrug-resistant staphylococci improvements are needed in several areas. However, these include improvement in vaccine delivery, development of combination vaccines, and increasing the effectiveness and utilization rates of existing vaccines. For several diseases that remain significant public health challenges throughout the world, vaccines have yet to be developed or made available. These much-needed vaccines, some of which are in clinical trials, are the focus of intensive research and will be the subject of this chapter.

Coming years will see a revolution in the manner vaccines are made, used and the diseases targeted for control or elimination. Vaccines have usually targeted infectious diseases. Efforts to develop vaccines against non-infectious diseases such as cancer, autoimmunity, allergies, and other conditions have been successful. Both preventive and therapeutic vaccines will improve outcome in a variety of chronic conditions.

NEWER TECHNOLOGIES IN VACCINE DEVELOPMENT

Vaccinology, as a branch of science, has a very short history. Variolation was practiced since ancient times. The first recorded history of variation was in the middle ages, in China, where air-dried pustules of smallpox were inhaled for protection against smallpox. Subsequently, Edward Jenner's observation that exposure of an individual to an agent that mimicked the disease, rather than exposing people to the disease directly, was protective, led to the production of the smallpox vaccine and eradication of smallpox from the world.[1]

The evolution of technologies for vaccines development[2] can be discussed here (**Fig. 10.1**).

Empirical Approach

This was based on the Pasteurian approach of isolate, inactivate (or attenuate) and inject. This approach resulted in the development of some highly successful vaccines, smallpox,

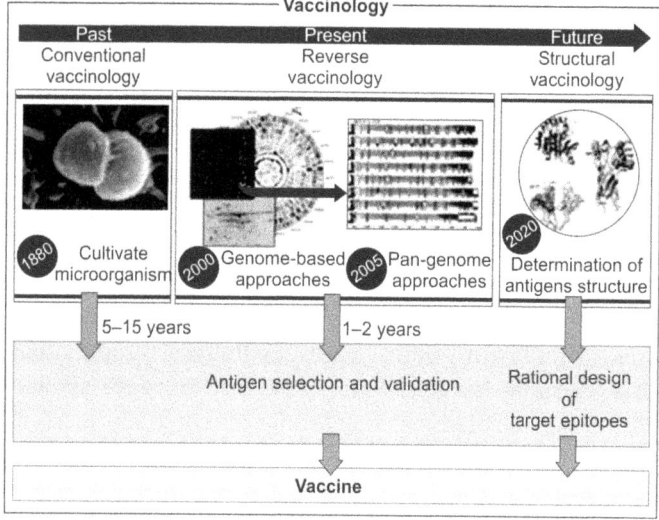

Fig. 10.1: Technologies in vaccine development. The past involved conventional approaches of cultivation of the microorganism in laboratory conditions, isolation of individual antigens, purification and testing for immunogenicity and safety. This method was empirical, laborious and took 5–15 years for development of a vaccine. The present, in the genomic era, involves choosing the most appropriate antigen from the virtual catalogue of all the potential vaccine candidates available in the genomic and pangenomic data of microorganisms and use of reverse vaccinology to produce a vaccine in 1–2 years. The future involves the use of structural vaccinology, to construct the most appropriate antigen and personalizing vaccines based on "vaccinomics".
Source: Reproduced with permission from Serruto D, Rappuoli R. FEBS Letters. Elsevier. 2006;580:2985-92.

rabies, polio and influenza. The development of cell culture techniques led to the development of many vaccines against poliomyelitis, measles, mumps, rubella, varicella, hepatitis A, and more recently rotavirus and influenza.

Recombinant DNA Technology

With the arrival of the "Genomic era", it was possible to isolate the gene for a protective antigen, clone it with the *Escherichia coli* or other mammalian cell lines and produce large quantities of the protective antigen. This technology led to the development of vaccines against Hep B, Lyme disease, pertussis and human papillomavirus (HPV).

Glycoconjugation Technology

Polysaccharide antigens are poorly immunogenic in children less than 2 years of age and do not induce a memory cell response and hence cannot be used in children less than 2 years of age. The discovery that conjugating the polysaccharide to a protein will result in a robust T-cell response led to the development of highly effective glycoconjugate vaccines against *Haemophilus influenzae type b (Hib)*, *Pneumococcus*, *Meningococcus*, and now *Salmonella*.

The characterization of the entire genome of the *H. influenzae* in 1995 spurred the "Genomic era" of vaccinology and now the genomes of over 2,000 bacteria and 3,000 viruses have been characterized. Once the complete genome sequence of the organism is available, high-throughput approaches can be used to screen for target molecules with desirable traits of a vaccine. Transcriptomics, functional genomics, proteomics, immunomics, structural genomics, and immunogenetics are other offshoots of the genomic era which are revolutionizing the way vaccines are made **(Fig. 10.2)**.

Reverse Vaccinology

The advent of genome sequencing technologies has revolutionized the field of vaccinology. With knowledge of the entire genome of a pathogen, it is possible to characterize the entire antigenic content, choose antigens which possess protective characteristics and test for their suitability as a vaccine. This is known as *reverse vaccinology*.[3] The first vaccine

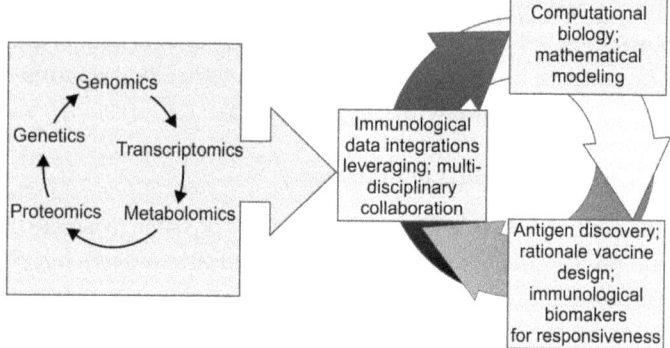

Fig. 10.2: Systems biology approaches for vaccine studies interactions and implications on translational research. Systems biology is a term used to describe the study of the interactions between the components of biological systems, and how these interactions give rise to the function and behavior of that system. This diagram illustrates the use of systems biology for vaccine development.
Source: Reproduced from Buonaguro, et al. BMC Systems Biology. 2011;5:146.

to be produced by this technology is the vaccine against the group B *Meningococcus*. Vaccines against group B *Streptococcus* (GBS), group A *Streptococcus* (GAS), *E. coli*, *Staphylococcus aureus,* and *Clostridium difficile* are in development utilizing the same technology.

NEXT GENERATION TECHNOLOGIES
Structural Vaccinology

Structural vaccinology (SV) is a new and emerging methodology of vaccine development in which immunogens are rationally engineered using available structural information. SV aims to identify protective B-cell epitopes on the antigens and optimize the antigens in terms of stability, epitope presentation, ease of production and safety. This is achieved by using a combination of human immunology, structural biology, and bioinformatics knowledge. A deeper characterization of the crystal structure of an antigen in complex with protective antibodies defines a structural epitope. This structural epitope is transplanted to scaffold proteins for structural stabilization and to design minimized antigens that retain only one or more key epitopes and eliminate the unnecessary components. This new class of antigens is called epitope-scaffolds. Epitope-scaffolds are grafted into heterologous protein scaffolds that support three-dimensional structure and provide conformational stabilization. This concept is being tested in vaccines against HIV.

The Systems Biology Approach to Vaccines Development[5]

Systems biology has been described as "an interdisciplinary approach that systematically describes the complex interactions between all the parts in a biological system, with a view to elucidating new biological rules capable of predicting the behavior of the biological system". It involves a combination of many scientific disciplines—biology, computer science, engineering, bioinformatics, physics, and others. The aims of systems biology are to evaluate vaccine-induced immune responses, identify response-specific signatures and assess their predictive value. Pulendran and colleagues, first applied this approach to study the immune response induced by the yellow fever vaccine. They could identify gene expression signatures in the blood a few days after vaccination that could predict, with up to 90% accuracy, the strength of the immune response to the yellow fever vaccine. Sékaly and colleagues made similar observations. Both studies showed a positive correlation between the early innate immunity-related events and protective vaccine response.

Carrying this concept further, Pulendran and colleagues studied the innate and adaptive immune responses in healthy adults, following administration of the inactivated and live-attenuated influenza vaccines. Their findings identify early innate response-related molecular signatures that predict with 90% accuracy later antibody titers. These gene expression signatures of early innate immune activation predict the ensuing adaptive immune responses. Moreover, the key genes in the predictive signatures are not all related to inflammatory immune responses.

The systems biology approach will enable to prospectively predict vaccine efficacy within a few days of administration. This may help in identifying "non-responders" in special populations. Another great advantage is its value in accelerating vaccine testing in clinical trials, wherein it will obviate the need for assessing the incidence of the target disease in vaccinated versus unvaccinated populations or subgroups of vaccinated populations.

DNA Vaccines

DNA vaccines[6] are vaccines which contain DNA that codes for specific proteins (antigens) from a pathogen. The DNA is injected into cells, resulting in *in situ* production of the target antigen. As these proteins are recognized as foreign, when they are processed by the host cells and displayed on their surface, the immune system is alerted, which then triggers immune responses, which results in the stimulation of both B- and T-cell responses. The advantages of this approach include the stimulation of both B- and T-cell responses, improved vaccine stability, the absence of any infectious agent and the relative ease of large-scale manufacture.

The low immunogenicity of the first-generation DNA vaccines was partly due to inefficient uptake of the plasmids by cells. The second-generation DNA vaccines are being delivered by efficient delivery systems and being adjuvanted by novel adjuvants.

Presently, there are no approved DNA vaccines for use in humans. A vaccine against West Nile virus (WNV) in horses and canine melanoma, which are DNA-based vaccines, are approved for clinical usage.

Viral Vector Vaccines

Recombinant viral vectors are being explored as delivery platforms for viral antigens.[7] They can express single or multiple heterologous antigens and induce highly efficient humoral and cytotoxic ($CD8^+$) T-cell responses, which are essential for effective viral vaccines. Viral vectors have intrinsic adjuvant properties, as they express pathogen-associated molecular patterns (PAMPs) which activate innate immunity. *Vaccinia virus* was the first virus to be developed as a vaccine vector and numerous others have since been explored as delivery vehicles for foreign immunogens. The replicative capacity of viral vectors is reduced or eliminated by targeted gene deletion (replication deficient viral vectors) which ensures safety for human use without loss of potency. Existing adaptive immune responses, prior or freshly induced, may render these viral vectors ineffective. This can be overcome by using higher tolerated doses or by heterologous prime boost regimens.

The *Vaccinia virus* and the adenovirus are the viral vectors most frequently used in viral vectored vaccines. Other viruses include adeno-associated virus, *cytomegalovirus, Sendai virus, Lentiviruses*, measles virus, and the *vesicular stomatitis virus* (VSV).[8] The most successful applications of viral-vector vaccines have been in the veterinary field, with at least 12 viral-vector vaccines currently licensed for veterinary use and many more under development. Highly immunogenic vaccine candidates, mainly based on adenovirus and poxvirus vectors, are now in Phase 1 and Phase 2 clinical trials for malaria, tuberculosis and influenza. Similar approaches are being adopted in the field of HIV and cancer vaccines.[8]

Newer Adjuvants

Adjuvants are substances added to vaccines to enhance the immunogenicity of highly purified antigens that have insufficient immune-stimulatory capabilities. Highly purified vaccine components frequently lack PAMPs, which results in poor stimulation of the initial innate immune response and negatively affect the subsequent adaptive response. Adjuvants can act like PAMPs, triggering the innate immune response through a variety of mechanisms and initiation of downstream adaptive immune activities.[9]

Some licensed adjuvants are as discussed under:
- *Aluminium salts* were first used in human vaccines in 1932, and was the only adjuvant in use in licensed vaccines for approximately 70 years. While it was widely believed the aluminium adjuvants act primarily to increase antibody production and are therefore suitable for vaccines targeting pathogens killed primarily by antibodies, recent evidence indicates that alum can activate the innate immune response by combining with the nucleotide-binding oligomerization domain (NOD)-like receptors (NLRs) and preferentially induce Th2 responses (characterized by antibody production).
- *MF59* is a water-in-oil squalene-based emulsion that is currently licensed as part of a flu vaccine for individuals >65 years old. The mechanisms of action of MF59 are not fully

understood. MF59 can stimulate macrophages, resident monocytes, and dendritic cells (DCs) to secrete several chemokines such as CCL4, CCL2, CCL5, and CXCL8 that in turn induce leukocyte recruitment and antigen uptake leading to migration to lymph nodes and triggering the adaptive immune response.

- *AS03* is an oil-in-water adjuvant emulsion that contains α-tocopherol, squalene, and polysorbate 80. AS03 stimulates the immune system by the activation of NF-κB, proinflammatory cytokine and chemokine production, recruitment of immune cells, mainly monocytes and macrophages, and induction of high antibody titers.
- *AS04* is a combination of MPL and aluminum salts which is currently part of two licensed vaccines, HPV-Cervarix and HBV-Fendrix. ASO4 exerts its biological actions by TLR4 activation, which leads to rapid (within 3–6 hours) production of cytokines and cell recruitment in the injected muscle and draining lymph node (LN). ASO4 also causes activation of NF-κB, production of proinflammatory cytokines and chemokines, and recruitment of monocytes and macrophages to the injection site, but specifically DCs. It induces a specific Th1 immune response.
- *AS01* contains two immune-stimulatory molecules, i.e. monophosphoryl lipid A (MPL) and the saponin QS21. MPL and QS21 which are formulated together in liposomes in the presence of cholesterol. It is a component of the RTS, S1 vaccine, licensed against malaria.
- *CpG 1018:* Oligonucleotides containing unmethylated CpG sequences are potent stimulators of the innate immune system through activation of Toll-like receptor-9. 1018 is a short (22-mer) oligonucleotide sequence containing CpG motifs. This is an adjuvant used in Heplisav-B, a newly licensed vaccine against hepatitis B10.
- *Virosomes:* A virosome is a reconstituted viral envelope possessing membrane lipids and viral glycoproteins, but devoid of viral genetic information. Two vaccines, the *influenza virus vaccine (Inflexal V)* and the hepatitis A virus (Epaxal) vaccine are approved for clinical usage. Both vaccines utilize virosomes derived from influenza virus represented by immuno-potentiating reconstituted

influenza virosomes (IRIV) harboring the influenza hemagglutinin (HA) protein.[10]
- *Immune potentiators:* Immune potentiators target innate immunity signaling pathways through pattern recognition receptors (PRRs) such as Toll-like receptors (TLRs), retinoid acid-inducible gene I (RIG-I)-like receptors (RLRs), and NLRs. In general, activation of PRRs by their agonists induces APC activation/maturation and cytokine/chemokine production that ultimately leads to adaptive immune responses. Examples of PRRs agonists include, poly(I:C), MPL, flagellin, imiquimod, resiquimod, CpG oligodeoxynucleotides (CpG ODN), and MDP.[10]

Edible Vaccines

A new approach for delivering vaccine antigens is the use of inexpensive, oral vaccines. Edible oral vaccines offer exciting possibilities for significantly reducing the burden of diseases such as hepatitis and diarrhea particularly in the developing world where storing and administering vaccines are often major problems. Even though they have some disadvantages like control of the "dosage" of the antigen that is present in the recombinant fruit or vegetable, they have many advantages as they trigger the immunity at the mucosal surfaces which is the body's first line of defense. To overcome the disadvantage of adequate dosage, stable plant lines that produce fruits and vegetables with relatively constant amounts of the antigen need to be developed. The hope is that edible vaccines could be grown in many of the developing countries where their need is more.

An edible vaccine is a genetically manipulated food-containing organisms or related antigens that may provide active immunity against infection. Edible vaccines against many microorganisms are being developed, with the goal of using them to vaccinate children in non-industrialized countries where there are obstacles to the use of traditional injectable vaccines.[11]

Needle-free Vaccine Delivery

The search for methods of vaccine delivery not requiring a needle and syringe has been accelerated by recent concerns regarding pandemic disease, bioterrorism, and disease eradication campaigns. Needle-free vaccine delivery could aid in these mass vaccinations by increasing ease and speed of delivery, and by offering improved safety and compliance, decreasing costs, and reducing pain associated with vaccinations. Jet injectors are needle-free devices that deliver liquid vaccine through a nozzle orifice and penetrate the skin with a high-speed narrow stream. They generate improved or equivalent immune responses compared with needle and syringe.[12] Powder injections, a form of jet injection using vaccines in powder form, may obviate the need for the cold chain. Transcutaneous immunization involves applying vaccine antigen and adjuvant to the skin, using a patch or micro-needles, and can induce both systemic and mucosal immunity. Mucosal immunization has thus far been focused on oral, nasal, and aerosol vaccines.

Select Vaccines

Anthrax Vaccine

Only vaccine for anthrax approved by US FDA, is the Biothrax. This is a sterile, milky-white suspension for intramuscular or subcutaneous injections made from cell-free filtrates of microaerophilic cultures of an avirulent, non-encapsulated strain of *Bacillus anthracis*. This vaccine will be very soon available in Indian market, marketed by Biological E Ltd, Hyderabad. In clinical use, however, this vaccine can be reactogenic and current efforts are aimed at rationalizing the clinical dosing regimen to reduce dosing frequency whilst enhancing immunogenicity by the inclusion of CpG, as NuThrax.

To achieve a more defined vaccine, the recombinant expression of protective antigen (PA) has been pursued and several candidates' rPA vaccines are currently in development and in clinical trials for safety.[13]

Cytomegalovirus Vaccine

The human cytomegalovirus (HCMV) is the most important infectious cause of congenital abnormalities and of infectious complications of transplantation. The biology of the infection is complex and acquired immunity does not always prevent reinfection. Nevertheless, vaccine development is far advanced, with numerous candidate vaccines being tested, both live and inactivated.

The vaccines in development include attenuated strain (Towne strain), recombinants with wild virus (Towne-Toledo), replication-defective virus, vectored vaccines, recombinant gB glycoprotein with adjuvant, soluble pentamers, DNA plasmids, self-replicating RNA, peptides, dense bodies and virus-like particles. No vaccines have entered Phase 3 trials.[14]

Group B Streptococcal Vaccine

One vaccine candidate is a fusion of highly immunogenic and protective protein domains from two surface proteins of group B *Streptococcus* (GBS) (N-terminals of Alpha C and Rib, GBS-NN). This protein is associated with serotypes Ia, Ib, II, III, IV, V, and VIII as well as cross-reactive proteins VI and VII). It is expected that this vaccine will protect against up to 95% of GBS isolates. More importantly, the Rib protein is expressed on all isolates of the hyper-virulent clone ST-17. Results from a phase 1 trial in 240 healthy adult women showed that all subjects immunized with one or two doses of GBS-NN showed an increase of over 30-fold in GBS-NN specific antibodies compared to pre-immune level.[15]

HIV Vaccines

The first experimental immunization of humans against HIV was started in November, 1986. Since then, more than 256 trials have been conducted and only one vaccine having reached Phase 3 trials. The HVTN 505 vaccine was abandoned because of lack of efficacy in Phase 2B trials and the Phase 3 trials of RV144 showed a disappointing 31.2% efficacy.[16]

Two vaccines are in Phase 2B trials:
1. *HVTN 705:* This trial is testing a prime-boost combination of an ALVAC vector and clade C Env protein. The vaccine regimen is comprised of two administrations of tetravalent Ad26 vaccine (four recombinant Ad26 vectors expressing mosaic inserts of HIV gag-pol or Env genes) at months 0 and 3, followed by two administrations of the same tetravalent rAd26 vaccine with soluble trimeric Clade C gp140 formulated in alum at months 6 and 12. The trial is expected to end in Dec, 2022.[17]
2. *HVTN 702:* This study will evaluate the preventive vaccine efficacy, safety, and tolerability of ALVAC-HIV (vCP2438) + bivalent subtype C gp120/MF59 in HIV-seronegative South

African adults over 24 months and potentially up to 36 months from enrollment. It commenced in Oct, 2016 and is expected to end in July, 2021. Participants will receive an intramuscular (IM) injection of ALVAC-HIV (vCP2438) at months 0 and 1, and an IM injection of ALVAC-HIV (vCP2438) + bivalent subtype C gp120/MF59 at months 3, 6, and 12.[17]

Herpes Simplex Virus Vaccines

Four vaccines, all therapeutic vaccines, have completed Phase 1 studies successfully and Phase 2 trials have been initiated. These are GEN-003 (Subunit vaccine: gD2/ICP4 with Matrix M2 adjuvant), HerpV (32-35-mer peptides, complexed with HSP, QS21 adjuvant), Codon optimized polynucleotide vaccine (DNA vaccine: gD2 codon-optimized/ubiquitin-tagged), and VCL-HB01/HM01 (DNA vaccine: gD2+/−UL46/Vaxfectin).[18]

Tuberculosis Vaccines

There are 2 types of tuberculosis (TB) vaccines—preventive and therapeutic. The preventive vaccines include priming vaccines and boosting vaccines. At present, around 14 TB vaccine candidates are in different phases of clinical trials. Three vaccines, VPM 1002, MIP and M, vaccae are in Phase 3 trials and three vaccines, M72-ASO1, DAR-901 and H56:IC31 are in Phase 2B trials.[19]

Malaria Vaccines

The RTS,S/AS01 vaccine, which is a hybrid molecule expressed in yeast, that consists of the tandem repeat tetrapeptide (R) and C-terminal T-cell epitope containing (T) regions of circumsporozoite protein (CSP) fused to the hepatitis B surface antigen (S), plus unfused S antigen with the adjuvant AS01, has entered clinical usage.

In Phase 3 studies which were completed 2014 and published in 2015.[20] Three-dose primary series reduced clinical malaria cases over the length of the study by 28% in young children (over a median follow-up of 48 months after first dose across trial sites) and 18% in infants (over a median follow-up of 38 months after first dose across trial sites). A booster dose of RTS,S, administered

18 months after completion of the primary series, reduced the number of cases of clinical malaria in young children (aged 5-17 months at first vaccination) by 36% over the entire study period and in infants (aged 6-12 weeks at first vaccination) by 26% over the study period. These results were achieved on top of existing malaria interventions, such as insecticide-treated mosquito nets (ITNs), which were used by approximately 80% of the trial participants.

Plasmodium falciparum sporozoites (PfSPZ) vaccine is a candidate malaria vaccine made of non-replicating irradiated whole sporozoites and developed by Sanaria. In a Phase 1 double-blind, randomized trial in 1993, 18-35-year adults from Mali, the vaccine was well-tolerated and safe. PfSPZ Vaccine showed significant protection in African adults against *Plasmodium falciparum* infection throughout an entire malaria season.[21]

No other candidate vaccines have reached Phase 2 trials.

Staphylococci Vaccines

Staphylococci are opportunistic pathogens, normally colonize the human anterior nares, skin, and gastrointestinal (GI) tract but rarely cause systemic infections in otherwise healthy individuals.

Nabi-StaphVax is a polysaccharide conjugate vaccine derived from *Staphylococcus aureus* capsular polysaccharides covalently bound to a carrier protein to induce polyclonal antibodies directed at multiple sites on the bacterial surface polysaccharide coat. The vaccine targets serotypes 5 and 8, which are responsible for 85-90% of S. aureus infections.[22]

Phase 1 and 2 studies have demonstrated safety and immunogenicity. Immune response has persisted for several years, and an optimal dose for healthy volunteers and for patients with end-stage renal disease has been established. A pivotal Phase 3 clinical trial showed the vaccine to be safe and 57% effective in reducing the incidence of life-threatening *S. aureus* bacteremia for 10 months following vaccination. There are six other staphylococcal vaccine projects underway based on polysaccharides, chimeric viruses, and conjugated epitopes on carriers.

Studies are also on for vaccine against multidrug-resistant *S. aureus* (MRSA).

Respiratory Vaccines

There are six programs devoted to development of respiratory syncytial virus vaccines, including live viruses, recombinant proteins, and DNA methods. There are three programs devoted to parainfluenza, virus vaccine development, and one parainfluenza virus vaccine is in clinical trials. No respiratory syncytial virus (RSV) vaccine is currently on the market, but diverse vaccine candidates, targeting different proteins within the RSV virion, are undergoing clinical trials. These include live-attenuated RSV vaccines, protein-based vaccine, viral vectors encoding RSV surface antigens, nucleic acid vaccines, and nanoparticle based vaccines.[23]

NovaVax, which is a RSV F-protein nanoparticle vaccine, is the only vaccine in phase 3 trial which is nearing completion.

Dengue Vaccines

Dengue vaccines offer an impending solution to control this major global health problem. Two new dengue vaccines are in Phase 3 trials, the NIH LAV, TetraVax-DV and the Takeda vaccine, TDV.[24]

The NIH LAV, TetraVax-DV is a live attenuated vaccine wherein the attenuation is based on a targeted 30-nucleotide (nt) deletion (D30) in the 30 non-translated region (NTR) of the dengue virus (DENV) genomes of the four monovalent vaccine viruses. A Phase 3 efficacy trial of TetraVax-DV is currently underway in several sites in Brazil, involving approximately 17,000 subjects including children, adolescents, and adults. The trial is expected to end in Dec, 2022. Panacea Biotec Ltd. of India has been granted license for development of this vaccine. Phase 1 trials are still to begin. Serum Institute of India Limited, which secured an independent license from NIH in 2015 to develop TetraVax-DV in India, is currently conducting preclinical toxicity studies.

Takeda's dengue vaccine (TDV) is a mixture of four monovalent chimeric live-attenuated vaccines (LAVs), with a backbone of an attenuated DENV-2 which has undergone serial passaging in primary dog kidney (PDK) cells. A large multicenter Phase 3 efficacy study in approximately 20,000 children, spread over several sites in the Philippines, Sri Lanka, Thailand, Brazil, Colombia, Dominican Republic, Nicaragua, and Panama, was initiated last year and is expected to be completed by December, 2021.

Other candidate vaccines are in Phase 1 and 2 trials.

Hepatitis C Virus Vaccine

Development of a Hepatitis C virus (HCV) vaccine is a challenging proposition due to virus diversity, limited models for testing vaccines, and an incomplete understanding of protective immune responses. Two main vaccine strategies are being explored in human trials, targeting either the cellular or humoral immune response.[25] Next-generation vaccines will likely involve a combination of these two strategies. Vaccines targeting the humoral responses, in human trials, are the recombinant E1E2 proteins adjuvanted with MF59 and recombinant E1 adjuvanted with alum.

Vaccines targeting the cellular immune response have used a prime-boost strategy, priming with a viral vectored human adenovirus 6 (Ad6) vaccine encoding certain parts of the HCV genome and boosting with a chimpanzee adenovirus type 3 (ChAd3) vaccine also encoding the same HCV genome. The NIAID vaccine uses the combination of ChAd3/MVA in a prime-boost strategy. None have entered Phase 3 trials.

FUTURE TRENDS IN IMMUNIZATION

With the development and use of successful vaccines against infections such as smallpox, polio, diphtheria, tetanus, and pertussis (DTP), Hib, and the Pneumococcus, focus has now shifted to vaccines against more complex organisms with complex structures and life cycles (malaria parasite, or successful immune evasion strategies (HIV, influenza viruses, TB). The modest efficacy and limitations of the recently introduced dengue vaccine, the limited success obtained with the most promising malaria vaccine RTS,S/AS01, prime boost HIV vaccine regimen and the failure of a new tuberculosis vaccine, all predict the difficult path ahead. However, many novel approaches to the development and delivery of new vaccines are being explored, as has been outlined above. Of the over 260 vaccines in different stages of development, 137 are against infectious diseases, 101 against cancers and the remaining against non-communicable diseases.

Pipeline Vaccines are Vaccines Against

- HIV vaccine
- Chikungunya vaccine
- *Escherichia coli* vaccine
- *Shigella* vaccine
- New oral cholera vaccine
- Malaria vaccine
- *Chlamydia trachomatis*
- Schistosomiasis
- Dengue illness
- New Japanese B encephalitis
- *Neisseria meningitidis*
- Hepatitis C
- Hepatitis E
- *Helicobacter pylori*
- Epstein-Barr virus
- New measles vaccine
- Group A *Streptococcus*
- Group B *Streptococcus*
- Leptospirosis.

VACCINE TIMELINE 1780–2020

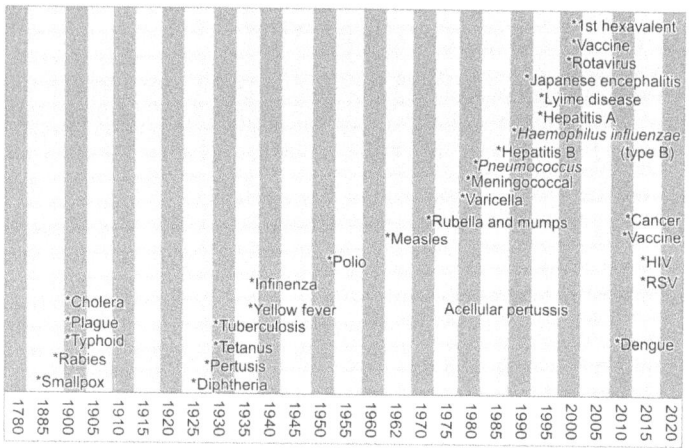

REFERENCES

1. Plotkin SA (Ed). History of Vaccine Development. New York, NY: Springer; 2011.
2. Finco O, Rappuoli R. Designing vaccines for the twenty-first century society. Front. Immunol. 2014;5:12. doi: 10.3389/fimmu.2014.00012.

3. Seib KL, Zhao X, Rappuoli R. Developing vaccines in the era of genomics: a decade of reverse vaccinology. Clin Microbiol Infect. 2012;18(Suppl 5):109-16.
4. Kulp DW, Schief WR. Advances in structure-based vaccine design. Curr Opin Virol. 2013;3(3):322-31. doi: 10.1016/j.coviro.2013.05.010.
5. Six A, Bellier B, Thomas-Vaslin V, Klatzmann D. Systems biology in vaccine design. Microb Biotechnol. 2012;5(2):295-304.
6. Ferraro B, Morrow MP, Hutnick NA, Shin TH, Lucke CE, Weiner DB. Clinical applications of DNA vaccines: current progress. Clin Infect Dis. 2011;53(3):296-302.
7. Ertl HC. Viral vectors as vaccine carriers. Curr Opin Virol. 2016;21:1-8.
8. Ura T, Okuda K, Shimada M. Developments in viral vector-based vaccines. Vaccines (Basel). 2014;2(3):624-41.
9. Mbow ML, De Gregorio E, Valiante NM, Rappuoli R. New adjuvants for human vaccines. Curr Opin Immunol. 2010;22:411-6.
10. Juliana de Souza Apostólico, Victória Alves Santos Lunardelli, Fernanda Caroline Coirada, Silvia Beatriz Boscardin, Daniela Santoro Rosa. Adjuvants: classification, modus Operandi, and Licensing. Journal of Immunology Research. Volume 2016, Article ID 1459394, 16 pages. [online] Available from: http://dx.doi.org/10.1155/2016/1459394.
11. Erna Laere, Anna Pick Kiong Ling, Ying Pei Wong, Rhun Yian Koh, Mohd Azmi Mohd Lila, Sobri Hussein. Plant-based vaccines: production and challenges. Journal of Botany. Volume 2016, Article ID 4928637, 11 pages. [online] Available from: http://dx.doi.org/10.1155/2016/4928637.
12. Larrañeta E, McCrudden MT, Courtenay AJ, et al. Microneedles: a new frontier in nanomedicine delivery. Pharm Res. 2016;33(5):1055-73.
13. Splino M, Patocka J, Prymula R, et al. Anthrax vaccines. Ann Saudi Med. 2005;25(2):143-9.
14. Plotkin SA, Boppana SB. Vaccination against the human cytomegalovirus. Vaccine. 2019;37(50):7437-42.
15. Heath PT. Status of vaccine research and development of vaccines for GBS. Vaccine. 2016;34(26):2876-9.
16. Giersing BK, Modjarrad K, Kaslow DC, Moorthya VS. Report from the World Health Organization's Product Development for Vaccines Advisory Committee (PDVAC) meeting, Geneva, 7-9th Sep 2015. Vaccine. 2016;34(26):2865-9.
17. Burton DR. Advancing an HIV vaccine; advancing vaccinology. Nat Rev Immunol. 2019;19(2):77-8. doi: 10.1038/s41577-018-0103-6.
18. Johnston C, Gottlieb SL, Wald A. Status of vaccine research and development of vaccines for herpes simplex virus. Vaccine. 2016;34(26):2948-52.
19. Global tuberculosis report 2018—WHO. [online] Available at: https://www.who.int/tb/publications/global_report/en/ [Assessed on June, 2019].
20. RTS,S Clinical Trials Partnership. Efficacy and safety of RTS,S/AS01 malaria vaccine with or without a booster dose in infants and children in Africa: final results of a phase 3, individually randomised, controlled trial. Lancet. 2015;386(9988):31-45.

21. Sissoko MS, Healy SA, Katile A, Omaswa F, Zaidi I, Gabriel EE, et al. Safety and efficacy of PfSPZ Vaccine against Plasmodium falciparum via direct venous inoculation in healthy malaria-exposed adults in Mali: a randomised, double-blind phase 1 trial. Lancet Infect Dis. 2017;17(5):498-509.
22. Giersinga BK, Dastgheyb SS, Modjarrad K, Moorthy V. Status of vaccine research and development of vaccines for Staphylococcus aureus. Vaccine. 2016;34:2962-6.
23. Neuzil KM. Progress toward a respiratory syncytial virus vaccine. Clin Vaccine Immunol. 2016;23(3):186-8. doi: 10.1128/CVI.00037-16.
24. Swaminathan S, Khanna N. Dengue vaccine development: Global and Indian scenarios. Int J Infect Dis. 2019;84S:S80-6.
25. Bailey JR, Barnes E, Cox AL. Approaches, progress, and challenges to hepatitis C vaccine development. Gastroenterology. 2019;156:418-30.

Vaccine Preventable Disease Surveillance

Mohit Vohra, Alok Gupta

INTRODUCTION

The French word *'Surveillance'* means watching with attention, suspicion and authority. The best *yard stick* to assess the impact of any immunization program is the vaccine preventable disease (VPD) surveillance. Government of India in collaboration with the World Health Organization (WHO), UNICEF, World Bank launched a single disease national VPD surveillance program to detect the prevalence of poliomyelitis, incidence of new cases and detection of old cases not notified. The program initiated in 1997 is working very well with active participation of private doctors apart from Government and Corporate Hospitals contribute to the success of the program.

TYPES OF VPD SURVEILLANCE

The type of surveillance for a specific disease depends on the attributes of that disease and the immunization program's objectives.

Active surveillance (Accelerated Disease Control) involves visiting health facilities, talking to healthcare providers and reviewing medical records to identify suspected cases of the disease under surveillance. This method is usually used when a disease is targeted for eradication or elimination, when every possible case must be found and investigated. Active surveillance is also used in outbreak investigations.

National passive surveillance involves passive notification through regular reporting of disease data by all facilities that see patients or test specimens. Passive surveillance is the most common method used to detect VPDs, the least expensive, and covers the widest geographical areas; however, it can be difficult to ensure completeness and timeliness of data collection.[1]

ACUTE FLACCID PARALYSIS SURVEILLANCE

Acute flaccid paralysis of any cause (Guillain-Barré syndrome (GBS), transverse myelitis (TM) and traumatic neuritis (TN) apart from other causes like Atonic Cerebral palsy, etc.) being important differential diagnosis for acute poliomyelitis.

The National Polio Surveillance Project Officers should be informed about any case of acute flaccid paralysis (AFP) that the practitioner encounters.

Surveillance systems which are sensitive are essential for polio eradication. They focus on the identification of any residual viruses and are vital for certification of eradication. It is done through these methods:
- Acute flaccid paralysis surveillance
- Environmental sampling
- Special surveillance.

Containment and Certification Process

Effective biocontainment of polioviruses is a fundamental step towards global certification and minimizing the longterm risks associated with poliovirus stocks.

Certification of Wild Poliovirus Eradication and Containment

The primary requirements for certifying a WHO region as free of wild poliovirus are:
- Absence of wild polioviruses for a minimum of 3 years in all countries of the region
- Presence of certification-standard surveillance in all countries, and
- Completion of phase I biocontainment activities for all facility-based wild poliovirus stocks.

Figures 11.1 to 11.13 provide maps and data that depict Global/India prevalence of wild/circulating vaccine-derived polio cases as on September 2016 and the recommendations of the India Experts Advisory Group (IEAG), about the strategies towards polio endgame in India. The important components of the recommendations include switch from tOPV to bOPV and the introduction of single dose of IPV along with third dose of DTwP and the emergency preparedness to contain possible polio spread and precautions to be taken at international borders as well as intensified surveillance network.

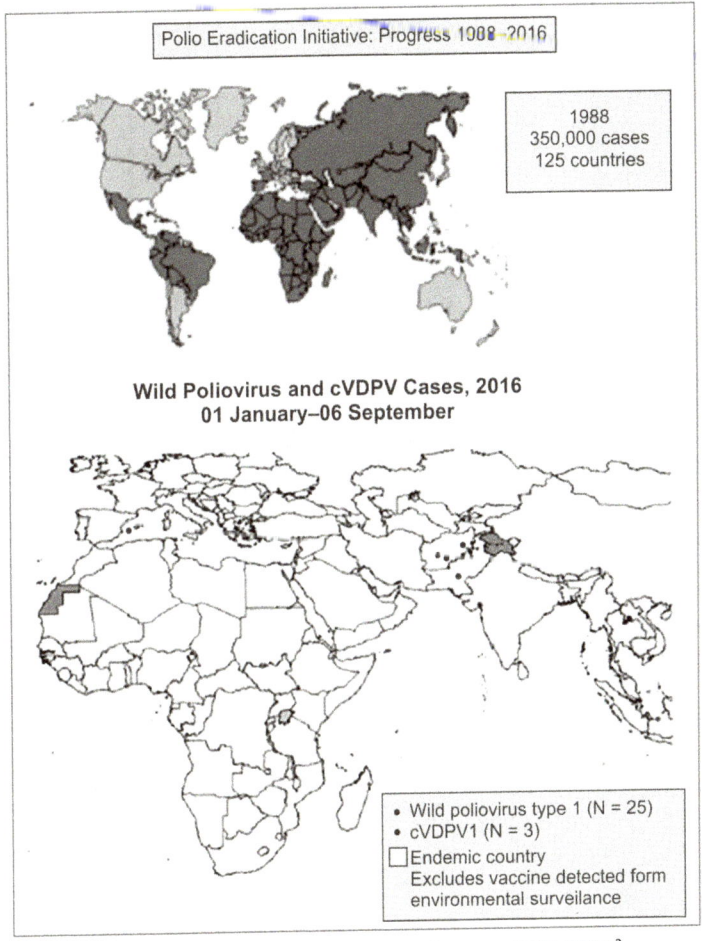

Fig. 11.1: Polio Eradication initiative: Progress 1988–2016.[2]
Source: http://www.who.int/topics/poliomyelitis/en/ (Accessed on Dec 16, 2016).

Country or territory[3]	Wild virus confirmed cases							Onset of most recent type 3	Onset of most recent type 1	Wild virus reported from other sources[2]						Date of most recent virus
	Total					01 Jan–27 Sep[1]				Total						
	2011	2012	2013	2014	2015	2015	2016			2011	2012	2013	2014	2015	2016	
Pakistan	198	58	93	306	54	32	14	18-04-12	27-07-16	136	89	66	127	84	33	20-08-16
Afghanistan	80	37	14	28	20	12	9	11-04-10	11-08-16				17	20		27-12-15
Nigeria	62	122	53	6	0	0	3	10-11-12	06-08-16	1	15	3	1			05-05-14
Somalia	0	0	194	5	0	0	0	NA	11-08-14							
Cameroon	0	0	4	5	0	0	0	15-10-09	09-07-14							
Equatorial Guinea	0	0	0	5	0	0	0	NA	03-05-14							
Iraq	0	0	0	2	0	0	0	NA	07-04-14							
Israel[4]	0	0	0	0	0	0	0	NA	NA			136	14			30-03-14
Syrian Arab Republic	0	0	35	1	0	0	0	NA	21-01-14							
Ethiopia	0	0	9	1	0	0	0	NA	05-01-14							
West Bank and Gaza	0	0	0	0	0	0	0	NA	NA				1			05-01-14
Kenya	1	0	14	0	0	0	0	NA	14-07-13			7				12-10-13
Egypt	0	0	0	0	0	0	0	NA	03-05-04			1				
Niger	5	1	0	0	0	0	0	19-01-11	15-11-12		2					06-12-12
Chad	132	5	0	0	0	0	0	10-03-11	14-06-12							
DRC	93	0	0	0	0	0	0	24-06-09	20-12-11							
CAR	4	0	0	0	0	0	0	09-08-09	08-12-11							
China	21	0	0	0	0	0	0	NA	09-10-11							
Guinea	3	0	0	0	0	0	0	03-08-11	03-11-09							
Côte d'Ivoire	36	0	0	0	0	0	0	24-07-11	06-08-09							

Contd...

Contd...

Vaccine Preventable Disease Surveillance

Country or territory[1]	Wild virus confirmed cases						Onset of most recent type 3	Onset of most recent type 1	Wild virus reported from other sources[2]						Date of most recent virus
	Total				01 Jan–27 Sep[1]				Total						
	2011	2012	2013	2014	2015	2016			2011	2012	2013	2014	2015	2016	
Angola	5	0	0	0	0	0	17-11-08	07-07-11							
Mali	7	0	0	0	0	0	23-06-11	01-05-10							
Congo	1	0	0	0	0	0	NA	22-01-11							
Gabon	1	0	0	0	0	0	NA	15-01-01							
India	1	0	0	0	0	0	22-10-10	13-01-11							10-11-10
Total	650	223	416	359	74	26			137	106	213	160	104	33	
Total wild virus type 1[5]	583	202	416	359	74	26									
Total wild virus type 3	67	21	0	0	0	0									
Tot. in endemic countries	341	217	160	340	74	26									
Tot. in non-end countries	309	6	256	19	0	0									
No. of countries (infected)	16	5	8	9	2	3									
No. of countries (endemic)	4	3	3	3	3[6]	3									

Countries in gray are endemic

[1]Data in WHO-HQ on 28th September 2015 for 2015 data and 27th September 2016 for 2016 data. [2]Wild viruses from environmental samples, contacts and other sources. [3]In March 2014, a serotype 1 wild poliovirus was detected in an environment specimen from Brazil, further investigation indicates this is an isolated event without evidence of circulation. [4]Results are based on L20B positive culture. Prior to reporting week 16, 2014, results were based on a combination of direct qRT-PCR on RNA from concentrated sewage and L20B positive culture. [5]Includes 1 case in 2012 with a mixture of W1W3 virus. [6]As of 27 September 2015, Nigeria no longer classified as endemic. NA—Most recent case had onset prior to 1999.

(Data in WHO-HQ as of 27 September 2016).

Fig. 11.2: Global wild poliovirus (2011–2016).

Source: http://www.who.int/topics/poliomyelitis/en/ (Accessed on Dec 16, 2016).

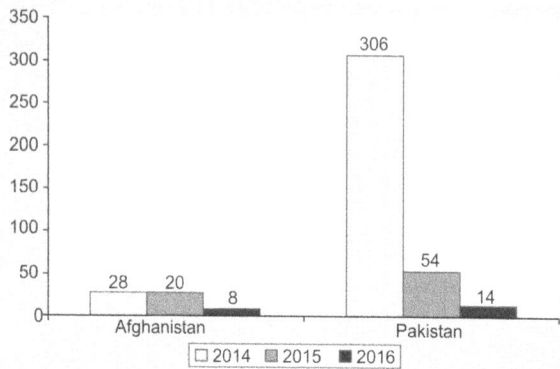

Fig. 11.3: WPV1 cases 2014–2016 of Afghanistan and Pakistan.
Source: http://www.who.int/topics/poliomyelitis/en/ (Accessed on Dec 16, 2016).

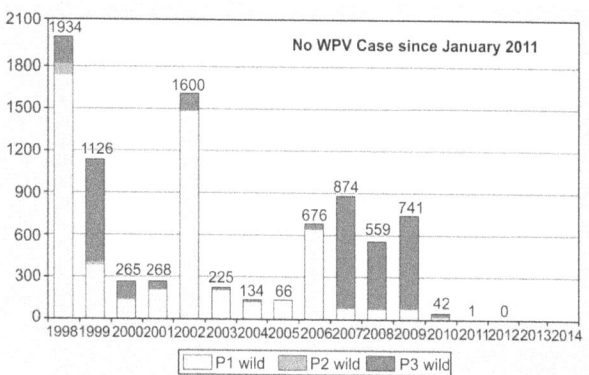

Fig. 11.4: Wild poliovirus cases, India.
Source: http://www.who.int/topics/poliomyelitis/en/ (Accessed on Dec 16, 2016).

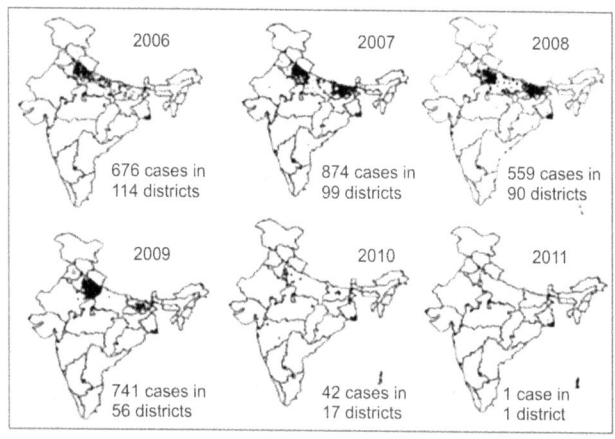

Fig. 11.5: Location of poliovirus, India (2006–2011).
Source: http://www.who.int/topics/poliomyelitis/en/ (Accessed on Dec 16, 2016).

Vaccine Preventable Disease Surveillance

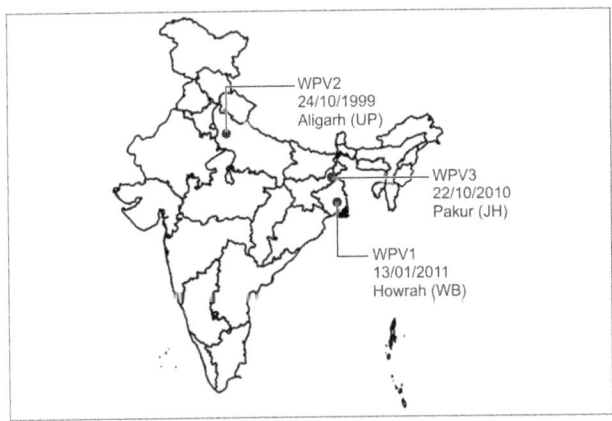

Fig. 11.6: Last wild polio virus cases by serotype, India.
Source: http://www.who.int/topics/poliomyelitis/en/ (Accessed on Dec 16, 2016).

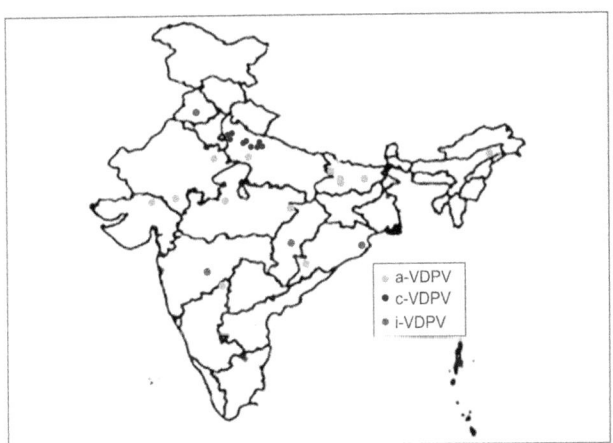

	Type 1		Type 2			Type 3	
Year	a	i	a	c	i	i	Total
2009	1	1	4	15			21
2010			1	3	1		5
2011			4		2	1	7
2012					1		1
2013					3		5
2014			2				3
2015			3		1		2
2016			1		1		1
Total	1	1	15	18	9	1	45

Fig. 11.7: Vaccine-derived poliovirus in AFP cases, India, 2009–2016.
Source: http://www.who.int/topics/poliomyelitis/en/ (Accessed on Dec 16, 2016).

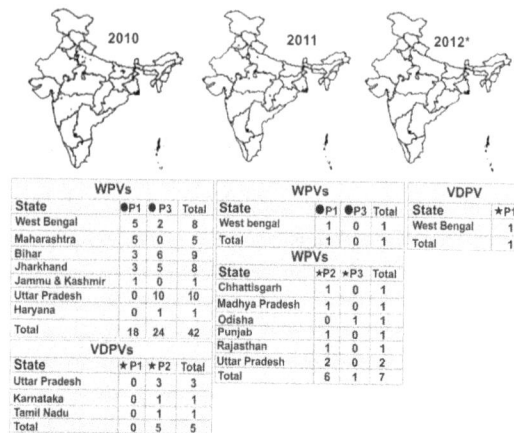

Fig. 11.8: Location of wild poliovirus and VDPV cases by type, India.
Source: http://www.who.int/topics/poliomyelitis/en/ (Accessed on Dec 16, 2016).

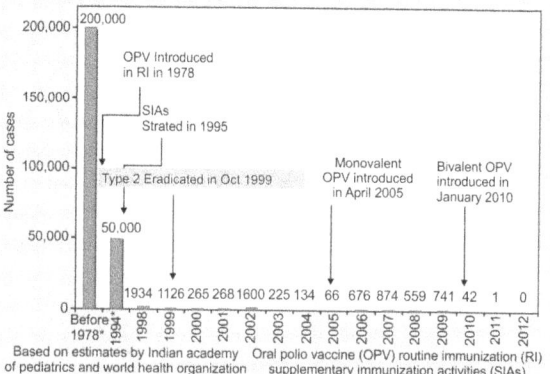

Fig. 11.9: History of polio in India (1978–2012).
Source: http://www.who.int/topics/poliomyelitis/en/ (Accessed on Dec 16, 2016).

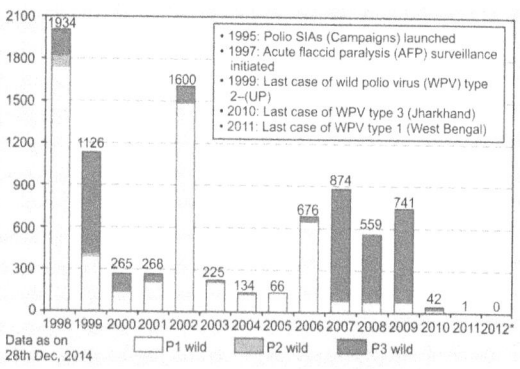

Fig. 11.10: Progress in India—A snapshot.
Source: http://www.who.int/topics/poliomyelitis/en/ (Accessed on Dec 16, 2016).

Vaccine Preventable Disease Surveillance

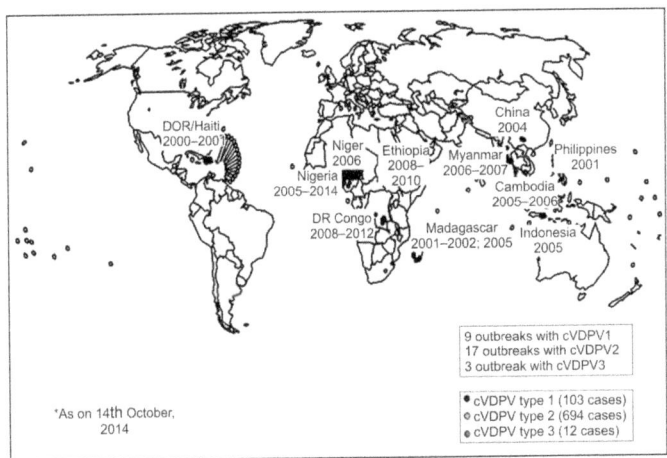

Fig. 11.11: 758 circulating vaccine-derived polio viruses, 2000–2014*
21 countries 24 outbreaks.
Source: http://www.who.int/topics/poliomyelitis/en/ (Accessed on Dec 16, 2016).

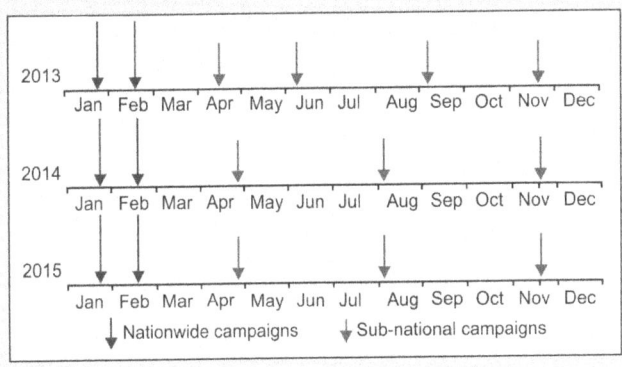

Fig. 11.12: Reaching every child during mass polio vaccination campaigns.
Source: http://www.who.int/topics/poliomyelitis/en/ (Accessed on Dec 16, 2016).

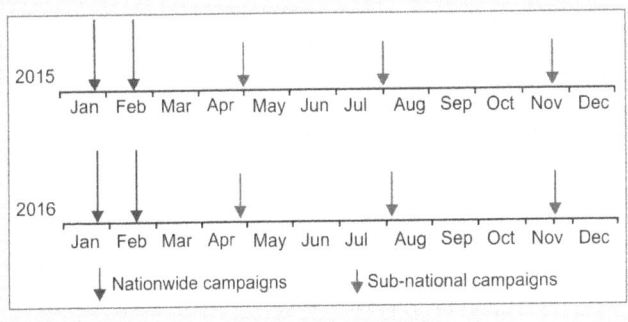

Fig. 11.13: Reaching every child during mass polio vaccination campaigns.
Source: http://www.who.int/topics/poliomyelitis/en/ (Accessed on Dec 16, 2016).

Polio Endgame Strategic Plan (2019–2023)[3]

Polio Endgame Strategy Plan 2019–2023

	Continue	Improve	Innovate	Polio Post-Certification Strategy
Polio Eradication and Endgame Strategic Plan 2013-2018	**Goal 1: Eradication**			**Detect and respond**
1. Detect and interrupt all poliovirus transmission	• Immunization campaigns • Stockpile management • AFP and environmental surveillance	• Community engagement • Accountability and supportive management • Surge capacity • Expand environmental surveillance network • Communication for eradication	• Regional hub for partnership support to endemic country teams • Expanded age groups for SIAs • Engagement of development and humanitarian actors for basic community needs • Rapid response team for outbreaks • Invest in antivirals and new IPV	Promptly detect any poliovirus in a human or in the environment and rapidly respond to prevent transmission
2. Strengthen immunization systems and withdraw oral polio vaccine	**Goal 2: Integration**			
3. Contain poliovirus and certify interruption of transmission	bOPV and IPV delivered as part of national immunization schedules	• Integration of polio surveillance with VPD surveillance • Engagement with CSOs to better reach communities • Joint delivery and/ or enhanced co-ordination between polio and other VPDs SIAs	• Joint accountability framework with Gavi and immunization partners for systematic collaboration • Formalized MoU between WHO emergency programme and GPEI to harmonize outbreak and emergency response • Immunization system recovery/ strengthening included in all outbreak response • *Harmonized data systems: POLIS and WIISE*	
4. Plan polio's legacy				

Contd...

Contd...

Goal 3: Certification and Containment

- Certification processes
- Poliovirus-essential facility certification process
- National containment surveys and inventories

- Containment guidance
- Communications (including VDPV plans)
- Data quality metrics

- Introduce genetically stable vaccine strains to eliminate the need to use and retain live poliovirus

Enabling Areas

- Increase female workers and leaders at all levels
- Promote staff rotations and incentive packages
- Establish focused support to polio transition activities

Protect population
Withdraw the oral live-attenuated polio vaccine (OPV) from use and immunize populations with inactivated polio vaccine (IPV) against possible re-emergence of any poliovirus

Contain polioviruses
Ensure potential sources of poliovirus are properly contained or removed

AFP: acute flaccid paralysis; SIA: supplementary immunization activities; bOPV: bivalent oral polio vaccine; VPD: vaccine-preventable disease; CSO: Civil Society Organization; MoU: Memorandum of Understanding; GPEI: global polio eradication initiative; POLIS: polio information system; WIISE: WHO immunization information system; VDPV: vaccine-derived poliovirus

Source: WHO

Year	Country/ Territory/ Region	AFP cases	Non polio AFP Rate	% Adequate Stool Collection	Pending	Wild poliovirus cases	cVDPV cases	Compatibles	Footnotes
2019	India	32524	10.29	87	3665	0	0	3	

Global Summary

Year	Country/ Territory/ Region	AFP cases	Non polio AFP Rate	% Adequate Stool Collection	Pending	Wild poliovirus cases	cVDPV cases	Compatibles	Footnotes
2019	Global total	82057	5.09	88	9937	96	117	72	

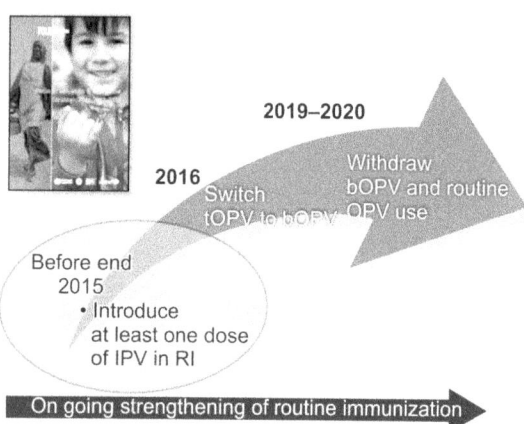

Fig. 11.14: Polio Endgame Strategy.
Source: http://www.who.int/topics/poliomyelitis/en/ (Accessed on Dec 16, 2016).

The Polio Eradication and Endgame Strategic Plan 2013–2018 is a comprehensive, long-term strategy that addresses what is needed to deliver a polio-free world by 2018 **(Fig. 11.14)**.

The plan was developed by the Global Polio Eradication Initiative (GPEI) in consultation with national health authorities, global health initiatives, scientific experts, donors and other stakeholders, in response to a directive of the World Health Assembly. This plan addresses the strategic approach to eradication all remaining polio disease—both due to wild poliovirus and due to circulating vaccine-derived poliovirus, management of polio infection risks in the post eradication era.

The Plan has four objectives:
1. Detection and interruption of all poliovirus transmission
2. Strengthen immunization systems and withdraw oral polio vaccine

3. Contain poliovirus and certify interruption of transmission
4. Plan polio's legacy

The major steps taken to achieve these objectives are:

Introduction of IPV → switch from tOPV to bOPV → OPV cessation.

Under this endgame plan to achieve and sustain a polio-free world, the use of oral polio vaccine (OPV) must eventually be stopped worldwide, starting with OPV that contains type 2 poliovirus (OPV type 2). At least one dose of inactivated polio vaccine (IPV) must be introduced as a risk mitigation measure.

- By end 2015, introduce at least 1 dose of IPV into all routine immunization systems, at least 6 months before the switch from trivalent oral polio vaccine (tOPV) to bivalent oral polio vaccine (bOPV, containing types 1 and 3 poliovirus).
- During 2016, switch from tOPV to bOPV, which does not contain type 2 virus, in routine immunization and polio campaigns.
- Plan for the eventual withdrawal of all OPV.

The tOPV to bOPV switch is necessary because:

- No wild poliovirus type 2 has been recorded over the past years and the risk of paralytic polio disease due to the type 2 component of OPV now outweighs its benefits.
- Since OPV is a live-attenuated vaccine, in rare cases, it can cause paralytic disease in two ways: as vaccine-associated paralytic poliomyelitis (VAPP) or in outbreaks of circulating vaccine-derived poliovirus (cVDPV). The vast majority of cVDPV outbreaks and a substantial proportion of the total VAPP cases are due to the type 2 component of OPV.
- Replacing tOPV with bOPV is key to ensuring the eradication of type 2 poliovirus.
- The switch from tOPV to bOPV will serve as a 'dry run' for the withdrawal of the other types of OPV.

IPV needs to be introduced on an accelerated timeline so that OPV type 2 can be withdrawn.

- IPV should be introduced at least 6 months before the switch from tOPV to bOPV, i.e. by the end of 2015. Countries using only OPV in their routine immunization programs should be prepared for a switch from tOPV to bOPV in 2016.

- The countries at highest risk for cVDPV emergence, wild poliovirus transmission and importations of either will be prioritized for earliest IPV introduction.
- Introducing at least 1 dose of IPV will ensure that a substantial proportion of the population is protected against type 2 polio after OPV type 2 withdrawal. It will also boost immunity to the remaining type 1 and 3 poliovirus serotypes.
- Introducing IPV will boost population immunity against polio and mitigate paralysis risks in the case of outbreaks by 'priming' the population against type 2 poliovirus and ensuring better immune responses to OPV, if needed.
- IPV introduction sets the stage for ending OPV use entirely in 2019–2020.

ENDGAME STRATEGIC PLAN: MILESTONES AND CHALLENGES

Achieving the globally synchronized cessation of routine immunization with type 2 oral poliovirus vaccine (OPV) faces a combination of logistical, communications, vaccine supply and programmatic challenges across a much greater geographic area given that over 125 countries were using trivalent OPV as of end2012. The recent availability (2009), and proven efficacy of bivalent OPV against the remaining wild polioviruses type 1 and 3 serotypes is central to the new endgame strategy **(Fig. 11.15 and Table 11.1)**.[4] While a sufficient and secure international supply of this product will by end2013 be available for an

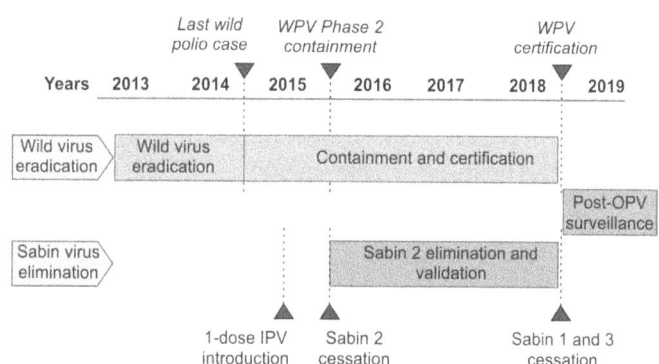

Fig. 11.15: Endgame milestones.
Source: http://www.who.int/topics/poliomyelitis/en/ (Accessed on Dec 16, 2016).

Table 11.1: Key dates of endgame strategic plan.

End-2014	Interruption of residual wild poliovirus transmission
During 2015/16	Synchronized switch of trivalent OPV with bivalent OPV globally
End-2018	Global certification
During 2019	bOPV cessation

Source: http://www.who.int/topics/poliomyelitis/en/ (Accessed on Dec 16, 2016).

eventual tOPV to bOPV switch globally, all countries relying on national tOPV production will need to develop and license a bivalent product.

As per the plan, there has been successful switch from tOPV to bOPV in April 2016 globally.

More complicated will be ensuring the availability of sufficient supplies of inactivated poliovirus vaccine (IPV)—at an affordable price—to allow all countries to introduce at least 1 dose of this product into their routine immunization programs in advance of the tOPVbOPV switch. As daunting are the logistical challenges of synchronously switching all OPV-using countries from tOPV to bOPV, withdrawing the tOPV field stocks, and safely destroying or containing residual vaccine virus. Accompanying this logistical work will be a significant communications effort for the parents whose children will receive the new vaccine schedule, and training of the health workers who must implement it.

OUTCOMES

The Polio Endgame Strategic Plan is designed to produce four major outcomes to complete the eradication and containment of all polioviruses:

1. Population immunity in infected and high-risk areas above the thresholds needed to interrupt circulating polioviruses and prevent reestablishment of imported or emergent viruses.
2. Global poliovirus surveillance and response capacity to rapidly detect and interrupt any emergent poliovirus.
3. Sabin 2 polioviruses removed from routine immunization programs in all OPV-using countries.

Table 11.2: Major activities to achieve the outcome.

Outcome	Major activities
High population immunity	- Routine immunization systems strengthening - National and subnational immunization days - IPV introduction - Community engagement and social - mobilization
Surveillance and response capacity	- Outbreak response and mop-ups - Stockpiles for emergency response - Acute flaccid paralysis surveillance - Environmental surveillance - New diagnostics and special studies
Sabin 2 poliovirus removal	- OPV cessation (type 2)
Poliovirus containment	- Biocontainment of residual polioviruses - Certification of eradication and containment

Source: http://www.who.int/topics/poliomyelitis/en/ (Accessed on Dec 16, 2016).

4. Appropriate biocontainment globally of all wild polioviruses, vaccine-related polioviruses and Sabin strain type 2 poliovirus.

The major activities outlined to achieve these outcomes are listed in **Table 11.2**:

- India has been polio free for more than three years.
- Poliovirus circulation is rapidly declining globally.
- Post-eradication policy issues are becoming more pressing.

Questions Which Arise to HCW?

- Is the emergency preparedness in the country adequate?
- Is poliovirus surveillance in India good enough to rapidly detect poliovirus circulation/importation?
- What additional steps should India take to mitigate the risk of importations?
- What are the next steps to finalize the timing of the IPV dose in the RI schedule in India?
- Are there other operational assessments required to optimize tOPVbOPV switch and IPV introduction?
- Are the proposed research studies sufficient to mitigate risks due to potential gaps in bOPV supply for RI and for IPV supply requirements for post-switch boosting?
- Are the areas that the polio network is currently supporting in routine immunization appropriate?

- Are there any additional areas that the program should be looking at to support broader immunization goals?
- How does the IEAG recommend transitioning the polio human resources and skills to benefit other programs, while maintaining a thorough response capacity for polio?

Maintaining Immunity (Table 11.3)

Recommendations: SIAs
- 2017 (Remainder of the year)
- Continue seroprevalence surveys to inform SIA strategy.

Recommendations: SIA Quality
- It is essential that the current high quality of the pulse polio campaigns be maintained to obtain the maximum possible benefit on population immunity
- State governments should ensure that full attention is paid to maintaining the highest possible quality of SIA rounds.

Detecting and Responding
- Is poliovirus surveillance in India good enough to rapidly detect poliovirus circulation/importation?
  Yes

Table 11.3: Seroprevalence against polioviruses (2007–2012).

	Moradabad, UP (2007)	AFP cases UP (2008–09)	Moradabad, UP (2009)	UP and Bihar (2010)	UP and Bihar (2011)	UP and Bihar (2012)
Age	6–7 months	6–11 months	6–7 months	6–7 months	6–7 months	6–7 months
Type 1	78%	96.5%	99%	98%	98.5%	95.2%
Type 2	56%	33.7%	75%	65%	85%	88.3%
Type 3	69%	42.6%	49%	77%	88.2%	81.8%
Median OPV doses tOPV (SIA +RI)	tOPV (SIA + RI)	2	Data not available	$P = 0.26$		
tOPV				3	3	3
						4
bOPV		0		0	3	5
						3
mOPV1		3		6	2	0
						0
mOPV3		2		0	0	0
						0

Source: http://www.who.int/topics/poliomyelitis/en/ (Accessed on Dec 16, 2016).

Recommendations: Surveillance

- Surveillance and laboratory: Human and financial resources must be ensured to maintain high performance.
- Continue field reviews and act on gaps
  - Rotational basis, particular attention to HR areas
- Conduct review of causes of AFP to identify any causes that may be amenable to intervention.
- Is emergency preparedness adequate?
  Yes

Recommendations: Emergency Response

- Ensure that national and state emergency response plans are undated every year.
- Conduct a simulation exercise '*Tabletop simulation*' at national and state levels at a least once a year to maintain the sharpness of the system.

Certification Process

Recommendations: Certification Process

- Urgently proceed with the inventory of laboratories in India to ensure that certification requirements can be met.
- Fast track the parallel active search process to rapidly identify those laboratories most likely to be holding poliovirus and ensure their status is known.
- Ensure the fast-track process includes all Indian vaccine suppliers and their associated facilities, and any other relevant private sector facilities.
- Given the complexity of this process, consider destroying or securing relevant WPV stocks as the process is implemented, i.e. Phase 2.

Certification of Wild Poliovirus Eradication and Containment

- The primary requirements for certifying a WHO region as free of wild poliovirus are:
  - Absence of wild polioviruses for a minimum of 3 years in all countries of the region,
  - Presence of certification-standard surveillance in all countries, and
  - Completion of phase I biocontainment activities for all facility-based wild poliovirus stocks.

- Reducing risk
- The current border postimmunization scheme is the most significant risk reduction strategy

Recommendations: Reducing Risk of Importation

- Immunization of travelers at border crossing points should continue until there is no longer an epidemiological risk.
- GoI should promote the current WHO polio immunization recommendations for travelers to and from endemic areas.
- The issue of immunization requirements for travelers from endemic areas should be revisited in late 2014 considering IHR discussions.

Preparing for the tOPV/bOPV Switch[5]

Recommendations: IPV Introduction Process

- The ICMR expert group should study the proposal for a routine single IM dose of IPV at the DPT3 contact to facilitate introduction in 2015 in advance of the global tOPV/bOPV switch.
- The ICMR Expert Group should finalize recommendations on the subject—considering the findings of the SAGE Polio Working Group meeting in June.

Recommendations: Mitigating Risk of Vaccine Supply Gaps

- The bOPV licensing study should be initiated immediately with all bOPV products to ensure security of supply and price for switch planning.
- An IPV boosting study should be conducted to compare IM versus ID delivery route to ensure the full range of affordable options are available.

Recommendations: Operational Assessments

- Government of India and partners should carry out a cold chain assessment taking into consideration requirements for all new vaccine introductions including IPV (**Figs. 11.16 and 11.17**).

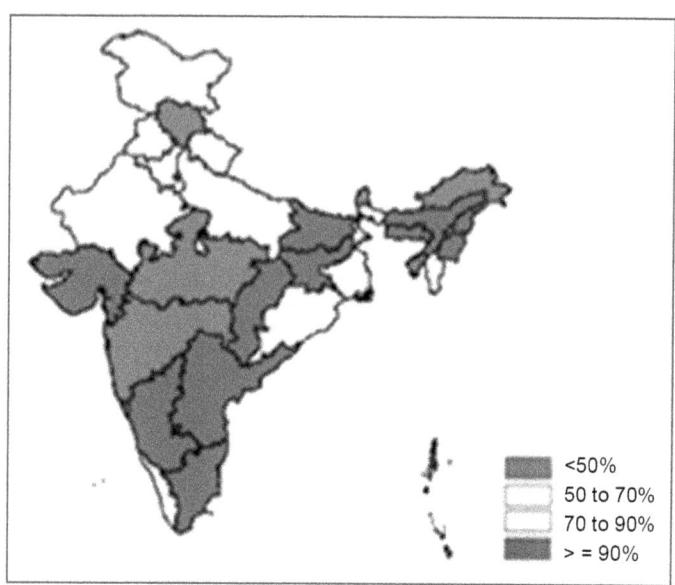

Fig. 11.16: About 66% of ~400,000 high-risk areas included in RI micro-plans during the last 6 months.
Source: http://www.who.int/topics/poliomyelitis/en/ (Accessed on Dec 16, 2016).

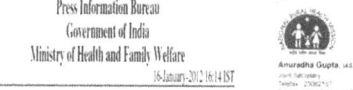

Fig. 11.17: 2012-2013 Year of Intensification of UIP.
Source: http://www.who.int/topics/poliomyelitis/en/ (Accessed on Dec 16, 2016).

Building on Polio

- Are the areas that the polio network is supporting appropriate?
  YES

2012-2013: Year of Intensification of UIP[6]

Recommendations

- The current process is a significant positive development and should be strengthened to ensure that it is effectively carried through.
- A comprehensive review of the impact of polio network support to broader immunization goals, particularly intensifying routine immunization, carried out in Q4 2013 to inform future plans.
- Surveillance for vaccine preventable diseases should be expanded based on the experience and structure of the AFP surveillance system.

Protecting the Investment

Government, partners, and donors must maintain the human, material, and financial infrastructure of polio eradication until the completion of the polio endgame

Recently, the concept has spread from a single disease to multiple disease surveillance entitled *Integrated Disease Surveillance Program.*

The country is having a network of 6 Regional Co-Ordinators (RC) 18 Sub-Regional Coordination (SRC) and 223 Surveillance Medical Officer (SMOs).

Expanded Indian National Rotavirus Surveillance Network[7]

To extend a nationwide rotavirus surveillance network in India, and to generate geographically representative data on rotaviral disease burden and prevalent strains.

Design: Hospital-based surveillance.

Setting: A comprehensive multicenter, multi-state hospital-based surveillance network was established in a phased manner involving 28 hospital sites across 17 states and two union territories in India.

Patients: Cases of acute diarrhea among children below 5 years of age admitted in the participating hospitals.

Results: During the 28-month study period between September 2012 and December 2014, 11898 children were enrolled and stool samples from 10207 children admitted with acute diarrhea were tested; 39.6% were positive for rotavirus. Highest positivity was seen in Tanda (60.4%) and Bhubaneswar (60.4%) followed by Midnapore (59.5%). Rotavirus infection was seen more among children aged below 2 years with highest (46.7%) positivity in the age group of 12–23 months. Cooler months of September–February accounted for most of the rotavirus-associated gastroenteritis, with highest prevalence seen during December–February (56.4%). 64% of rotavirus-infected children had severe to very severe disease. G1P was the predominant rotavirus strain (62.7%) during the surveillance period.

Conclusion: The surveillance data highlights the high rotaviral disease burden in India. The network will continue to be a platform for monitoring the impact of the vaccine.

INTEGRATED DISEASE SURVEILLANCE PROGRAM

Integrated Disease Surveillance Program (IDSP) is intended to be the backbone of public health delivery system in the country. IDSP is being initiated by the Ministry of Health and Family Welfare (MOHFW) with funding from the World Bank (WB). It is expected to provide essential data to monitor progress of ongoing disease control programs and will be able to detect early warning signals of impending outbreaks and help initiate an effective response in a timely manner. Integrating and decentralizing surveillance activity is one of the main components of the program. IDSP is expected to monitor a limited number of conditions based on state perceptions for which public health response is available. The conditions selected initially include important communicable disease. Since more than 70% of the health care is provided by the private sector overall (more in some states and in urban regions)—a strategy for the participation private health providers in the formal and informal sectors is crucial to the success of the program. Currently, there are several fragmented efforts on surveillance by the public health system of the country particularly in polio, leprosy, Tuberculosis (TB) and a few districts covered by NPSP. Except for polio surveillance success of private sector participation in disease surveillance has been limited in the public-sector program.

REPORTING REQUIREMENT OF IDSP[8]

Diseases under Surveillance by Health Providers

Vector-borne disease	1. Malaria
Water-borne disease	2. Acute diarrheal disease (Cholera)
	3. Typhoid
Respiratory diseases vaccine	4. Tuberculosis
Preventable diseases	5. Measles
Diseases under eradication	6. Polio
Other international commitments	7. Plague, Yellow fever
Unusual clinical syndromes (Causing death/hospitalization)	8. Meningoencephalitis/Respiratory distress Hemorrhagic fevers, other undiagnosed conditions
State-specific diseases	9. Dengue
	10. Japanese B encephalitis
	11. Leptospirosis

Method of Surveillance

- *Regular Surveillance:* In IDSP, the private health provides have been designated to be providing sentinel data for disease surveillance. Sentinel surveillance system is likely to be sensitive to changing pattern of diseases and able to report emerging epidemics in the country. Any health provider catering to a relatively large number of cases of the diseases can be considered as a sentinel center. Sentinel center data will not include all cases in the area. However, if one or more sentinel centers have been carefully selected, it will include sufficiently large number of cases for epidemiological analysis. Data from sentinel centers are usefully able to determine trends in the incidence of the reported disease.
- *Participate in Identifying emerging epidemics through Rumor registry:* Rumor registry is being maintained by the PHC/CHC officers and also by the district hospital. The medical officer needs early warning of emerging diseases. It is expected that early warning of emerging diseases will be obtained through information gathered from public, private practitioners both informal and formal types, teachers, panchayat members and ward members. Media and NGOs also can play an important role in surveillance through active participation in rumor registry.

REPORTING FORMAT FOR SENTINEL SITES[9]

I. District code number: *Unique identifier for reporting unit: Patients treated*

II. Suspected diseases/Syndromes	OPD	IPD	Total	Death
	<5 or >5	<5 or >5	<5 or >5	<5 or >5
1. Acute watery diarrhea/cholera		M F T		
2. Fever >7 days/Typhoid		M F T		
3. AFP <in less than 15 years of age/polio		M F T		
4. Fever with rash/Measles		M F T		
5. Fever/Malaria		M F T		
6. Cough >3 weeks/Tuberculosis		M F T		
7. Unusual syndromes causing death or hospital admission		M F T		
8. Fever with bleeding/Dengue		M F T		
9. Fever with altered consciousness or convulsions/JE		M F T		
10. Others specify		M F T		

M: Male, F: Female, T: Total

If no cases are seen '0' will be marked against the corresponding disease and the results submitted to the DSO or MO of PHC/CHC. Each sentinel site will record 1-3 disease conditions by prior agreement but will sent regular weekly report including zero reporting.

PRIVATE SECTOR COLLABORATION IN TUBERCULOSIS CONTROL PROGRAM[10]

National Tuberculosis Control Program (NTCP) in the earlier phase did not have any private sector units participating in the TB program. However, Revised National Tuberculosis Control Program (RNTCP) has envisaged incorporating private sector into the program. Over the last few years, there are a few large hospitals in the private sector who have been included as DOTS centers under RNTCP. A typical example is CMC Hospital Vellore, Tamil Nadu, India. However, it can be said that reporting from most of these centers are very poor and there is no systems in place to monitor their participation.

Quality Control

A manual is available under RNTCP program for TB surveillance. This is available at all district TB centers. This manual is made by central TB division of Ministry of Health and Family Welfare (MOHFW). The manual provides data formats and specifies the method of reporting required from the participating units. No special training program has been carried out for the private sector units participating in the RNTCP since the selected units have already trained personnel.

Method of Recruitment

No specific method has been evolved to integrate private sector in RNTCP. The existing private sector units have come on their own and the government is trying to understand the significance of this to the program. Recently, there has been an emphasis to include private sector units in the program.

Incentives

No incentives are being given to private sector units to participate in DOTS program. Those units which are included in NTCP get their regular supply of TB drugs for the program. Separate guidelines are available for childhood and adult TB cases.

IAP INFECTIOUS DISEASE SURVEILLANCE PROGRAM[11]

For the past 10 years, *IAP Infectious Disease Surveillance Program* of collecting disease surveillance data from members is working successfully. Though the reported case count is just the tip of the iceberg, Members of IAP have been sensitized about the importance of VPD surveillance and the program is picking up gradually. The Government of India has shown interest in collaborating with IAP in strengthening the VPD Surveillance Program, viz. IAP IDsurv.

LEARNING POINTS

- Disease surveillance is an important epidemiological necessity to plan strategies for existing and future control and eradication of VPDs.
- All practitioners should notify the VPDs and other infectious diseases treated by them to the local health authority.
- IAP members can contribute to IAPs IDsurv program by reporting diseases treated by them in office practice.
- All hospitals should report notifiable diseases to the IDSP program. In the reporting form.

REFERENCES

1. https://www.who.int/immunization/monitoring_surveillance/burden/VPDs/en/.
2. American Academy Pediatrics Polio Virus Infections. In: Pickering LK (Ed). 2016 Red Book: Report of the Committee on Infectious Diseases, 30th edn. Elk Grove Village, IL, American Academy of Pediatrics.
3. http://polioeradication.org/wp-content/uploads/2019/06/english-polio-endgame-strategy%20016;56,992-3.
4. http://www.who.int/topics/poliomyelitis/en/ (Accessed on Dec 16, 2016).
5. Immunization Strengthening Project—Training Level Module for Mid-level Managers. Vaccine Preventable Diseases, Vaccines and Surveillance of VPDs II. Govt of India, Ministry of Health and Family Welfare, New Delhi; 2001;47-50.
6. India Experts Advisory Group (IEAG): Recommendations on strategies for Polio Endgame, May, 2013.
7. Mehendale S, Venkatasubramanian S, Girish Kumar CP, Kang G, Gupte MD, Arora R. Expanded Indian National Rotavirus Surveillance Network in the Context of Rotavirus Vaccine Introduction. Indian Pediatr. 2016;53:575-81.
8. Thomas K. Integrated disease surveillance program—private sector collaboration; Lecture Notes IDSP Workshop, Chennai, Oct. 2003.

9. Thacker N, Thacker D. VPD Surveillance; Chapter on Immunization in Frequently Asked Questions. In: Parthasarathy A, Borker A, Gupta A, Dharmapalan D (Eds). Pediatric and Adolescent Practice. Jaypee Brothers Medical Publishers: New Delhi, 2015.
10. Seth V. Revised National Tuberculosis Control Program (RNTCP) including indirectly observed treatment. In: IAP Textbook of Pediatrics, 5th edn. Parthasarathy A, Menon PSN, Nair MKC, P Gupta (Eds). Jaypee Brothers Medical Publishers: New Delhi. 2009.pp.342-9.
11. Vashishtha VM, Thacker N. National Immunization Days—vital component of eradication strategy. In: IAP Textbook of Pediatrics, 6th edn, A Parthasarathy, PSN Menon, MKC Nair, P Gupta (Eds). Jaypee Brothers Medical Publishers: New Delhi, 2015.pp.359-62.

CHAPTER 12

WHO Position Papers on Vaccines in NIP and IAP Schedules

Alok Gupta

WHO POSITION PAPER ON BCG VACCINES: FEBRUARY, 2018

This position paper replaces the 2004 WHO position paper on Bacillus Calmette-Guérin (BCG) vaccine and the 2007 WHO revised BCG vaccination guidelines for infants at risk for human immunodeficiency virus (HIV) infection. It incorporates recent developments in the tuberculosis (TB) field, provides revised guidance on the immunization of children infected with HIV, and re-emphasizes the importance of the birth dose. This position paper also includes recommendations for the prevention of leprosy.

Background

Tuberculosis

The causative agent of TB is the bacterium *Mycobacterium tuberculosis*. In children, TB occurs most commonly in those aged <5 years. While TB typically affects the lungs, it may also affect other sites of the body (extrapulmonary TB). HIV infection, malnutrition, tobacco use, and diabetes are predisposing factors for TB. Multidrug-resistant TB (MDR-TB) is caused when bacteria do not respond to the two most powerful first line anti-TB drugs. Globally, 1.7 billion people are estimated to be infected with *M. tuberculosis* and in 2016, 1.7 million people died from TB, including 400,000 among people infected with HIV.

Leprosy

Leprosy is caused by *Mycobacterium leprae* and mainly affects the skin and peripheral nerves, if it presents with deformities it can result in lifelong disability. Cases tend to occur in clusters and mainly affect adults but can also occur in children. More than 200,000 cases were reported in 2016, including 12,819 new cases with visible deformities.

Buruli Ulcer and Other Nontuberculous Mycobacterial Infections

Buruli ulcer (BU) is caused by *Mycobacterium ulcerans*. In 2016, 1,864 new cases of BU were reported from 11 countries. Other nontuberculous mycobacterial (NTM) infections can cause a wide spectrum of diseases and are treated by combinations of antibiotics.

Bacillus Calmette-Guérin Vaccines

Bacillus Calmette-Guérin is a live-attenuated bacterial vaccine derived from *Mycobacterium bovis*. Several BCG vaccines, based on different strains, are available worldwide. While BCG has demonstrated significant effectiveness, protection has not been consistent against all forms in all age groups. BCG has also shown effectiveness in preventing leprosy (RR from 20–80%) and Buruli ulcer (RR of 50% in Africa region).

WHO Recommendations

Bacillus Calmette-Guérin vaccination is recommended in countries or settings with a high incidence of TB and/or high leprosy burden as well as where BU occurs. A single dose should be given to all healthy neonates at birth. If the vaccine cannot be administered at birth, it should be given at the earliest opportunity thereafter.

Countries with low incidence of TB or leprosy may choose to selectively vaccinate high-risk neonates. Additionally, countries with declining rates of TB are encouraged to evaluate the epidemiology of TB and leprosy and consider a switch to selective risk group vaccination.

The standard dose of BCG vaccine is and intradermal (ID) injection of 0.05 mL of the reconstituted vaccine for infants <1 year, and 0.1 mL for those >1 year. BCG vaccine can be safely co-administered with other routine childhood vaccines including the hepatitis B birth dose. BCG multi-dose vials should be used despite any wastage. Studies have shown minimal or no evidence of any additional benefit of repeat BCG vaccination against TB or leprosy. Therefore, revaccination is not recommended even if the tuberculin skin testing (TST) reaction or result of an IFN-γ release assay (IGRA) is negative.

Vaccination of Older Age Groups, Special Populations, Contraindications, and Precautions

Older age groups: BCG vaccination of unvaccinated, TST-negative or IGRA-negative school children is recommended for those coming from or moving to high incidence/burden settings, as well as older groups at risk through occupational exposure.

Pregnant: As a precaution, BCG vaccination is not recommended during pregnancy.

Immunocompromised and HIV-infected person: BCG vaccination is contraindicated for immunocompromised persons and for patients undergoing immunosuppressive treatment. Infants exposed to immunosuppressive treatment in utero or via breastfeeding should not receive BCG. Children who are HIV-infected should not receive BCG vaccination. However, if HIV-infected individuals, including children, are receiving antiretroviral therapy (ART), are clinically well and immunologically stable they should be vaccinated with BCG.

Neonates born to women of unknown HIV status should be vaccinated. However, neonates with unknown HIV status born to HIV-infected women should be vaccinated if they have no clinical evidence suggestive of HIV infection, regardless of whether the mother is receiving ART. Additionally, neonates with HIV infection should delay BCG vaccination until ART has been started and are immunologically stable.

Neonates born to mothers with pulmonary TB: BCG vaccination is recommended if an infant is asymptomatic, has no immunological evidence of TB, and is HIV-negative.

Further Monitoring and Research Needs

To better understand the safety and effectiveness of BCG vaccination at different ages and in different populations, especially of HIV-infected children including those receiving ART, reporting of TB cases is encouraged. Additionally, further evidence is needed on programmatic strategies of BCG vaccination, such as timeliness of vaccination and wastage.

There is also a need for development of vaccines that provide greater protection than BCG on all forms of TB for all age groups including persons infected with HIV. The development of more effective vaccines against leprosy is also encouraged.

WHO POSITION PAPER ON POLIO VACCINES: MARCH, 2016

Background

This position paper on polio vaccines published in the 25 March, 2016 WHO Weekly Epidemiological Record (Vol. 91, 12), replaces the previous 2014 WHO polio position paper, and summarizes recent developments in the field. It integrates new information related to the addition of a dose of IPV for countries currently using exclusively OPV, in the context of the global switch from trivalent to bivalent OPV.

Poliomyelitis is an acute communicable disease caused by any of three poliovirus serotypes (types 1, 2 or 3). In the pre-vaccine era when poliovirus was the leading cause of permanent disability in children, almost all children became infected by polioviruses, with on average 1 in 200 susceptible individuals developing paralytic poliomyelitis.

Two types of poliovirus vaccines are available, inactivated poliovirus vaccine (IPV) introduced in 1955 and the live-attenuated oral poliovirus vaccine (OPV) introduced in the early 1960s. Worldwide, sustained use of polio vaccines since 1988 has led to a precipitous drop in the global incidence of poliomyelitis by >99% and the number of countries with endemic polio from 125 to just 2 in 2015 (Afghanistan and Pakistan). Globally, the last case of poliomyelitis caused by naturally circulating wild-strain polio viruses type 2 (WPV2) occurred in India in 1999. No case due to wild-strain polio viruses type 3 (WPV3) has been detected since 10 November, 2012. In 2015, 73 polio cases were reported, all due to WPV1, which represents the lowest number for any calendar year on record.

The effectiveness of OPV in controlling poliomyelitis and eliminating the circulation of wild polioviruses (WPVs) is amply demonstrated by the sharp decline in the number of poliomyelitis cases following the introduction of OPV in both industrialized and developing countries. The only rare serious adverse events associated with OPV are the occurrence of vaccine-associated paralytic poliomyelitis (VAPP) and the emergence of vaccine-derived polioviruses (VDPVs). The eradication of indigenous WPV2 in 1999, coupled with the continuing emergence of neurovirulent circulating type 2 vaccine-derived polioviruses (cVDPV2s) as well as vaccine-associated paralytic poliomyelitis

(VAPP), led to the recommendation that there should be coordinated global cessation of use of the type 2 component of OPV and a switch from tOPV to bOPV.

WHO Position

In the current position paper, WHO recommends that all children worldwide should be fully vaccinated against polio, and every country should seek to achieve and maintain high levels of coverage with polio vaccine in support of the global commitment to eradicate polio.

WHO no longer recommends an OPV-only vaccination schedule. For all countries currently using OPV only, at least one dose of IPV should be added to the schedule. In polio-endemic countries and in countries at high risk for importation and subsequent spread, WHO recommends a bOPV birth dose (a zero dose) followed by a primary series of three bOPV doses and at least one IPV dose.

The primary series consisting of three bOPV doses plus one IPV dose can be initiated from the age of 6 weeks with a minimum interval of 4 weeks between the bOPV doses. If one dose of IPV is used, it should be given from 14 weeks of age (when maternal antibodies have diminished, and immunogenicity is significantly higher) and can be co-administered with a bOPV dose. The primary series can administered according to the regular schedules of national immunization programs, for example at 6, 10, and 14 weeks (bOPV1, bOPV2, bOPV3+IPV), or at 2, 4, and 6 months (bOPV1, bOPV2+IPV, bOPV3 or bOPV1, bOPV2, bOPV3+IPV). Both OPV and IPV may be co-administered with other infant vaccines.

For infants starting the routine immunization schedule late (age >3 months) the IPV dose should be administered at the first immunization contact along with bOPV and the other routinely recommended vaccines. In countries with high vaccination coverage (e.g. 90–95%) and low importation risk (neighboring countries and major population movement all having similarly high coverage) an IPV-bOPV sequential schedule can be used when VAPP is a significant concern.

Where a sequential IPV-bOPV schedule is used, the initial administration of one or two doses of IPV should be followed by ≥2 doses of bOPV to ensure both enough levels of protection in the intestinal mucosa and a decrease in the burden of VAPP.

For sequential IPV–bOPV schedules, WHO recommends that IPV be given at 2 months of age (e.g. a 3-dose IPV–bOPV–bOPV schedule), or at 2 months and 3–4 months of age (e.g. a 4-dose IPV–IPV–bOPV–bOPV schedule) followed by at least two doses of bOPV.

An IPV-only schedule may be considered in countries with both sustained high immunization coverage and the lowest risk of both WPV importation and transmission. A primary series of three doses of IPV should be administered beginning at 2 months of age. If the primary series begins earlier (e.g. with a 6, 10, and 14-week schedule) then a booster dose should be given after an interval of ≥6 months (for a 4-dose schedule).

To mitigate the risk of undetected transmission, WHO recommends that endemic countries and countries with a high risk of WPV importation should not switch to an IPV-only or a sequential IPV-bOPV schedule at this time. The 3 bOPV+1 IPV schedule as currently recommended should be adopted and supplemental immunization activities should continue to support intensive efforts to eliminate poliovirus transmission. A sequential IPV-bOPV schedule or IPV-only schedule can be considered in order to minimize the risk of VAPP, but only after a thorough review of local epidemiology.

Polio vaccine (IPV or bOPV) may be administered safely to asymptomatic HIV-infected infants. HIV testing is not a prerequisite for vaccination. bOPV is contraindicated in severely immunocompromised patients. These populations can safely receive IPV. Before traveling abroad, persons residing in countries with active transmission of a wild or vaccine-derived poliovirus should have completed a full course of polio vaccination in compliance with the national schedule, and received one dose of IPV or bOPV within 4 weeks to 12 months of travel, in order to boost intestinal mucosal immunity and reduce the risk of poliovirus shedding. Travelers to infected areas should be vaccinated according to their national schedules.

All healthcare workers worldwide should have completed a full course of primary vaccination against poliomyelitis.

WHO POSITION PAPER ON HEPATITIS B VACCINES: JULY, 2017

This position paper, published in July 2017, replaces the corresponding WHO position paper on hepatitis B vaccines published in the Weekly Epidemiological Record in 2009. In particular, the recommendations stress the importance of birth-dose vaccination for all infants as the most effective intervention for preventing hepatitis B virus (HBV)-associated disease worldwide. The recommendations also address target groups and appropriate schedules for vaccination, and the paper provides updated information on hepatitis B vaccines and their storage, transport, and deployment.

Background

Hepatitis B virus is transmitted by exposure of mucosal membranes or non-intact skin to infected blood or other specific body fluids (saliva, semen, and vaginal fluid). In 2015, the global prevalence of HBV infection was estimated at 3.5%, with about 257 million persons living with chronic HBV infection. An estimated 887,220 persons died due to HBV infection—337,454 due to hepatocellular carcinoma, 462,690 due to cirrhosis, and 87,076 due to acute hepatitis. A substantial burden of chronic HBV infection persists because birth-dose coverage is still low, estimated at 39% globally. Most of this burden results from infections acquired in infancy through perinatal or early childhood exposure, as infection acquired at an early age is more likely to become chronic than infection acquired later in life.

Vaccines

Hepatitis B vaccines are available as monovalent formulations and in combination with other vaccines, including diphtheria-tetanus–pertussis (DTP), *Haemophilus influenzae* type b (Hib), and inactivated poliovirus (IPV). Yeast-derived recombinant vaccines are the most widely used. Hepatitis B vaccines are very effective, as evidenced by the dramatic decrease in the incidence of hepatocellular carcinoma (HCC, 60.1%), mortality due to fulminant hepatic failure (76.3%), and mortality due to chronic liver diseases (92.0%) in Taiwan over the decades since vaccine introduction. A study in Alaska estimated that approximately 90% of vaccinees remained protected for at least 30 years; however, additional longer-term studies should be conducted to explore lifelong vaccine effectiveness and the need for booster doses in different subgroups of the population. Additionally, the Global Advisory Committee on Vaccine Safety (GACVS) has confirmed the excellent safety profile of the hepatitis B vaccine. It is also cost-effective, and the triple elimination strategy for mother-to-child transmission of HIV, hepatitis B and syphilis, in particular, increases the cost-effectiveness of hepatitis B vaccination.

WHO Position

Hepatitis B vaccination is recommended for all children worldwide, and all national programs should include a monovalent hepatitis B vaccine birth dose, ideally within 24 hours. Although effectiveness declines progressively in the days after birth, after 7 days, a late birth dose can still be effective in preventing horizontal transmission and therefore remains beneficial. For this reason, WHO recommends that all infants receive the late birth dose during the first contact with healthcare providers at any time up to the time of the next dose of the primary schedule.

The available hepatitis B vaccines may be used interchangeably within immunization programs. However, allergy to yeast is considered a contraindication to immunization with yeast-produced hepatitis B vaccine. Hepatitis B vaccines may be co-administered at different anatomical sites with other vaccines—in particular, monovalent hepatitis B vaccine can be co-administered with OPV and BCG at birth.

Either (i) a 3-dose schedule of hepatitis B vaccine, with the first dose (monovalent) being given at birth and the second and third (monovalent or as part of a combined vaccine) given at the same time as the first and third doses of DTP-containing vaccine; or (ii) four doses, where a monovalent birth dose is followed by three (monovalent or combined vaccine) doses, usually given with other routine infant vaccines is appropriate. The interval between doses should be at least 4 weeks. There is no evidence to support the need for a booster dose. For catch-up vaccination, priority should be given to younger age groups since the risk for chronic infection is the highest in these cohorts. Catch-up vaccination is a time limited opportunity for prevention and should be considered based on the available resources and priority.

Vaccination of groups at highest risk of acquiring HBV infection is recommended. These include patients who frequently require blood or blood products, dialysis patients, diabetes patients, recipients of solid organ transplantation, persons with chronic liver disease including those with hepatitis C, persons with HIV infection, persons interned in prisons, persons who use injecting drugs, household and sexual contacts of persons with chronic HBV infection, men who have sex with men, persons with multiple sexual partners, as well as healthcare workers and others who may be exposed to blood, blood products or other potentially infectious body fluids during their work. To obtain optimal immune responses to vaccination, it is essential that HIV-positive individuals are vaccinated as early as possible in the course of the HIV infection. In immunocompromised individuals, including patients with chronic renal failure, chronic liver disease, celiac disease, and diabetes, the immune response following vaccination is often reduced. Hepatitis B vaccine can be administered safely to pregnant and lactating women. A birth dose of hepatitis B vaccine can be given to low birth weight and premature infants. For these infants, the birth dose should not count as part of the primary 3-dose series; the three doses of the standard primary series should be given according to the national vaccination schedule.

Reporting and monitoring systems should be strengthened to improve the quality of data on the birth dose. To monitor accurately the delivery of doses given within 24 hours of birth, these doses should be recorded as a "timely birth dose" of hepatitis B vaccine to differentiate them from birth doses given later ("late birth dose"). Serological surveys of HBV surface antigen (HBsAg) prevalence, representative of the target population, will serve as the primary tool to measure the impact of vaccination and verify achievement of the hepatitis B control goals.

WHO POSITION PAPER ON DIPHTHERIA VACCINES: AUGUST, 2017

This position paper, published in August, 2017, replaces the corresponding WHO position paper on diphtheria vaccines published in the Weekly Epidemiological Record in 2006. In particular, it provides revised recommendations on the optimal number of doses and timing of diphtheria vaccination, as well as guidance on the alignment of vaccination schedules for different antigens included in routine childhood immunization programs, considering the widespread use of combination vaccines.

Background

Throughout history, diphtheria has been one of the most feared infectious diseases globally causing devastating epidemics with high case-fatality rates, mainly affecting children. Transmission of *Corynebacterium diphtheria* occurs from person-to-person through droplets and close physical contact. Infection can cause respiratory or cutaneous diphtheria. Morbidity and mortality are mediated by the diphtheria toxin. Respiratory diphtheria usually occurs after an incubation period of 2–5 days. The onset is usually relatively slow and characterized by mild fever and an exudative pharyngitis initially with progression of symptoms over 2–3 days. In classic cases, the exudate organizes into a pseudomembrane that gradually forms in the nose, pharynx, tonsils, or larynx. The pseudomembrane may extend into the nasal cavity and the larynx causing obstruction of the airways, which is a medical emergency that often requires tracheotomy. In rare cases, systemic diphtheria can occur damaging heart, kidneys, and/or peripheral nerves. Diphtheria antitoxin (DAT), if administered in time, is highly effective and the gold standard for diphtheria treatment. However, global access to DAT is limited as most manufacturers have ceased production.

Vaccines

In the 1940s, diphtheria toxoid, tetanus toxoid and pertussis antigens were combined in the diphtheria-tetanus-pertussis (DTP) vaccine used widely for childhood immunization throughout the world. DTP may also be combined with additional vaccine antigens, such as hepatitis B surface antigen (HBsAg) and Hib conjugates as pentavalent vaccines, and with inactivated polio vaccine (IPV) as hexavalent vaccines. Tetanus diphtheria (Td, low-dose diphtheria toxoid) formulations and tetanus-diphtheria-acellular pertussis (Tdap) formulations are licensed for use from 5 years of age and 3 years of age, respectively. After the 3-dose primary series of DTP-containing vaccine, 94–100% of children have protective anti-diphtheria antibody levels >0.01 IU/mL, but booster doses are needed to ensure continuing protection. The effectiveness of the vaccine can be seen in outbreak settings—most recent data on vaccine effectiveness stem from the epidemic in the 1990s in countries of the former Soviet Union. Case-control studies showed that three or more doses of diphtheria toxoid induced 95.5% (95% CI: 92.1-97.4%) protective effectiveness among children aged <15 years. Protection increased to 98.4% (95% CI: 96.5-99.3%) after five or more doses of this vaccine. Diphtheria toxoid is one of the safest vaccines available.

WHO Position

All children worldwide should be immunized against diphtheria. Every country should seek to achieve timely vaccination with a complete primary series plus booster doses. A primary series of three doses of diphtheria toxoid-containing vaccine is recommended, with the first dose administered as early as 6 weeks of age. Subsequent doses should be given with an interval of at least 4 weeks between doses. The third dose of the primary series should be completed by 6 months of age if possible. The diphtheria booster doses should be given in combination with tetanus toxoid using the same schedule, i.e. at 12-23 months of age, 4-7 years of age, and 9-15 years of age, using age-appropriate vaccine formulations.

Opportunities should be taken to provide or complete the 3-dose diphtheria toxoid-containing vaccine series for children aged ≥1 year, adolescents and adults who were not vaccinated, or incompletely vaccinated, during infancy. For previously unimmunized children aged 1-7 years, the recommended primary schedule is three doses with a minimum interval of 4 weeks between the first and the second dose, and an interval of at least 6 months between the second and third dose, using DTP-containing vaccine. Using Td or Tdap combination vaccine, the recommended schedule for primary immunization of older children (>7 years), adolescents and adults is three doses with a minimum interval of 4 weeks between the first and the second dose, and an interval of at least 6 months between the second and a third dose. Two subsequent booster doses using Td or Tdap combination vaccines are needed with an interval of at least 1 year between doses. To further promote immunity against diphtheria, the use of Td rather than tetanus toxoid is recommended during pregnancy to protect against maternal and neonatal tetanus in the context of prenatal care, and when tetanus prophylaxis is needed following injuries.

As diphtheria toxoid is almost exclusively available in fixed combinations with other antigens, immunization programs will need to harmonize immunization schedules between diphtheria, tetanus and pertussis. Diphtheria toxoid-containing vaccine can also be co-administered with other childhood and adolescence vaccines.

Vaccination during pregnancy is not necessary to protect neonatal infants against diphtheria, but diphtheria-containing vaccines combined with pertussis and tetanus can be used to protect young infants against tetanus and pertussis. Diphtheria toxoid-containing vaccines can be used in immunocompromised persons including HIV-infected individuals. All healthcare workers should up to date with immunization as recommended in their national immunization schedules. Travelers are generally not at special risk of diphtheria unless they travel to an endemic country or outbreak setting. They should be immunized as recommended in their national immunization schedules. Efficient national surveillance and reporting systems, with district-level data analysis, are essential in all countries.

Further studies, including serosurveys, are required to generate information on the duration of protection and the possible need for booster doses in older age groups.

WHO POSITION PAPER ON PERTUSSIS VACCINES: SEPTEMBER, 2015

Background

The 2015 updated position paper on pertussis vaccines replaces the 2010,pertussis position paper. The main revisions in this position paper concern the guidance on the choice of pertussis vaccine—whole-cell pertussis (wP) or acellular pertussis (aP) vaccine—reflecting the updated guidance published in 2014, and incorporating recent evidence on the use of additional strategies, particularly vaccination during pregnancy, for prevention of early infant mortality.

Pertussis (whooping cough) is an important cause of death in infants worldwide and continues to be a public health concern despite high vaccination coverage. In 2013, according to WHO estimates, pertussis was still causing around 63,000 deaths in children aged <5 years. Two types of pertussis vaccines are available—wP vaccines and aP vaccines. The wP vaccines were introduced widely in industrialized countries in mid-20th century. Starting in the 80s, many high-income countries have replaced wP with aP vaccines, as a means of decreasing the reactogenicity of the vaccine.

Studies to date indicate that aP vaccines are more effective than low-efficacy wP vaccines (wP vaccines shown to be suboptimal are no longer in use) but may be less effective than the highest-efficacy wP vaccines.

Recent modeling studies as well as data from a baboon model of pertussis suggest faster waning of protection with aP primary series and limited impact on infection and transmission. Although the reasons for the resurgence of pertussis in several countries were found to be complex and varied by country, the shorter duration of protection and probable lower impact of aP vaccines on infection and transmission are likely to play critical roles.

WHO Position

The main aim of pertussis vaccination is to reduce the risk of severe pertussis in infants and young children. All children worldwide, including HIV-positive individuals, should be immunized against pertussis. Every country should seek to achieve early and timely vaccination and maintain high coverage (≥90%) at all levels (national and subnational).

Protection can be obtained after a primary series of vaccination with either wP or aP vaccine. Although local and systemic reactogenicity are more commonly associated with wP-containing vaccines, both vaccines have excellent safety records.

A switch from wP to aP vaccines for the primary schedule should only be considered if additional periodic booster or maternal immunization can be assured and sustained. National programs currently administering wP vaccination should continue to use wP vaccines for primary vaccination series. National programs currently using aP vaccine may continue using this vaccine but should consider the need for additional booster doses and additional strategies such as maternal immunization in case of resurgence of pertussis.

The following vaccine dosing schedules and ages of administration are recommended:

- WHO recommends a 3-dose primary series, with the first dose administered as early as 6weeks subsequent doses should be given 4–8 weeks apart, at age 10–14 weeks and 14–18weeks, last dose of the recommended primary series should ideally be completed by 6months.
- For those who have not completed the primary schedule, vaccine may be given later than 6 months of age, at any age and at the earliest opportunity.
- National programs using alternate primary vaccination schedules with adequate surveillance should continue using these schedules and continue to monitor disease trends.

This schedule should provide protection for at least 6 years for countries using wP vaccine. For countries using aP vaccine, protection may decline appreciably before 6 years of age. Only aP-containing vaccines should be used for vaccination of persons aged ≥7 years.

Although a booster dose in adolescence has been shown to decrease disease in adolescents, this is not generally recommended as a means of controlling disease in infants. Introduction of adolescent and/or adult boosters should only be done after assessment of local epidemiology. When a country implements a program for adults, vaccination of healthcare workers should be prioritized, especially those with direct contact with pregnant mothers and infant patients.

Vaccination of pregnant women is likely to be the most cost-effective additional strategy for preventing disease in infants too young to be vaccinated and appears to be more effective and favorable than cocooning. National programs may therefore consider the vaccination of pregnant women with one dose of Tdap in the 2nd or 3rd trimester and at least 15 days before the end of pregnancy were despite high infant coverage there would still be some infant mortality.

Data regarding simultaneous administration of DTaP or DTwP containing vaccines with other childhood vaccines indicate no interference with the response to any other antigens. When two injections are given concomitantly, they can be given in different limbs.

There is an urgent need to improve surveillance and assessment of disease burden particularly in low- and middle-income countries and to assess the impact of infant immunization, with particular focus on fatalities in infants <1 year of age and on hospital surveillance.

WHO POSITION PAPER ON TETANUS VACCINES: FEBRUARY, 2017

Background

This position paper replaces the previous 2006 WHO position paper on tetanus toxoid (TT) vaccines. It incorporates recent developments in the field of tetanus prevention and provides revised guidance on the optimal timing of recommended tetanus vaccine booster doses.

Tetanus is an acute infectious disease caused by toxigenic strains of the bacterium *Clostridium tetani*. The spores of *C. tetani* are present in the environment irrespective of geographical location; they enter the body through contaminated skin wounds or tissue injuries including puncture wounds. The disease may occur at any age and case-fatality rates are high even where intensive care is available. Most reported tetanus cases are birth-associated, occurring in low income countries among insufficiently vaccinated mothers and their newborn infants, following unhygienic deliveries and abortions and poor postnatal hygiene, and cord care practices.

Tetanus toxoid vaccine was first produced in 1924 and used extensively for the first time among soldiers during World War II. Since then, immunization programs using TT-containing vaccines (TTCVs) have been highly successful in preventing maternal and neonatal tetanus (MNT) as well as injury-associated tetanus.

The disease remains an important public health problem in many parts of the world where immunization programs are suboptimal, particularly in the least developed districts of low-income countries.

WHO Position

The aims of tetanus vaccination are—(1) to achieve global elimination of MNT and (2) to ensure lifelong protection against tetanus in all people by attaining and sustaining high coverage of six doses (three primary plus three booster doses) of

TTCV through routine childhood immunization schedules. All children worldwide should be immunized against tetanus.

WHO recommends a 3-dose primary series, with the first dose of TTCV administered as early as 6 weeks of age. Subsequent doses should be given with a minimum interval of 4 weeks between doses. The third dose of the primary series should ideally be completed by 6 months of age.

WHO recommends that immunization programs ensure that three TTCV booster doses are provided. These should be given at: 12–23 months of age; 4–7 years of age; and 9–15 years of age. Ideally, there should be at least 4 years between booster doses.

Opportunistic catch-up for adolescents and adults could include the delivery of TTCV with other vaccination campaigns such as HPV vaccination for adolescent girls, during voluntary medical male circumcision services for adolescent and adult males or during routine entry into military services.

Pregnant women and their newborn infants are protected from birth-associated tetanus if the mother received six doses (documented by card, immunization registry and/or history) before the time of reproductive age. Vaccination history should be verified in order to determine whether a dose of TTCV is needed in the current pregnancy.

In countries where MNT remains a public health problem, pregnant women for whom reliable information on previous tetanus vaccinations is not available should receive at least two doses of TTCV, preferably Td, with an interval of at least 4 weeks between doses and the second dose at least 2 weeks before the birth. To ensure protection for a minimum of 5 years, a third dose should be given at least 6 months later. A fourth and fifth dose should be given at intervals of at least 1 year, or in subsequent pregnancies, in order to ensure lifelong protection.

Pregnant women who have received only three doses of TTCV during childhood without booster doses should receive two doses of TTCV at the earliest opportunity during pregnancy with a minimal interval of 4 weeks between doses and the second dose at least 2 weeks before giving birth. To provide lifelong protection, a sixth dose would be needed at least 1 year after the fifth dose.

Women who received four TTCV doses during childhood or pre-adulthood need only one booster dose, which should be given at the first opportunity. To provide lifelong protection, a sixth dose would be needed at least 1 year after the fifth dose.

In countries that have not achieved Maternal and Neonatal Tetanus Elimination (MNTE) status (<1 neonatal tetanus case per 1,000 live births in every district), the "high-risk" approach should be part of the elimination strategy. This approach targets all women of reproductive age in high-risk districts and consists of three campaign-style vaccination rounds to provide three doses of TTCV, irrespective of previous vaccination status, with an interval of at least 4 weeks between doses one and two, and at least 6 months between doses two and three. Ensuring clean delivery and cord care practices are important complementary activities to prevent maternal and neonatal tetanus.

WHO POSITION PAPER ON *HAEMOPHILUS INFLUENZAE* TYPE B VACCINATION: JULY, 2013

Haemophilus influenzae type b (Hib) is a vaccine preventable cause of death and serious disease(meningitis and pneumonia) in infants and young children.

In the year 2000, before widespread introduction of Hib vaccine in resource-poor countries, Hib was responsible for at least 8.13 million cases of serious disease in children aged 1-59 months(uncertainty range 7.33-13.2 million cases) and 371,000 deaths (uncertainty range 247,000-527,000). By 2008, when 136 WHO Member States had introduced the vaccine, it is estimated that Hib caused 203,000 deaths in children aged <60 months (uncertainty range 136,000-281,000).

Hib bacteria are carried in the human nasopharynx from where they can be transmitted to other humans via droplets from nasopharyngeal secretions. Only a very small proportion of those who harbour Hib will develop clinical disease; however, those who carry Hib in the nasopharynx are important disseminators of the organism. Vaccination remains the only effective means of preventing Hib disease and is becoming increasingly important as Hib antibiotic resistance grows.

In view of their demonstrated safety and efficacy, *WHO recommends the inclusion of* conjugate Hib vaccines in all infant immunization programs. The use of Hib vaccines should be part of a comprehensive strategy to control pneumonia including exclusive breastfeeding for6months, handwashing with soap, improved water supply and sanitation, reduction of household air pollution, and improved case management at community and health facility levels.

Recommended Schedule

WHO recommends that any one of the following Hib immunization schedules may be followed:
- Three primary doses without a booster (3p);
- Two primary doses plus a booster (2p+1);
- Three primary doses with a booster (3p+1).

In countries where the peak burden of severe Hib disease occurs in young infants, providing three doses of vaccine early in life may confer a greater benefit.

Booster Dose

In some settings (e.g. where the greatest disease morbidity and mortality occur later, or where rate reductions of disease are not fully sustained after the routine use of Hib vaccine), it might be advantageous to give a booster dose by following either a 2p+1 or 3p+1 schedule.

Age at First Dose

Because serious Hib disease occurs most commonly in children aged between 4 months and 18 months, immunization should start from 6 weeks of age, or as early as possible thereafter.

Interval between Doses

The interval between doses should be at least 4 weeks if three primary doses are given, and at least 8 weeks if two primary doses are given. Booster doses should be administered at least 6months after completion of the primary series.

Interrupted Schedule/Late Commencement

If the schedule has been interrupted, vaccination should be resumed without repeating the previous dose. Children who start vaccination late, but are aged under 12 months, should complete the vaccination schedule (e.g. have three primary doses or two primary doses plus a booster). When a first dose is given to a child older than 12 months of age, only one dose is recommended. Hib vaccine is not required for healthy children after 5 years of age.

Contraindications/Precautions

The Hib conjugate vaccine is contraindicated in people with known allergies to any component of the vaccine. There are no other known contraindications or precautions.

Surveillance

Continuous high-quality surveillance for Hib disease is needed to monitor the impact and changes in disease epidemiology over time. Surveillance should cover not only the age group targeted for immunization but also older age groups in order to document the impact of vaccination on age patterns of disease and identify the need for, and timing of, booster doses.

Managing Resurgence

Some countries have observed increases in disease incidence several years after vaccine introduction, but these increases have been very small relative to the overall Hib disease reductions following vaccine introduction. Increases in the incidence of Hib cases should be investigated promptly and include documentation of the age, Hib vaccination status, time since last Hib vaccine dose, and HIV status of individuals infected.

WHO POSITION PAPER ON PNEUMOCOCCAL CONJUGATE VACCINES IN INFANTS AND CHILDREN UNDER 5 YEARS OF AGE: FEBRUARY, 2019

This position paper, published in February 2019, replaces the corresponding WHO position paper on pneumococcal vaccines published in the Weekly Epidemiological Record in 2012. The focus of this position paper is use of pneumococcal conjugate vaccine (PCV) in infants and children <5 years of age; a separate position paper on vaccination of older age groups with conjugate and polysaccharide vaccines will be developed after consideration by SAGE. The present position paper includes data on the effects of the 10- and 13-valent PCVs (PCV10 and PCV13) published up to June 2017 and specifically addresses the dosing schedule, product choice and the value of catch-up vaccination in children under 5 years of age.

Background

Pneumococcal infections can lead to serious invasive diseases such as meningitis, septicemia and pneumonia, as well as milder but more common illnesses such as sinusitis and otitis media. There are >90 known serotypes of *S. pneumoniae*. The distribution of serotypes that cause disease varies over time and by age, disease syndrome, disease severity, geographical region and the presence of antimicrobial-resistant genes. Of the estimated 5.83 million deaths among children <5 years of age globally in 2015, 294,000 [uncertainty range (UR), 192,000–366,000] were estimated to be caused by pneumococcal infections. Before the introduction of pneumococcal conjugate vaccines (PCVs) in the different WHO regions, 6–11 serotypes accounted for ≥70% of all invasive pneumococcal disease (IPD). The reported mean annual incidence of IPD in children aged <2 years was 44.4/100,000 per year in Europe and 167/100,000 per year in the United States of America. In comparison, the annual incidence of IPD in children <2 years in Africa ranged from 60/100,000 in South Africa to 797/100,000 in Mozambique. On average, about 75% of cases of IPD and 83% of cases of pneumococcal meningitis occur in children aged <2 years, but the incidence and age distribution of cases may vary by country, study method and socioeconomic status within countries. Case fatality rates from IPD in children can be high, ranging up to 20% for septicemia and 50% for meningitis in low- and middle-income countries (LMICs).

Vaccines

Two polysaccharide-protein conjugate vaccines have been on the market since 2009—the 10-valent (PCV10) and the 13-valent (PCV13) vaccines. Previously, a 7-valent pneumococcal conjugate vaccine (PCV7) was available. Both PCV10 and PCV13 have been shown to be safe and effective and to have both direct (in vaccinated individuals) and indirect (in unvaccinated individuals living in communities with vaccinated children) effects against pneumococcal disease caused by vaccine serotypes when used in a 3-dose schedule (either 2p+1 or 3p+0) or in a 4-dose schedule (3p+1). After the third dose of each schedule (post-booster for 2p+1 and post-primary for 3p+0), the 2p+1 schedule resulted in higher geometric mean concentrations (GMCs) but a similar percentage of responders as compared with a 3p+0 schedule for most serotypes, except for serotype 6B, for which the percentage of responders was higher with the 2p+1 schedule.

Both PCV10 and PCV13 induce antibodies against the serotypes common to both vaccines (1, 4, 5, 6B, 7F, 9V, 14, 18C, 19F, and 23F). Although the mean antibody response to the common serotypes differed with the 2 products, in general, they induced comparable immunogenicity. PCV13 has three additional serotypes, 3, 6A, and 19A. PCV13 induces an immune response to serotype 3; PCV10 contains neither serotype 3 nor any cross-reactive serotype, and immunogenicity against serotype 3 is not measured in studies of this vaccine. Both PCV10 and PCV13 induce an antibody response to serotype 6A, which is included in PCV13 but not in PCV10. Both PCV10 and PCV13 induce an antibody response against serotype 19A.

WHO Position

WHO recommends the inclusion of PCVs in childhood immunization programs worldwide. Use of pneumococcal vaccine should be complementary to other disease prevention and control measures, such as appropriate case management, promotion of exclusive breastfeeding for the first 6 months of life and reducing known risk factors such as indoor air pollution and tobacco smoke.

For administration of PCV to infants, WHO recommends a 3-dose schedule administered either as 2p+1 or as 3p+0, starting as early as 6 weeks of age. In choosing between the 2p+1 and 3p+0 schedules, countries should consider programmatic factors, including timeliness of vaccination and expected coverage. The 2p+1 schedule has potential benefits over the 3p+0 schedule, when programmatically feasible, as higher antibody levels are induced in the second year of life, which may be important in maintaining herd immunity, although no high-quality evidence is available. If the 3p+0 schedule is used, a minimum interval of 4 weeks should be maintained between doses. If the 2p+1 schedule is selected, an interval of ≥8 weeks is recommended between the two primary doses, but the interval may be shortened if there is a compelling reason to do so, such as timeliness of receipt of the second dose and/or achieving higher coverage when a

4-week interval is used. The booster dose should be given at 9–18 months of age, according to programmatic considerations; there is no defined minimum or maximum interval between the primary series and the booster dose.

Previously unvaccinated or incompletely vaccinated children who recover from IPD should be vaccinated according to the recommended age-appropriate regimens. Interrupted schedules should be resumed without repeating the previous dose.

Both PCV10 and PCV13 have substantial impacts against pneumonia, vaccine-type IPD and nasopharyngeal (NP) carriage. There is at present insufficient evidence of a difference in the net impact of the two products on overall disease burden. PCV13 may have an additional benefit in settings where disease attributable to serotype 19A or serotype 6C is significant. The choice of product to be used in a country should be based on programmatic characteristics, vaccine supply, vaccine price, the local and regional prevalence of vaccine serotypes and antimicrobial resistance patterns. Once a PCV vaccination program has been initiated, product switching is not recommended unless there are substantial changes in the epidemiological or programmatic factors that determined the original choice of product, e.g. an increasing burden of serotype 19A.

If a series cannot be completed with the same type of vaccine, the available PCV product should be used. Restarting a series is not recommended, even for the primary series. Wherever possible, catch-up vaccination at the time of introduction of PCV should be used to accelerate its impact on disease in children aged 1–5 years, particularly in settings with a high disease burden and mortality.

PCVs should not be given to individuals with a history of anaphylactic reactions or severe allergic reactions to any component of the vaccine. HIV-positive infants and preterm neonates who have received their three primary vaccine doses before 12 months of age may benefit from a booster dose in the second year of life.

Traveling children are generally not at special risk of pneumococcal disease unless they travel to an outbreak setting. They should follow the vaccine recommendations for the general population and ensure they are up to date with their vaccinations before traveling.

While a comprehensive surveillance system for pneumococcal disease is recommended, countries without such a system in place should not wait to introduce PCV vaccines.

WHO recommends that the epidemiological impact of PCV be carefully monitored in sustained, high-quality sentinel and population-based surveillance for pneumococcal disease and in periodic NP carriage surveys.

Additional research should be conducted on—(1) further assessment of vaccine impact, duration of protection and indirect effects of different dosing schedules; (2) serotype replacement; (3) further establishment of serotype-specific immune correlates of protection against IPD in different transmission settings; (4) the epidemiology of pneumococcal outbreaks, particularly epidemics of serotype 1 disease, including use of PCV to prevent or respond to outbreaks; (5) the impact of PCV on antimicrobial use and resistance; and (6) comparison of a 1-dose versus a 2-dose catch-up schedule for children >12 months of age.

WHO POSITION PAPER ON ROTAVIRUS VACCINES

Background

Rotaviruses (RVs) are globally the leading cause of severe, dehydrating diarrhea in young children. Most children have been infected by these highly contagious viruses by the age of 5 years. Most of the severe rotavirus gastroenteritis (RVGE) episodes occurs in low-income countries and affects infants under 1 year of age. WHO estimates that in 2008 there were approximately 453,000 RVGE-associated child deaths. In most low-income countries in Asia and Africa, the rotavirus epidemiology is characterized by episodes of relatively intense viral circulation against a background of year-round transmission. However, in high income countries in temperate climates, a distinct winter seasonality is typically observed.

Rotaviruses belong to the *Reoviridae* family. The outermost layer of these viruses contains the proteins VP7 and VP4 which stimulate the production of neutralizing antibodies. In human rotaviruses, at least 12 different VP7 antigens (G-types) and 15 different VP4 antigens (P-types) have been identified. Currently, five G-P combinations (G1P[8], G2P[4], G3P[8], G4P[8], and

G9P[8]) account for approximately 90% of all human rotavirus infections.

Rotaviruses damage the enterocyte lining of the small intestinal villi, leading to reduced absorptive capacity and diarrhea. The wide clinical spectrum of rotavirus disease ranges from transient loose stools to severe diarrhea and vomiting causing dehydration, electrolyte disturbances, shock and, in untreated cases, death. The cornerstones of treatment of severe RVGE are fluid replacement and zinc supplementation. An etiological diagnosis of rotavirus gastroenteritis requires laboratory confirmation.

Currently available vaccines are based on live, oral, attenuated rotavirus strains of human and/or animal origin that replicate in the human gut. Two rotavirus vaccines are marketed internationally—the monovalent (RV1) and the pentavalent (RV5). RV1 originates from a human strain, whereas RV5 contains five reassortants developed from rotaviruses of human and bovine origin.

Many randomized controlled trials have shown that both RV1 and RV5 are 80-90% efficacious against severe RVGE in countries with very low or low child and adult mortality, and 40-60% efficacious in countries with high child mortality and high or very high adult mortality. In most cases, vaccination in infancy provides protection against severe RVGE for at least 2 years. Breastfeeding and prematurity (<37 weeks' gestation) do not significantly impair the response to the rotavirus vaccines.

In large controlled trials, no differences were observed between the vaccine groups and the placebo groups in terms of serious adverse events. However, in some, but not all settings, post-marketing surveillance has detected a small increased risk of intussusception (about 1-2/100,000 infants vaccinated) shortly after the first dose. Still, the benefits that rotavirus vaccination provides, through prevention of severe diarrhea and death from rotavirus infection, far exceed the risk of intussusception.

WHO Recommendations

Rotavirus vaccines should be included in all national immunization programs and considered a priority, particularly in countries with high RVGE-associated fatality rates, such as in south and south-eastern Asia and sub-Saharan Africa. The use of rotavirus vaccines should be part of a comprehensive strategy to control diarrheal diseases.

Plans for introduction of rotavirus vaccines should consider the epidemiology of the disease by age, the coverage and actual age at vaccination and also include an evaluation of the estimated public health impact and potential risks. It is important to establish the baseline incidence of intussusception. Proper planning and training of staff to conduct pharmacovigilance should take place before the vaccine is introduced. Also, caregivers should be adequately counseled to recognize danger signs of dehydration or intussusception.

The first dose of rotavirus vaccine should be administered as soon as possible after 6 weeks of age. RV1 should be administered in a 2-dose schedule at the time of DPT1 and DPT2, and RV5 in a 3-dose schedule at the time of the DTP1, DTP2, and DTP3 contacts. Both vaccines are given orally with an interval of at least 4 weeks between doses.

Infants should receive rotavirus vaccine together with DTP regardless of the time of vaccination. Rotavirus vaccination of healthy children aged over 2 years is not considered necessary. Rotavirus vaccinations can be administered simultaneously with other routine infant vaccines.

Apart from a very low risk of intussusception, the current rotavirus vaccines are safe and well-tolerated. Major contraindications for rotavirus vaccination are severe allergic reaction after a previous dose and severe immunodeficiency. Precautions for use of rotavirus vaccination include a history of intussusception or intestinal malformations, chronic gastrointestinal disease, and severe acute illness. Vaccination should be postponed when the child has ongoing acute gastroenteritis or fever with moderate-to-severe illness.

WHO POSITION PAPER ON MEASLES VACCINE: APRIL, 2017

This position paper replaces the 2009, WHO position paper on measles. It incorporates the most recent developments in the field of measles and includes removal of introduction criteria for the routine second dose of measles-containing vaccine (MCV2), guidance on when to vaccinate infants from 6 months of age, and guidance on re-vaccination of HIV-infected children receiving highly active antiretroviral therapy (HAART).

Background

Measles is one of the most contagious diseases of humans, and in the absence of vaccination, about 95% of individuals would be infected with measles virus by 15 years of age. In 2015, worldwide measles vaccination coverage with the first and second dose had reached 85% and 61%, respectively. In 2015, there were an estimated 134,200 measles deaths globally, representing a 79% decline since 2000.

Several live-attenuated measles vaccines are currently available, either as monovalent vaccine or as measles-containing vaccine combinations (MCVs) with one or more of rubella (R), mumps (M), and varicella (V) vaccines. The measles vaccines that are now internationally available are safe, effective, and may be used interchangeably in immunization programs.

WHO Position

Reaching all children with two doses of measles vaccine should be the standard for all national immunization programs. In addition to the first routine dose of MCV (MCV1), all countries should include a second routine dose of MCV (MCV2) in their national vaccination schedules regardless of the level of MCV1 coverage. Countries aiming at measles elimination should achieve ≥95% coverage with both doses equitably to all children in every district. Measles vaccines are recommended for all susceptible children and adults for whom measles vaccination is not contraindicated.

Where risk of measles mortality among infants remains high, MCV1 should be administered at 9 months of age. These countries should administer the routine dose of MCV2 at age 15-18 months. The minimum interval between MCV1 and MCV2 is 4 weeks. In countries with low risk of measles infection among infants (i.e. near elimination), MCV1 may be administered at 12 months and the optimal age for delivering routine MCV2 is based on programmatic considerations that achieve the highest coverage of MCV2. Every opportunity (e.g. whenever children come in contact with health services) should be taken to vaccinate all children who missed one or both MCV routine doses, particularly those <15 years of age.

A supplementary dose of MCV should be given to infants from 6 months of age:

- During a measles outbreak as part of intensified service delivery;
- During campaigns where the risk of measles among infants <9 months of age is high;
- For internally displaced populations, refugees, and populations in conflict zones;
- For individual infants at high risk of contracting measles;
- For infants traveling to countries experiencing measles outbreaks;
- For infants known to be HIV-infected or exposed.

MCV administered before 9 months of age should be considered a supplementary dose 1 and recorded as "MCV0". Children who receive a MCV0 dose should also receive MCV1 and MCV2 at the recommended ages according to the national schedule. In countries with moderate to weak health systems, regular measles immunization campaigns can protect children who do not have access to routine health services. Campaigns should be conducted before the number of pre-school children susceptible to measles approaches the equivalent of one birth cohort. For large countries and countries which are close to measles elimination, a more extensive assessment of the accumulation of susceptible persons and timing of campaigns should be carried out at the subnational level. Countries should integrate their surveillance, demographic, survey and seroprevalence data together with vaccination coverage information, history of MCV and RCV use, and local knowledge to determine the age distribution of susceptibility (age-specific immunity gaps) and hence the target age range(s) for measles and MR campaigns. Campaigns should continue until >90–95% vaccination coverage has been achieved at the national level for both MCV1 and MCV2, as determined by accurate coverage data for a period of at least 3 consecutive years.

All HCWs and any staff who are in contact with patients should be immune to measles. Documentation of immunity should be required before signing an employment contract or entering into a training program. Susceptible individual traveling to measles-endemic areas are considered at risk of contracting measles and should be offered vaccine from 6 months of age.

MCVs should not be given to individuals with a history of anaphylactic reactions or severe allergic reactions to any component of the vaccine (e.g. neomycin or gelatin) or those with any form of severe immunosuppression. Mild, concurrent infections are not a contraindication to vaccination. As a precautionary measure, MCVs should be avoided during pregnancy. Inadvertent administration of MCV during pregnancy is not a reason for terminating the pregnancy.

Measles vaccination should be routinely given to potentially susceptible, asymptomatic HIV-infected children and adults. In areas with high incidences both of HIV-infection and measles, the first measles immunization may be offered as early as 6 months of age (recorded as MCV0). Two additional doses of measles vaccine should be administered to these children according to the national immunization schedule. An additional dose of MCV should be administered to HIV-infected children receiving HAART following immune reconstitution (e.g. when the $CD4^+$ T-lymphocyte count reaches 20–25% or when $CD4^+$ T-lymphocyte monitoring is not available, children should receive an additional dose of MCV 6–12 months after initiation of HAART).

As countries approach elimination, they should intensify surveillance and move towards weekly reporting to the WHO regional offices. To determine if a country or a WHO region has achieved elimination, the regional verification commission should consider five lines of evidence (on disease epidemiology, population immunity, quality of surveillance, sustainability of the program, and genotyping evidence). These lines of evidence should be evaluated together to establish the case for elimination.

WHO POSITION PAPER ON RUBELLA VACCINES PUBLISHED IN WER JULY, 2011

Rubella is an acute, viral disease traditionally affecting children and young adults. The virus is transmitted by the respiratory route, replicates in the nasopharyngeal mucosa and local lymph nodes and spreads by viremia to different organs. The incubation period ranges from 12–23 days.

Although usually a mild self-limited illness, rubella during early pregnancy may result in miscarriage, fetal death or congenital ophthalmic, auditory and/or cardiac defects known as congenital rubella syndrome (CRS). The period of highest risk of CRS (up to 90% of cases) is from just before conception and during the first 8-10 weeks of gestation. Serious manifestations of CRS include meningoencephalitis, hepatosplenomegaly, hepatitis, and thrombocytopenia. Surviving infants may face developmental disabilities. Maternal rubella is rarely associated with fetal defects after the 16th week of pregnancy.

Before the introduction of rubella vaccine, the incidence of CRS varied from 0.1-0.2 per 1,000 live births during endemic periods, and from 0.8-4 per 1,000 live births during rubella epidemics. Large-scale rubella vaccination during the past decade has drastically reduced or practically eliminated rubella and CRS in many countries.

Most rubella vaccines are based on the live, attenuated RA 27/3 strain. Other live-attenuated rubella-vaccines include the Takahashi, Matsuura, TO-336, or BRD-2 strains.

Rubella containing vaccines (RCVs) are available either as monovalent formulations or, more commonly, in combinations with vaccines against measles (MR), measles and mumps (MMR), or measles, mumps, and varicella (MMRV). The immune response to rubella antigens is not affected by the other vaccine components.

RCVs are administered subcutaneously or intramuscularly, usually at age 12-15 months, but may be administered to children aged 9-11 months and to older children, adolescents and adults. Although one dose of rubella vaccine probably induces life-long protection, in most countries using the MR or MMR vaccines a second dose is offered at 15-18 months or 4-6 years, as indicated for protection against measles and mumps.

In clinical trials, 95-100% of susceptible persons aged ≥12 months develop rubella antibodies after a single dose of the vaccine. In outbreak situations the effectiveness of different rubella vaccines has been estimated at 90-100%. RA 27/3-containing vaccines have eliminated rubella and CRS from the western hemisphere and in European countries with high vaccination coverage.

Adverse reactions following vaccination with RA27/3-containing rubella vaccine are mild, particularly in children. However, in susceptible adult women, transient arthralgias and arthritis are relatively common. No causal link has been demonstrated between RCVs and chronic joint disease, Crohn's disease, ulcerative colitis, or autism. Furthermore, no cases of CRS have been reported in more than 1,000 susceptible women who unknowingly were vaccinated in early stages of pregnancy. However, because of a theoretical, but never demonstrated teratogenic risk, rubella vaccination of pregnant women should be avoided, and those planning a pregnancy are advised to avoid pregnancy for 1 month following rubella vaccination.

Rubella vaccination is contraindicated for people with a history of an anaphylactic reaction to components of the vaccine and for persons suffering from severe immunodeficiency.

There are two general approaches to the use of rubella vaccine: The first focuses exclusively on reducing CRS by immunizing adolescent girls and/or women of childbearing age; the second approach aims at interrupting viral transmission and thereby eliminating rubella as well as CRS.

For CRS reduction alone, adolescent and adult females should be vaccinated through either routine services or supplementary immunization activities (SIAs). This option will provide direct protection to women of childbearing age; however, the impact of this strategy is limited by the coverage achieved and the age groups targeted. In the absence of a program that ensures vaccination of infants and young children, rubella will continue to circulate, resulting in ongoing exposure of pregnant women and the associated risk of CRS.

For the elimination of rubella and CRS, the preferred approach is to begin with MR vaccine or MMR vaccine in a campaign targeting a wide range of ages, immediately followed by the introduction of MR or MMR vaccine into the routine program. All subsequent follow-up campaigns should use MR vaccine or MMR vaccine. In addition, countries should make efforts to reach women of childbearing age by immunizing adolescent girls or women of childbearing age, or both, either through routine services or mass campaigns.

Measles-vaccine delivery strategies provide an opportunity for synergy and a platform for advancing rubella and CRS elimination. All countries that are providing two doses of measles vaccine using routine immunization or SIAs, or both, should consider including RCVs in their immunization program.

Sustained low coverage of rubella immunization in infants and young children can result in increased susceptibility among women that may increase the risk of CRS above levels during the pre-vaccine era ("paradoxical effect"). Therefore, countries should achieve and maintain immunization coverage of ≥80% with at least one dose of an RCV delivered through routine services or regular SIAs.

The need to document the impact of rubella vaccination requires laboratory-supported surveillance for rubella and CRS, and molecular epidemiology. Immunization coverage should be monitored by age and locality and supplemented by seroprevalence surveys where necessary to determine age-specific susceptibility to rubella and direct vaccination activities. Antenatal serological screening is a practical tool in this context.

WHO POSITION PAPER ON VARICELLA AND HERPES ZOSTER VACCINATION: JUNE, 2014

Varicella (chickenpox) is an acute, highly contagious disease with worldwide distribution caused by the varicella zoster virus (VZV). In temperate climates most cases occur before the age of 10 years. The epidemiology is less well understood in tropical areas, where a relatively large proportion of adults in some countries are seronegative.

The estimated global burden of disease-specific mortality caused by varicella is considerably lower than that due to other major infectious diseases such as measles, pertussis, rotavirus, or invasive pneumococcal disease. Based on conservative estimates, the global annual varicella disease burden would include 4.2 million severe complications leading to hospitalization and 4,200 deaths. Despite the routine use of measles and pertussis vaccination, the age-standardized death rates (per 100,000 cases) in 2010 was 0.1 (95% CI: 0.0–0.7) for varicella compared to 1.7 (95% CI: 0.6–4.1) for measles and 1.1 (95% CI: 0.0–5.5) for pertussis. In the pre-vaccine era in high-income developed countries, case fatality rates for varicella were approximately 3 per 100,000 cases compared to 1–3 per 1,000 cases for measles.

While mostly a mild disorder in childhood, varicella tends to be more severe in adults. It is characterized by an itchy, vesicular rash, usually starting on the scalp and face, initially accompanied by fever and malaise. The disease may be fatal, especially in neonates and immunocompromised individuals. Complications include VZV-induced pneumonitis or encephalitis and invasive group A streptococcal infections.

The transmission of VZV is via droplets, aerosol or direct contact, or indirectly by touching freshly soiled contaminated items. Patients are usually contagious from a few days before onset of the rash until the rash has crusted over.

Following infection, the virus remains latent in neural ganglia; upon subsequent reactivation, usually much later in adult life, VZV may cause herpes zoster (HZ) commonly known as shingles, a disease affecting mainly immunocompromised individuals and elderly people. The clinical manifestation is a unilateral vesicular rash, characteristically restricted to a single dermatome, which is usually accompanied by radicular pain along that dermatome. Patients experience significant pain and discomfort that may last for weeks, months or even years in severe cases, diminishing the quality of life.

No causal treatment is available for varicella or HZ, though live attenuated vaccines are available for the prevention of varicella and for the prevention of HZ.

WHO Position

There is strong scientific evidence that varicella vaccine is safe and effective in preventing varicella related morbidity and mortality in immunocompetent individuals. WHO recommended that routine childhood immunization against varicella could be considered in countries where the disease has an important public health impact. Resources should be sufficient to support sustained vaccine coverage ≥80%. Settings where varicella vaccine coverage levels are less than 80% are at risk of an increase of severe disease and mortality in adults.

Those countries deciding to introduce routine childhood varicella immunization, should administer vaccination at 12–18 months of age. The number of doses administered is dependent on the goal of the vaccination program. One dose is sufficient to reduce mortality and severe morbidity from varicella. Two doses induce higher effectiveness and should therefore be recommended in countries where the programmatic goal is, in addition to decreasing mortality and severe morbidity, to further reduce the number of cases and outbreaks.

Due to the increase in severity of varicella in immunocompromised, certain groups of immunocompromised should be considered for VZV vaccination. Limited data on the immunization of healthcare workers (HCW) are available, yet countries should consider vaccination of nonimmunized healthcare workers without a history of varicella with two doses of varicella vaccine, even in absence of varicella vaccination in the routine immunization schedule, if the risk of severe varicella in the population in direct contact with the HCW is high (e.g. immunocompromised).

Herpes zoster vaccine is safe and demonstrated clinical protection against herpes zoster, postherpetic neuralgia and other serious herpes zoster complications. To date no data are available on long term protection induced by the vaccine. Due to limited data and the unknown burden of disease in most countries, initial evidence of waning of protection over time and uncertainty of the optimal age for vaccination SAGE could not make any recommendation about routine HZ vaccination at this time.

WHO POSITION PAPER ON TYPHOID VACCINES: MARCH, 2018

This position paper published in March 2018, replaces the WHO position paper on typhoid vaccines published in 2008. It re-emphasises the importance of vaccination to control typhoid fever and presents the WHO recommendations on the use of a new generation of typhoid conjugate vaccine.

Background

Typhoid fever is an acute generalized infection, caused by an enteric bacterium, *Salmonella enteric* serovar Typhi, generally termed *Salmonella typhi* (*S. typhi*). Global estimates of typhoid fever burden range between 11 and 21 million cases and approximately 128,000–161,000 deaths annually. Children are disproportionately affected by typhoid fever, with peak incidence known to occur in individuals aged 5 to <15 years of age.

If the circulating *S. typhi* strains are susceptible, acute typhoid fever and carriage of *S. typhi* can be effectively treated with antibiotics. The emergence of antimicrobial resistant strains of *S. typhi* and subsequent trends over the past few decades and recent outbreak of ceftriaxone-resistant typhoid in Pakistan demonstrate the importance of understanding local resistance patterns to enable the selection of appropriate antibiotics.

Currently three types of typhoid vaccines are licensed for use—(1) typhoid conjugate vaccine (TCV); (2) unconjugated Vi polysaccharide (ViPS) vaccine; and (3) live-attenuated Ty21a vaccine. The second and third types have been recommended by WHO since 2008 for endemic and epidemic settings.

WHO Position

WHO recommends programmatic use of typhoid vaccines for the control of typhoid fever. All typhoid vaccination programs should be implemented in the context of other efforts to control the disease. TCV is preferred at all ages in view of its improved immunological properties, use in younger children and longer duration of protection. TCV should be prioritized in countries with high burden of disease or antimicrobial resistance. Countries may also consider the routine use of ViPS vaccine in those ≥2 years, and Ty21a vaccine for those >6 years.

WHO recommends a 0.5 mL single dose of TCV in children from 6 months and in adults up to 45 years in endemic regions. WHO also encourages routine programmatic administration of TCV at the same time as other vaccines, at 9 months or in the second year of life. When ViPS is used, a single dose of the vaccine should be administered intramuscularly or subcutaneously from 2 years. For Ty21a, a 3-dose oral immunization schedule, administering the vaccine every second day, is recommended above 6 years. Catch-up vaccination with TCV up to 15 years of age is recommended when feasible and supported by epidemiologic data. Catch-up vaccination of multiple age cohorts is likely to accelerate impact.

WHO recommends vaccination in response to confirmed outbreaks of typhoid fever and in humanitarian emergencies depending on the risk assessment in the particular setting.

The potential need for revaccination with TCV is currently unclear. When ViPS or Ty21a vaccine is used, revaccination is recommended every 3 years for ViPS, and every 3-7 years in most endemic settings for Ty21a or every 1-7 years for travelers from non-endemic to endemic areas, depending on national policies.

Vaccination of Special Populations, Contraindications, and Precautions

Typhoid conjugate vaccine and ViPS vaccines are contraindicated for individuals with known hypersensitivity to any component of the vaccine. Ty21a should not be administered to persons taking antibiotics. Certain antimalarials exhibit activity against Ty21a. Ty21a may be taken with chloroquine but should not be taken until 8–24 hours after administration of mefloquine.

Typhoid vaccination should be considered for professional food handlers in typhoid endemic areas, travelers from non-endemic going to endemic areas and clinical microbiology laboratory staff with a recognized risk of occupational exposure. Data are currently lacking on typhoid vaccine use in pregnant women, however, there are no theoretical safety concerns for ViPS and TCV. Use of the live-attenuated Ty21a vaccine during pregnancy should be avoided.

Immunocompromised persons, including those with HIV infection, should receive TCV or ViPS vaccine. Ty21a vaccine can be administered to HIV-infected, immunologically stable individuals with a CD4 percent >25% for children aged <5 years or CD4 count ≥200 cells/mm^3 if aged ≥5 years.

Administration of Typhoid Vaccines

Typhoid conjugate vaccine is administered by intramuscular injection and ViPS is administered by intramuscular or subcutaneous route. Both vaccines should be injected into the anterolateral aspect of the thigh for infants or into the deltoid muscle for older children and adults.

Monitoring and Research Priorities

WHO recommends: (1) Post-licensure monitoring of effectiveness and safety of TCV especially in special population groups; (2) use of Brighton Collaboration case definitions; and (3) analysis of non-specific effects of vaccination. WHO also recommends that endemic countries strengthen the surveillance of typhoid fever in all age groups, and monitor antimicrobial resistant strains before and after introduction of vaccines.

Research priority should focus on vaccination policy and programs, particularly in the following areas—identifying at risk populations; risk of transmission and strategies to identify and treat carriers; correlate(s) of protection for typhoid vaccines; co-administration with other vaccines; safety and immunogenicity in special populations; duration of protection for a single dose of TCV and need for revaccination; whether the tetanus toxoid carrier protein of the Vi-TT conjugate vaccine provides protection equivalent to a booster dose of tetanus vaccine; and the impact of different TCV strategies including target age ranges for routine and catch-up vaccination as well as the impact of vaccination for outbreak control.

WHO POSITION PAPER ON VACCINES AGAINST INFLUENZA: NOVEMBER, 2012

This position paper is concerned mainly with vaccines and vaccination against seasonal (epidemic) influenza.

Influenza A and B viruses are globally important human respiratory pathogens causing epidemics, usually during the winter season, and out-of-season sporadic cases and outbreaks. Influenza A viruses may also cause worldwide pandemics. Subtypes of influenza A viruses are determined by either hemagglutinin (HA) or neuraminidase (NA) activity. Minor mutations causing small changes ("antigenic drift") in the HA gene enable the virus to evade immune recognition, resulting in seasonal influenza outbreaks during inter-pandemic years.

The annual attack rate of influenza is estimated at 5–10% in adults and 20–30% in children. Influenza is typically characterized by fever, cough, sore throat, runny nose, headache, muscle and joint pain and malaise. In young children, impaired respiration, dehydration, altered mental status, and irritability signify serious disease. Secondary bacterial pneumonia is a frequent complication of influenza, particularly in risk groups. Etiology-specific diagnosis of influenza requires laboratory confirmation.

Risk groups for severe influenza include pregnant women, children aged <5 years, the elderly, and individuals with underlying health conditions such as HIV-AIDS, asthma, or chronic heart or lung diseases. Infected healthcare workers may transmit influenza virus to individuals at risk of severe disease.

Currently available vaccines for the control of seasonal influenza are safe and efficacious and have the potential to prevent significant annual morbidity and mortality. Their antigenic composition is revised twice annually to ensure optimal vaccine efficacy against prevailing strains for the northern and southern hemispheres.

Seasonal influenza vaccines include two influenza A-strains and one influenza B strain. Both trivalent inactivated influenza vaccines (TIVs) for intramuscular injection and trivalent live-attenuated influenza vaccines (LAIVs) for intranasal application are available. TIVs include formulations containing an adjuvant or an increased antigen concentration for use mainly in the elderly, and in some countries an intradermally administered TIV is licensed. Recently, a quadrivalent LAIV (2A- and 2B-strains) became available.

TIVs are the only vaccines licensed for children aged 6–24 months, for persons aged ≥50 years, and for pregnant women. Non-pregnant individuals aged 2–49 years may receive either TIV or LAIV. When the vaccine strains closely match the circulating influenza viruses, efficacy rates of TIV and LAIV against laboratory-confirmed influenza in healthy individuals <65 years of age typically range from 70% to 90%, whereas efficacy is at best modest in individuals aged ≥65 years, and in those with underlying medical conditions.

WHO Position and Recommendations

Internationally available vaccines for the control of seasonal influenza are safe and efficacious and have the potential to prevent significant annual morbidity and mortality.

Country-specific information about risk groups, disease burden and cost-effectiveness are important to aid national policy makers and health program planners in making informed decisions about target groups and timing for vaccination.

For countries considering the initiation or expansion of programs for seasonal influenza vaccination, WHO recommends that pregnant women should have the highest priority. Additional risk groups to be considered for vaccination, in no particular order of priority, are children aged 6–59 months, the elderly, individuals with specific chronic medical conditions, and healthcare workers.

Countries with existing influenza vaccination programs targeting any of these additional groups should continue to do so and incorporate immunization of pregnant women into such programs.

Children <6 months of age should be protected against influenza through vaccination during pregnancy and vaccination of close contacts. Because of their high burden of severe disease, children 6-23 months of age are a target group for influenza immunization. Compared with younger children, those 2-5 years of age are at lower risk, but respond better to vaccination with TIV and in particular with LAIV.

Persons ≥65 years of age have the highest risk of mortality from influenza, and are an important target for vaccination, although the vaccines are in general less effective in elderly people. Vaccination of healthcare workers should be considered as part of a broader infection control policy for healthcare facilities.

Influenza vaccination is recommended every year, particularly for high-risk groups. TIV is administered intramuscularly (except for intradermal formulations). Children aged 6 through 35 months should receive a pediatric dose and previously unvaccinated children aged <9 years should receive two injections administered at least 4 weeks apart. A single dose of the vaccine is appropriate for children aged ≥9 years and healthy adults. LAIV is given as nasal spray, one dose only, but children aged 2-8 years should normally receive two doses, at least 4 weeks apart.

Successful introduction of influenza vaccines to healthy younger populations, including pregnant women and young children, will require effective educational programs and communication. For pregnant women year-round availability of the most recent influenza vaccines is essential.

Influenza surveillance platforms are critical for monitoring and communicating the impact of introducing seasonal influenza vaccination. Strengthening of seasonal influenza programs will assist in programmatic preparedness for pandemic vaccine introduction.

WHO POSITION PAPER ON HEPATITIS A VACCINES: JULY, 2012

The current document replaces the 2000, WHO position paper on hepatitis A vaccines. Hepatitis A virus (HAV) is transmitted primarily via the faecal/oral route and the incidence of hepatitis A is strongly correlated with access to clean water and adequate sanitation. According to WHO estimates, 212 million cases of acute hepatitis A occurred in 2005.

In low-income regions, exposure to HAV tend to occur before the age of 5 years, when HAV infection is usually asymptomatic. In high-income regions, the risk of acquiring HAV infection is low. In most middle-income regions there is a mix of intermediate and low prevalences and here, a substantial proportion of adolescents and adults are susceptible. HAV infection in these age groups is associated with a higher rate of severe clinical manifestations and hence, transition from high to intermediate endemicity may result in increased incidence of clinically significant disease and mortality from hepatitis A.

Other groups at high risk of HAV exposure and disease include travelers to areas of high endemicity, men who have sex with men, and injection drug users. Groups at risk of serious clinical outcome, once infected, include the elderly and immunocompromised individuals.

The clinical manifestations of acute viral hepatitis typically include nonspecific symptoms such as malaise, fatigue, anorexia, vomiting, abdominal discomfort, and diarrhea. Elevated levels of liver enzymes, the appearance of dark urine and sometimes clay-colored stools and jaundice are characteristic manifestations. Hepatitis A resolves completely in >99% of the cases. Rare fatalities (0.1% in children <15 years of age and 2.1% in adults ≥40 years of age) are associated mainly with the development fulminant hepatitis.

Two types of hepatitis A vaccines are currently used worldwide—(1) formaldehyde inactivated vaccines and (2) live-attenuated vaccines. Following immunization, a positive test for total anti-HAV antibodies is considered to signify immunity to hepatitis A.

1. *Inactivated hepatitis A vaccines*, alone or in fixed combinations, are widely used internationally. These vaccines are licensed for use in persons ≥12 months of age and the manufacturers recommend a 2-dose schedule with 6–12 (up to 18–36) months interval between the two doses. Inactivated hepatitis A vaccines are interchangeable and can be administered simultaneously with any other routinely used vaccine.

In general, two doses of inactivated hepatitis A vaccine induce protective efficacies of 90–95%, or more. The median predicted duration of protection has been estimated at 45 years. High vaccine efficacy can be achieved also with one single dose of inactivated hepatitis A vaccine: 6 years after implementation of country-wide, annual immunization with a single dose of vaccine to 12-months old children in Argentina, no hepatitis A cases has been detected among vaccinated individuals. Studies among adult travelers confirm that one dose of hepatitis A vaccine induces immunological memory and in most cases, anti-HAV antibodies that persist throughout 4–11 year periods of observation.

High efficacy of post-exposure prophylaxis against hepatitis A using one single dose of inactivated vaccine within 2 weeks of exposure is documented. Cumulative global experience from the use of several hundred million doses of inactivated hepatitis A vaccines testify to their excellent overall safety profile.

2. *Live-attenuated hepatitis A vaccines* are manufactured in China. One dose of this vaccine is used in children aged ≥1 year in several national immunization programs. Controlled trials conducted among large numbers of children 1–15 years of age have shown up to 100% efficacy for pre-exposure prophylaxis and 95% efficacy for post-exposure prophylaxis. Anti-HAV antibodies were detected in 72–88% of the vaccinees 15 years after vaccination. No substantial safety concerns have been identified during these trials. However, live-attenuated vaccines are not recommended for use in pregnant women and in immune compromised patients.

Estimates of cost-effectiveness of hepatitis A vaccination in high- and middle income countries show lower ratios for universal vaccination as compared to more targeted vaccination. Universal vaccination was found to be particularly cost-effective in children in high incidence areas.

WHO concludes that both inactivated and live-attenuated hepatitis A vaccines are safe and highly immunogenic and that in most cases, these vaccines will generate long-lasting, possibly life-long, protection against hepatitis A both in children and adults.

- Vaccination against HAV should be part of a comprehensive plan for the prevention and control of viral hepatitis. If indicated on the basis of age-specific epidemiological studies and consideration of cost-effectiveness, vaccination against hepatitis A should be integrated into the national immunization schedule for children aged ≥1 year.
- In highly endemic countries, where natural immunity is acquired in young age, large-scale vaccination programs are not recommended. In contrast, countries in transition from high to intermediate endemicity may experience an increased incidence of clinically significant disease and mortality from hepatitis A. In these settings, large-scale hepatitis A vaccination is likely to be cost-effective and is therefore encouraged. To control community-wide outbreaks, a single dose regimen of hepatitis A vaccine has been most successful when vaccination was started early and high coverage of multiple age-cohorts was achieved.

In low endemicity settings, targeted vaccination of high-risk groups should be considered. In certain risk groups such as the elderly or immunocompromised individuals, hepatitis A vaccines may be less efficacious and protection of shorter duration than in healthy young individuals.

Currently, inactivated HAV vaccines are licensed for intramuscular administration in a 2-dose schedule. Apart from a severe allergic reaction to the previous dose, there is no contraindication to their use. Inactivated hepatitis A vaccines should also be considered for pregnant women at definite risk of HAV infection.

Compared to the classical two-dose schedule, one single dose of inactivated hepatitis A vaccines is similarly efficacious, less expensive and easier to implement. Therefore, countries may consider the use of a single-dose schedule of this vaccine. However, in risk groups for hepatitis A, a two dose vaccination schedule is preferred.

The live-attenuated vaccine is administered as a single dose. As a rule, live vaccines should not be used in pregnancy or in severely immunocompromised patients. The use of hepatitis A vaccine rather than passive prophylaxis with immune globulin should be considered for both pre- and post-exposure prophylaxis.

WHO POSITION PAPER ON VACCINES AGAINST HUMAN PAPILLOMAVIRUS: MAY, 2017

This position paper published in May 2017, replaces the corresponding document published in October, 2014. It incorporates recent developments concerning human papillomavirus (HPV) vaccines, including the licensure of a nonavalent (9-valent) vaccine and recent data on vaccine effectiveness, and provides guidance on the choice of vaccine. New recommendations are proposed regarding vaccination strategies targeting girls only or both girls and boys, and vaccination of multiple birth cohorts.

Epidemiology and Virology

Persistent infection by oncogenic HPV types is a prerequisite for the development of cervical cancer, which each year hits about 528,000 women and causes 266,000 deaths worldwide. The viral types 16 and 18 HPV are the most common types in invasive cervical cancer, accounting for about 70% of all cervical cancers. In total, 85% of cervical cancer cases occur in the less developed regions and mortality rates vary as much as 18-fold between industrialized and developing countries. Other manifestations of HPV infection include vaginal, vulvar, penile, oropharyngeal and anal cancers. In addition, HPV types 6 and 11 cause anogenital warts and recurrent respiratory papillomatosis. HPV is mainly transmitted sexually. Cervical cancer occurs only in a small fraction of those infected and takes a decade or more to develop. Properly implemented screening and treatment programs contribute to the low mortality observed in some countries.

Vaccines

Three prophylactic HPV vaccines, directed against high-risk HPV types, are currently available and marketed in many countries worldwide for the prevention of HPV-related disease: the quadrivalent vaccine was first licensed in 2006, the bivalent vaccine in 2007 and the nonavalent vaccine in 2014. The bivalent vaccine contains non-infectious protein antigens for HPV 16 and 18, the qudrivalent against noninfectious protein antigens for HPV 6, 11, 16, and 18 and the nonvalent noninfectious protein antigens for HPV 6, 11, 16, 18, 31, 33, 45, 52, and 58.

Current evidence suggests that from the public health perspective the bivalent, quadrivalent and nonavalent vaccines offer comparable immunogenicity, efficacy and effectiveness for the prevention of cervical cancer, which is mainly caused by HPV types 16 and 18. All three HPV vaccines have an excellent safety profiles.

By 31 March, 2017, globally 71 countries (37%) had introduced HPV vaccine in their national immunization program for girls, and 11 countries (6%) also for boys.

WHO Recommendations

Recognizing the importance of cervical cancer and other HPV related diseases as global health problems, WHO recommends that routine HPV vaccination should be included in national immunization programs.

For the prevention of cervical cancer, the WHO recommended primary target population for HPV vaccination is girls aged 9–14 years, prior to becoming sexually active. The current evidence supports the recommendation for a 2-dose schedule with adequate spacing between the first and second dose (min: 6-month interval) in those aged 9–14 years. An interval no greater than 12–15 months is suggested in order to complete the schedule promptly and before becoming sexually active. If the interval between doses is shorter than 5 months, a third dose should be given at least 6 months after the first dose. Individuals older than ≥15 years and older and HIV infected/immunocompromised should receive a 3-dose schedule (0, 1–2, 6 months).

Current evidence suggests that from the public health perspective the bivalent, quadrivalent and nonavalent vaccines offer comparable immunogenicity, efficacy and effectiveness for the prevention of cervical cancer, which is mainly caused by HPV types 16 and 18.

The choice of HPV vaccine should be based on:
- Assessment of locally relevant data;
- The scale of the prevailing HPV-associated public health problem (cervical cancer, other anogenital cancers, or anogenital warts);
- The population for which the vaccine has been approved;
- Unique product characteristics, such as price, supply, and programmatic considerations.

The initial vaccination of multiple cohorts of girls aged 9–14 years is recommended when the vaccine is first introduced. Vaccination targeting multiple age cohorts of girls aged between 9 and 18 years together at time of HPV vaccine introduction would result in faster and greater population impact than vaccination of single age cohorts, due to the estimated increase in direct protection and herd immunity.

Vaccination of secondary target populations, e.g. females aged ≥15 years or males, is only recommended if feasible, affordable, cost-effective and does not divert resources from vaccinating primary target population or from effective cervical cancer screening programs. HPV vaccines should be introduced as part of a coordinated and comprehensive strategy to prevent cervical cancer and other diseases caused by HPV. The introduction of HPV vaccine should not undermine or divert funding from developing or maintaining effective screening programs for cervical cancer. Opportunities should be sought to link the introduction of HPV vaccination to other vaccinations carried out at this age (e.g. diphtheria and tetanus vaccination) and programs targeting young people.

HPV vaccine can be co-administered with other non-live and live vaccines using separate syringes and different injection sites. Efforts should be made to administer the same vaccine for all doses.

However, if the vaccine used for prior dose(s) is unknown or unavailable, either of the HPV vaccines can be administered to complete the recommended schedule.

HPV vaccine can be administered safely to immunocompromised and/or HIV-infected individuals. HPV vaccination of pregnant women should be avoided due to lack of data, though no adverse effects in mother or offspring have been observed. If a young female becomes pregnant after initiating the vaccination series, the remaining dose(s) should be delayed until after the pregnancy is completed. Breastfeeding is not a contraindication for HPV vaccination.

WHO POSITION PAPER ON VACCINATION AGAINST YELLOW FEVER

Yellow fever (YF) is a mosquito-borne viral disease of humans and other primates, currently endemic in 44 countries in the tropical regions of Africa and South America. According to WHO estimates from the early 1990s, 200,000 cases of YF, with 30,000 deaths, are expected globally each year, the majority occurring in sub-Saharan Africa. Large scale YF vaccination has been very effective. However, where mass vaccination campaigns have ceased and coverage has not been sustained, the disease has recurred, resulting in major outbreaks.

All current commercially available YF vaccines are live attenuated viral vaccines from the 17D lineage. YF vaccines are given as a single dose (0.5 mL) and the manufacturers recommend that the vaccine be injected either subcutaneously or intramuscularly.

Healthy individuals rarely fail to develop neutralizing antibodies after vaccination. Clinical trials have found that 80–100% of vaccine recipients develop protective levels of neutralizing antibodies within 10 days and 99% do so within 30 days. Protection appears to last at least 20–35 years and probably for life.

There are three types of serious adverse events following immunization with YF vaccine: (1) Immediate severe hypersensitivity or anaphylactic reactions; (2) YF vaccine-associated neurologic disease (YEL-AND); and (3) YF vaccine-associated viscerotropic disease (YEL-AVD). To date, all reported and published cases of YEL-AND and YEL-AVD have been described in primary vaccines. The reporting rate of YEL-AVD is highest among persons aged ≥70 years but also higher in people aged ≥60 years.

WHO Position

Yellow fever vaccination is performed to:
- Protect populations living in areas subject to endemic and epidemic disease;
- Protect travelers visiting these areas;
- Prevent international spread by viremic travelers.

A single dose of YF vaccine is sufficient to confer sustained life-long protective immunity against YF disease. A booster dose is not necessary.

Endemic Countries

- Endemic countries should introduce YF vaccine into their routine immunization programs, giving it to children at age 9–12 months at the same time as the measles vaccine.

- Preventive mass vaccination campaigns are recommended where vaccination coverage is low.
- Vaccination should be provided to everyone aged ≥9 months in any area with reported cases.
- Countries with *areas* at-risk of YF disease should introduce YF vaccine into their immunization programs.

Travelers

Yellow fever vaccine should be offered to all unvaccinated travelers aged >9 months, traveling to and from at-risk areas, unless they belong to groups for whom it is contraindicated.

HIV-infected Individuals

- Yellow fever vaccine may be offered to asymptomatic HIV-infected persons with CD4 T-cell counts ≥200 cells/mm^3.
- Yellow fever vaccine may be administered to all clinically well children—HIV testing is not required.

Pregnant Women

A risk-benefit assessment should be undertaken for all pregnant and lactating women noting that:
- In YF endemic areas, or during outbreaks, the benefits of YF vaccination are likely to far outweigh the risk of potential transmission of vaccine virus to the fetus or infant.
- Pregnant women and nursing mothers should be counseled on the potential benefits and risks of vaccination, noting that the benefits of breastfeeding far outweigh alternatives.
- Vaccination is recommended, if indicated, for pregnant or breastfeeding women traveling to endemic areas when such travel cannot be avoided or postponed.

Contraindications

- Yellow fever vaccine is contraindicated in children aged <6 months. It is not recommended for those aged 6–8 months, *except* during epidemics.
- Severe hypersensitivity to egg antigens.
- Severe immunodeficiency such as primary immunodeficiencies, thymus disorder, symptomatic HIV infection or CD4 T-cell values <200 per mm^3, malignant neoplasm treated with chemotherapy, recent hematopoietic stem cell

transplantation, drugs with known immunosuppressive or immunomodulatory properties, and current or recent radiation therapies.

Precautions

Individuals aged over 60 years: The overall risk of adverse effects is higher in primary vaccinees ≥60 years of age, but remains low. A risk benefit assessment should be performed, taking into consideration the following:
- The risk of acquiring YF disease (e.g. location, season, duration of exposure, occupational and recreational activities, and local rate of virus transmission in the potential area of exposure).
- The risk of a potential adverse event following immunization (e.g. age, underlying medical conditions, and medications being taken).

Co-administration

- Yellow fever vaccine may be administered simultaneously with other vaccines.
- Oral polio vaccine may be given at any time in relation to YF vaccination.

Surveillance

- Yellow fever control strategies should include sound epidemiologic surveillance, supported by appropriate diagnostic facilities, for both YF disease and adverse events following immunization.
- Surveillance and clinical studies should be used to identify specific risk groups (such as infants or HIV-infected patients) that may benefit from a second or booster dose.

Research Priorities

- Additional data is needed on YF vaccine safety and immunogenicity including persistence of immunity in HIV-positive adults and children.
- Well-designed and adequately-powered studies are needed to assess co-administration of YF vaccine with other live vaccines, including MMR, and to assess the safety and immunogenicity of YF vaccine in pregnant women and in people aged ≥60 years.

WHO POSITION PAPER ON RABIES VACCINES AND IMMUNOGLOBULINS: APRIL, 2018

The April, 2018 position paper replaces the 2010, WHO position paper on rabies vaccines. It presents new evidence in the field of rabies and the use of rabies vaccines, focusing on programmatic feasibility, simplification of vaccination schedules and improved cost-effectiveness.

The recommendations concern the two main immunization strategies, namely vaccination for post-exposure prophylaxis (PEP) and vaccination for pre-exposure prophylaxis (PrEP) **(Fig. 12.1)**. The following sections summarize the main points of the updated WHO position as endorsed by the Strategic Advisory Group of Experts (SAGE) on immunization at its meeting in October, 2017.

Background

Rabies is a viral zoonotic disease responsible for an estimated 59,000 human deaths and over 3.7 million disability-adjusted life years (DALYs) lost every year. Rabies is almost invariably fatal once clinical signs occur, as a result of acute progressive encephalitis. Rabies occurs mainly in underserved populations,

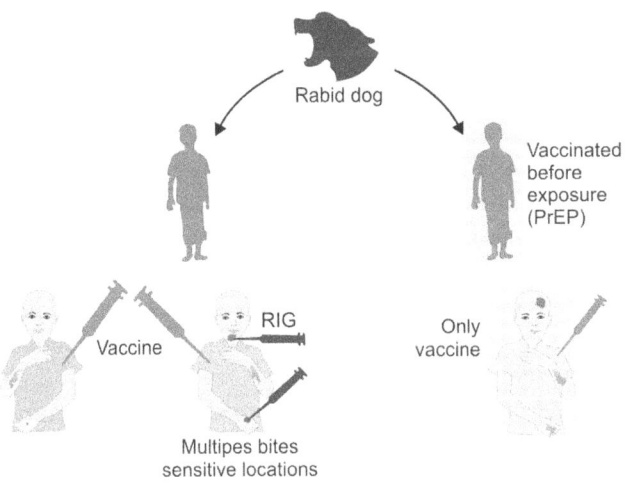

Fig. 12.1: WHO recommends two main immunization strategies for the prevention of human rabies: post-exposure prophylaxis (PEP) and pre-exposure prophylaxis (PrEP).

both rural and urban. Most cases occur in Africa and Asia, with approximately 40% of cases in children aged <15 years. Mass vaccination campaigns targeting dogs is the principal strategy for rabies control by interrupting rabies virus (RABV) transmission between dogs and reducing transmission to humans and other mammals. Human-to-human transmission of rabies has never been confirmed, except extremely rarely as a result of infected tissue and organ transplantation. The primary diagnosis of rabies relies on clinical presentation and history of exposure to a suspect rabid animal or RABV.

Rabies vaccines can be administered by two different routes, ID or IM, and according to different schedules.

WHO Position

Administration of Rabies Vaccines

For both PEP and PrEP, vaccines can be administered by either the ID or IM route. For all age groups ID injection sites are the deltoid region and either the anterolateral thigh or suprascapular regions. The recommended site for IM administration is the deltoid area of the arm for adults and children aged ≥2 years, and the anterolateral area of the thigh for children aged <2 years. Rabies vaccine should not be administered IM in the gluteal area. One ID dose is 0.1 mL of vaccine and one IM dose is an entire vial of vaccine, irrespective of the vial size.

Post-exposure Prophylaxis

Post-exposure prophylaxis consists of the following steps:
- All bite wounds, scratches and RABV-exposure sites should be attended to as soon as possible after the exposure; thorough washing and flushing of the wound for approximately 15 minutes, with soap or detergent and copious amounts of water, is required. Where available, an iodine-containing, or similarly viricidal, topical preparation should be applied to the wound.
- A series of rabies vaccine injections should be administered promptly after an exposure.
- RIG should be administered for severe category III exposures. Wounds that require suturing should be sutured loosely and only after RIG infiltration into the wound.

Table 12.1: PEP recommendations by category of exposure.

	Category I exposure	Category II exposure	Category III exposure
Immunologically naive individuals of all age groups	Wash exposed skin surfaces No PEP required	*Wound washing and immediate vaccination:* • 2-sites ID on days 0, 3 and 7, or • 1-site IM on days 0, 3, 7 and between day 14 and 28, or • 2-sites IM on days 0 and 1-site IM on days 7 and 21 RIG is not indicated	*Wound washing and immediate vaccination:* • 2-sites ID on days 0, 3 and 7, or • 1-site IM on days 0, 3, 7 and between day 14 and 28, or • 2-sites IM on days 0 and 1-site IM on days 7 and 21 RIG administration is recommended
Previously immunized individuals of all age groups	Wash exposed skin surfaces No PEP required	*Wound washing and immediate vaccination:** • 1-site ID on days 0 and 3, or • At 4-sites ID on day 0, or • At 1-site IM on days 0 and 3 RIG is not indicated	*Wound washing and immediate vaccination:** • 1-site ID on days 0 and 3, or • At 4-sites ID on day 0, or • At 1-site IM on days 0 and 3 RIG is not indicated

*Except if complete PEP already received within <3 months previously.

WHO recommends PEP for category II and III exposures **(Table 12.1)**.

The WHO rabies exposure categories are:
- *Category I:* Touching or feeding animals, animal licks on intact skin (no exposure);
- *Category II:* Nibbling of uncovered skin, minor scratches or abrasions without bleeding (exposure);
- *Category III:* Single or multiple transdermal bites or scratches, contamination of mucous membrane or broken skin with saliva from animal licks, exposures due to direct contact with bats (severe exposure).

Intradermal PEP schedules are cost- and dose-sparing and cost-effectiveness increases with numbers of patients seen in clinics. If a repeat exposure occurs within 3 months of completion of PEP, only wound treatment is required, neither vaccine nor RIG are needed.

Changes in rabies vaccine product and/or the route of administration during the same PEP course are acceptable, if unavoidable, to ensure PEP course completion. Should a vaccine dose be delayed for any reason, the PEP schedule should be resumed (not restarted). Individuals with documented immunodeficiency should be evaluated on a case-by-case basis and receive a complete course of ID or IM PEP, including RIG.

Rabies immunoglobulin administration (RIG): RIG provides passive immunization and is administered only once, as soon as possible after the initiation of PEP and not beyond day 7 after the first dose of vaccine. Correctly administered, RIG neutralizes the virus at the wound site within a few hours.

eRIG is less costly than hRIG, both have shown similar clinical outcomes in preventing rabies. As eRIG products are now highly purified, skin testing before administration is unnecessary and should be abandoned.

To confer the maximum public health benefit, WHO recommends the following:

- The maximum dose is 20 IU (hRIG) and 40 IU (eRIG) per kg body weight. There is no minimum dose.
- Infiltrate as much as possible into the wound; the remainder of the calculated dose of RIG does not need to be injected IM at a distance from the wound but can be fractionated in smaller, individual syringes to be used for other patients, aseptic retention given.

If RIG is not available, thorough, prompt wound washing, together with immediate administration of the first vaccine dose, followed by a complete course of rabies vaccine, is highly effective in preventing rabies. Vaccines should never be withheld, regardless of the availability of RIG.

If a limited amount of RIG is available, RIG allocation should be prioritized for exposed patients based on the following criteria—multiple bites, deep wounds, bites to highly innervated parts of the body (such as head, neck, and hands), severe immunodeficiency, the biting animal is a confirmed or probable rabies case, and bites, scratches or exposures of mucous membranes caused by a bat.

Pre-exposure Prophylaxis

Pre-exposure prophylaxis is the administration of several doses of rabies vaccine before exposure to RABV. PrEP is recommended for individuals at higher risk due to occupation. PrEP should be considered in sub-populations living in remote, rabies endemic areas, where access to PEP is difficult, the dog bite incidence is >5% per year or vampire bat rabies is known to be present.

The immune response to subsequent rabies vaccine boosters such as PEP when exposed, can be recalled very effectively even decades after PrEP.

For immunologically naive individuals of all age groups WHO recommends the following PrEP schedules: a 2 sites ID or a 1-site IM vaccine administration on days 0 and 7.

A routine PrEP booster or serology for neutralizing antibody titers is recommended only if a continued, high risk of rabies exposure remains.

Individuals with documented immunodeficiency should be evaluated on a case-by-case basis and best receive an ID or IM PrEP schedule as above, plus a third vaccine administration between days 21 and 28. Additionally, in the event of an exposure, a complete PEP course, including RIG, is recommended.

WHO POSITION PAPER ON VACCINES AGAINST JAPANESE ENCEPHALITIS

Background

This 2015 updated position paper on Japanese encephalitis (JE) vaccines replaces the 2006, JE position paper; it focuses on new information concerning the availability, safety, immunogenicity, and effectiveness of JE vaccines and the duration of protection they confer.

Japanese encephalitis is a vector-borne zoonotic viral disease. JE virus (JEV) is the leading cause of viral encephalitis in Asia. Currently, an estimated three billion people live in the 24 countries, mainly in the WHO South-East Asia and

Western Pacific Regions, considered at risk of JE. It is estimated that 67,900 severe clinical cases of JE occur annually despite widespread availability of vaccine, with approximately 13,600–20,400 deaths. There is no specific antiviral treatment for JE. Most JEV infections are asymptomatic, and severe disease is estimated to occur in about one case per 250 JEV infections. While traditionally considered a childhood disease, JE can occur at all ages.

JE vaccines fall into four classes—(1) inactivated mouse brain-derived vaccines, (2) inactivated Vero cell-derived vaccines, (3) live-attenuated vaccines, and (4) live-recombinant (chimeric) vaccines. Protection against JEV is associated with the presence of sufficient levels of neutralizing antibodies. The accepted immunological surrogate of protection is a serum neutralizing antibody titer of at least 1:10 as determined in a 50% plaque reduction neutralization assay (PRNT50). The available evidence demonstrates that all four classes of vaccines elicit protective levels of neutralizing antibody. Vaccine effectiveness data for live attenuated vaccine suggest over 95% effectiveness five years postvaccination. The WHO Global Advisory Committee on Vaccine Safety (GACVS) has reviewed data on two inactivated Vero cell-derived vaccines, the live-attenuated vaccine and the live recombinant vaccine, and all were found to have acceptable safety profiles. Available data do not raise concerns for those previously vaccinated with mouse brain-derived vaccine subsequently receiving any of the three newer JE vaccines.

Data on the population impact of vaccination programs show significant reductions in JE cases. When high coverage is achieved and sustained in populations at risk of disease, JE in humans can be virtually eliminated while the virus remains in circulation in animal reservoirs. It has been demonstrated that a variety of JE vaccination strategies are cost-effective or highly cost-effective.

WHO Position

JE vaccination should be integrated into national immunization schedules in all areas where JE is recognized as a public health priority. Even if the number of JE-confirmed cases is low, vaccination should be considered where there is a suitable environment for JEV transmission. Adjunctive interventions, such as bednets and mosquito control measures, should not divert efforts from childhood JE vaccination.

The most effective immunization strategy in JE endemic settings is a one-time campaign in the primary target population, as defined by local epidemiology (typically children aged <15 years) followed by incorporation of JE vaccine into the routine childhood immunization program. This approach has a greater public health impact than either of these approaches alone, as campaigns rapidly reduce disease incidence in a broader age group of susceptible individuals. Older groups may be considered for vaccination if the disease burden in such groups is sufficiently high.

The following vaccine dosing schedules and ages of administration are recommended:

- *Inactivated vero cell-derived vaccine*: Primary series according to manufacturer's recommendations (these vary by product), generally two doses at 4-week intervals starting the primary series at ≥6 months of age in endemic settings
- *Live-attenuated vaccine:* Single dose administered at ≥8 months of age
- *Live-recombinant vaccine:* Single dose administered at ≥9 months of age

The need for a booster dose in endemic settings has not been clearly established for any of the vaccines listed above. Preferably, inactivated mouse brain-derived vaccines should be replaced by these newer generation JE vaccines.

Despite a lack of comprehensive immunogenicity/ effectiveness and safety data for all possible combinations of JE and other routine vaccines, co-administration for programmatic reasons seems acceptable, even in the context of mass campaigns.

Strengthened surveillance is needed to assess the burden of JE, inform vaccination strategies, identify breakthrough cases, monitor vaccine safety, and monitor the impact and effectiveness of JE vaccines and assess the potential need for booster doses to close gaps in immunity. All JE-endemic countries are encouraged to carry out at least sentinel surveillance with laboratory confirmation of JE.

Long-term immunogenicity studies are needed to inform optimal dosing schedules for long-term protection, which may vary by location (based on natural boosting or other factors). Vaccine effectiveness and impact studies are also important.

WHO POSITION PAPER ON MENINGOCOCCAL, A CONJUGATE VACCINE: UPDATED GUIDANCE, FEBRUARY, 2015

Background

A position paper on meningococcal vaccines was published in 2011 and its recommendations remain valid. This update adds to the previous recommendations specifically concerning routine immunization of infants and young children in the African meningitis belt with meningococcal A conjugate vaccine.

Since publication of the meningococcal vaccine position paper, preventive mass campaigns in 17 of the 26 countries in the African meningitis belt have been, or are in the process of being, implemented, and over 217 million persons have received monovalent MenA conjugate vaccine. A study in Chad provides evidence of the impact of the MenA conjugate vaccine on the incidence of serogroup A invasive disease and carriage.

Two licensed formulations of the vaccine are available: MenAfriVac, containing 10 μg of purified meningococcal A polysaccharide antigen conjugated with tetanus toxoid (PsA-TT) for use in those aged 1–29 years, and MenAfriVac 5 μg, containing 5 μg of PsA-TT for use in infants and children aged 3–24 months.

Current Evidence on Schedule and Dosing

Two double-blind randomized controlled studies of monovalent MenA conjugate vaccine have been conducted in Ghana and Mali that show that both formulations of MenA conjugate vaccine are immunogenic in a 1-dose schedule for those aged 9–24 months or in a 2-dose schedule for those aged 3–9 months. Duration of protection beyond 27 months after the final dose is unknown.

The reactogenicity profile of MenA conjugate vaccine given concomitantly with routinely administered vaccines was shown to be similar to that of the concomitantly-given routine vaccines alone, with a comparable safety profile. Both clinical studies provide evidence that the two MenAfriVac formulations were well tolerated and safe.

WHO Updated Recommendations

WHO emphasizes the importance of completing mass vaccination campaigns in individuals aged 1-29 years in all countries in the African meningitis belt, and the need to conduct high quality surveillance and vaccine program evaluation in those countries. The following recommendations are additional to those in the 2011 position paper.

WHO recommends that countries completing mass vaccination campaigns introduce meningococcal A conjugate vaccine into the routine childhood immunization program within 1-5 years following campaign completion, along with a one-time catch-up campaign for birth cohorts born since the initial mass vaccination and which would not be within the age range targeted by the routine immunization program. In areas where coverage with meningococcal A conjugate vaccine is less than 60%, periodic campaigns could be considered to complement routine vaccination, as herd protection may not be sufficient to protect those who are not immunized.

WHO recommends a 1-dose schedule with vaccine administration by deep intramuscular injection, preferably in the anterolateral aspect of the thigh at 9-18 months of age based on local programmatic and epidemiologic considerations. Any children who miss vaccination at the recommended age should be vaccinated as soon as possible thereafter. If in a specific context there is a compelling reason to vaccinate infants younger than 9 months, a 2-priming dose infant schedule should be used starting at 3 months of age, with doses at least 8 weeks apart. MenAfriVac 5 µg should be used for routine immunization of those 3-24 months of age. MenAfriVac 10 µg should be used for catch-up and periodic campaigns from 12 months of age onwards unless bridging studies have been conducted and show that MenAfriVac 5 µg can be used in older age groups. The need for a booster dose has not been established.

Data on co-administration with other vaccines has been evaluated and found to be acceptable for diphtheria toxoid, tetanus toxoid, whole cell pertussis, hepatitis B, Hib, oral poliovirus, yellow fever, measles and rubella vaccines. No evidence exists for co-administration with rotavirus vaccine, pneumococcal conjugate vaccine or inactivated polio vaccine; however, absence of data should not discourage coadministration.

Vaccination of pregnant women is safe, as assessed in a well-conducted observational study, and they should be vaccinated if in the age range targeted by the mass vaccination campaigns.

BIBLIOGRAPHY

1. https://www.who.int/immunization/documents/positionpapers/en/ (Accessed on Dec 05, 2019).

ANNEXURES

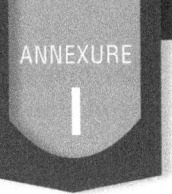

ANNEXURE I

Frequently Asked Questions on Immunization

Alok Gupta, Mohit Vohra

IMMUNIZATION: GENERAL

1. What is the basic difference between immunization and vaccination?

Ans. The Greek word '*immune*' means '*to be protected*'. The process of offering protection to the individual through active or passive method is called 'immunization'. The act of administering the vaccine by the recommended route is known as 'vaccination'.

2. Is the interval of 4 weeks (28 days) mandatory between every immunization contact? Is it correct to give BCG vaccine at 2 weeks followed by OPV/DPT at 6 weeks of age?

Ans. Yes, for vaccines requiring multiple primary doses only (e.g. HB, DPT, OPV and Hib), minimum 4 weeks' interval is mandatory between 1st and 2nd, and 2nd and 3rd doses. For instance, hepatitis B vaccine is recommended within 12 hours after birth to prevent perinatal transmission along with hepatitis B immunoglobulin. BCG vaccine may be given either at birth or anytime within 2 weeks. Thereafter ideally DPT, OPV, Hib, HB, IPV, rotavirus, PCV vaccines can be given at 6, 10, 14 weeks (Rabies vaccine is an exception where 4–5 doses were given in 4 weeks' period).

3. Is local massage indicated at the site of injection in intramuscular (IM), subcutaneous (SC) and intradermal (ID) immunization?

Ans. Make sure that you do not enter a blood vessel, which is very rare if vaccine is administered at the recommended site. A gentle pressure for a few seconds will suffice. Hot or cold-water fomentations are also not advisable. No local massage is needed.

4. (A) How soon can immunization be given after stopping steroid therapy in nephrotic syndrome (or in other

immune-competent children)? and (B) After blood transfusion/whole/partial, how soon immunoglobulins be given?

Ans. (A) Basically, question relates to steroid therapy in various settings (As recommended by Red Book 2018 AAP):

  i. *Topical therapy or local injection of corticosteroids:* Skin ointments or aerosol not contraindication for vaccination. If prolonged application results in immunosuppression, 1-month interval is needed.

  ii. *Physiologic maintenance dose of corticosteroids:* Live as well as other antigens can be safely given.

  iii. High doses of systemic corticosteroids given daily or on alternate days for fewer than 14 days, with the above schedule, can receive live vaccines immediately after stopping treatment. Some experts advocate 2 weeks' interval.

  iv. In the same schedule if given for more than 14 days, an interval of 1 month is desirable for live vaccine administration.

  v. Children with a disease are considered to have a suppressed immune response and who are receiving systemic corticosteroids should not be given live virus vaccines except in special circumstances.

(B) **Table AI.1**, adapted from Redbook 2018 AAP, is self-explanatory.

Suggested intervals between immunoglobulin administration and measles immunization (MMR or monovalent measles vaccine)

Table AI.1: Intervals between immunoglobulin administration and measles immunization.

Indication for immunoglobulin	Route	Dose U or mL	mg, IgG/mg	Interval months
Tetanus (as TIg)	IM	250U	–10	3
Hepatitis A prophylaxis (as Ig), contact prophylaxis	IM	0.02 mL/kg	3.3	3
International travel	IM	0.06 mL/kg	10	3
Hepatitis B prophylaxis (as HBIg)	IM	0.06	10	3

Contd...

Contd...

Indication for immunoglobulin	Route	Dose U or mL	Dose mg, IgG/mg	Interval months
Measles prophylaxis (as Ig) standard	IM	0.25 mL/kg	40	5
Immunocompromised host	IM	0.50 mL/kg	80	6
Varicella prophylaxis (as VZIG)	IM	125 U/10 kg (maximum 625 U)	20–39	5
Blood transfusion				
Washed RBC	IV	10 mL/kg	Negligible	0
RBCs, adenine-saline added	IV	10 mL/kg	10	3
Packed RBCs	IV	10 mL/kg	20–60	5
Whole blood	IV	10 mL/kg	80–100	6
Plasma or platelet products	IV	10 mL/kg	160	7
Replacement (or therapy) of immune deficiencies (as IgIV)	IV		300–400	8
ITP (as IgIV)	IV	—	400	8
RSV-IgIV	IV	—	750	9
ITP	IV	—	1000	10
ITP or Kawasaki disease	IV	—	1600–2000	11

5. Considering that even with live vaccines the immunity lasts for about 20 years, should we give second dose of MMR varicella vaccines in adolescence, if only one dose for these vaccines have been administered in early childhood?

Ans. Yes. The second dose is routinely recommended at 4-6 years of age in children who had already received the first dose at 15 months of age. However, in 'Catchup 'immunization, the second dose can be given at 4-6 weeks' interval also. The second dose thus given offers lifelong protection against all three diseases, viz. measles, mumps and rubella. The current recommendation of IAP is to administer three doses of MMR vaccine is, first dose at 9 months, second dose at 15 months and third dose at 4-6 years. The minimum interval between the 2nd and 3rd dose should be 4 weeks and the second dose should not be given before 12 months of age.

BCG VACCINE

1. If the child does not develop a scar after BCG vaccination what to do?

Ans. Ordinarily, it takes about 10–12 weeks for the scar formation. Non-formation of scar does not mean that BCG has not taken up. In 10–12% of vaccinated infants, scar formation may not take place at all. There are tests to confirm BCG take, viz. lymphocyte migration inhibition test (LMIT), phytohemagglutination assay (PHA), etc. Normally, no test is needed to check BCG take-up.

2. Can we give BCG to HIV infected/AIDS inflicted children or adolescents?

Ans. Yes, in both situations. Though live vaccines are contraindicated in AIDS cases, BCG must be given as TB in a child with AIDS in endemic region is much more dangerous as it has the tendency for multidrug resistance.

3. Do you recommend BCG vaccine after infancy?

Ans. Yes. It can be given up to 5 years of age if not given earlier. Tuberculin testing may be done to rule out any preexisting infection with *Mycobacterium tuberculosis*.

ORAL POLIO VACCINE

1. If an adolescent has not received OPV previously should it be given and what is the schedule?

Ans. In India, the upper limit for OPV is only up to 5 years based on epidemiology of polio incidence. IAP does not recommend adolescent polio immunization. However, it is mandatory for Hajj Pilgrims and all people traveling to or from polio endemic countries as Pakistan and Afghanistan.

2. Will extra doses of OPV given during pulse polio immunization (PPI) harm the child?

Ans. No, the PPI doses are given only with the objective of interrupting the transmission of the wild polio virus. There will not be any immunological overload.

3. Is vaccine associated paralytic polio (VAPP)/Polio cases due to circulating vaccine derived polio viruses (cVDPV) a concern for India?

Ans. No. VAPP has not emerged as a problem in India both in the National Immunization Program and in office practice as thought of initially as a theoretical possibility. However, in some parts of India, polio cases due to circulating vaccine derived poliovirus (cVDPV) have been reported. In 2019 as of 11th December, it is gratifying to note that No cases due to cVDPVs has been reported for the years 2011-19. The last reported cVDPV cases were 15 cases in 2009 and 3 cases in 2010 in few states where tOPV was administered for routine immunization. However, now switch over to bOPV from tOPV is complete and to administer single dose of IPV along with 3rd dose of DTwP, as strategy towards maintaining India 'Polio Free' due to wild/vaccine derived.

4. What is provocative polio?

Ans. In areas endemic for polio, if you give an intramuscular injection including DTP/IPV, etc. during the incubation period, when the child is incubating the polio virus infection, the injection will provoke the onset of muscle paralysis resulting in paralytic poliomyelitis. Hence, IM injections must be strictly avoided especially during spurt/epidemic of polio cases where poliomyelitis is still endemic. Since India has been certified 'Polio Free' in 2014, this will no more be a problem in our country.

5. How to use bOPV and IPV in office practice?

Ans. Due to global shortage of IPV full 0.5 mL IM doses cannot be given as standalone IPV is available in Indian Government Health centers, where fractional IPV (fIPV) 0.1 mL ID is given at 6 and 14 weeks or single 0.5 ml IM dose at 14 weeks. bOPV is given at Birth, 6-10-14 weeks and during 2nd year. In office practice, bOPV is given at birth and then IPV is given as combination vaccines at 6-10-14 weeks and in 2nd year with 1st booster.

HEPATITIS B VACCINE

1. What is the prevalence of hepatitis B in India?

Ans. India falls into intermediate category of HBsAg prevalence with a carrier rate of 4.2%, which means there are an estimated 40 million carriers in India. About 60-70% of acute hepatitis in adults, 20-25% of acute hepatitis in children, 60-70% of chronic hepatitis, 50% of chronic liver disease, 20-30% of cases of fulminant hepatitis and

80% of pediatric cases of primary liver cell carcinoma are due to HBV infection. It is estimated that 20-30% of the total population shows some serological markers of past infection with HBV.

2. What is the natural history of hepatitis B?

Ans. HBV infection in <10yearold child is mostly silent. Younger the age at which the infection occurs, milder is the clinical course. However, the chance of becoming a chronic carrier is higher. If a newborn is infected, he rarely suffers but has 90% chances of becoming a carrier, 25% of the newborn will develop chronic liver disease by the 3rd or 4th decade of life. Some will go on to develop liver carcinoma.

Adults infected with HBV develop acute hepatitis and most of them recover. About 5-10% develop chronic carrier state. Again, of these carriers, 30% will develop chronic liver disease and some will develop carcinoma of liver, 1-2% of patients with HBV infection develop fulminant hepatitis which carries >80% mortality.

3. What are the modes of transmission of HBV?

Ans. Vertical transmission occurs from HBsAg positive pregnant women to their babies during the perinatal period. It mainly occurs due to material blood infecting the baby. The risk of transmission is 30% if the mother is HBeAg negative and 70-90% if HBeAg positive (10% of pregnant mothers who are HBsAg positive are also HBeAg positive in India). Horizontal transmission occurs due to close contact, e.g. amongst family members or at daycare centers, 50-70% of the carrier pool is contributed by horizontal transmission. Parenteral route can also lead to spread via blood and blood products, contaminated needles, surgical instruments, IV drug abuse, tattooing, acupuncture needles, ear piercing, etc. In developed countries, sexual transmission is a common route.

4. What is the dose and schedule of HB immunization?

Ans. Dose depends on the age of the child. For a child <20-year-old, 10 µg/dose is advocated and for a child >20 years, the dose is 20 µg/dose. It is given IM in the anterolateral aspect of thigh, or in the deltoid muscle in older children. Gluteal region should not be used as the muscle mass is large in that area which can lead to poor sero-response.

Schedule consists of giving 3 doses at birth, 6 weeks and 14 weeks. It is preferable to start the vaccination as early as possible within 12 hours of birth, in which case the 2nd dose can be given at 6 weeks along with OPV, DPT, Hib and 3rd dose can be given at 14 weeks, along with OPV DPT Hib vaccines. And 0-1-6 months is the most preferred schedule.

As a routine antenatal screening for HBsAg is advised. If mother is HBsAg positive, the first dose of vaccine should ideally be given within 12 hours of birth along with HBIg. If mother is tested to be HBsAg negative the vaccine can be given at 6, 10, 14 weeks also either as monovalent or in combination formulation.

5. What is the efficacy of HB vaccine?

Ans. The efficacy is excellent. Anti-HBsAg antibody levels of >10 mIU/mL are considered as protective. This is achieved in >95-98% of vaccines after 3 doses. Some workers claim that the protection lasts for a lifetime in most of the vaccines especially when the immunization is started at birth. No further boosters are necessary.

6. What if the child comes late for subsequent doses?

Ans. If the gap between the first and the second dose is less than 6 months and that between 2nd and 3rd dose is less than 1 year, there is no need to restart the course. Instead just complete the remaining doses as per original schedule. However, such delays are not desirable as the child remain unprotected till the course of 3 doses is completed.

7. What about vaccine failure?

Ans. Vaccine failure can occur due to poor storage and poor cold chain maintenance. True vaccine failure occurs in less than 2-3% of vaccinees. It can be due to immune compromised state of the host like patients with leukemia and hemodialysis patients. In such cases using double the dose and additional 1-2 doses may help them. Yet, as low as 25-30% of cases of leukemia have been shown to seroconvert and they may have to be given passive prophylaxis using HBIg. Other reason for vaccine failure is infection with surface mutant strains which will escape neutralization by surface antibody and lead to infection inspite of presence of HBsAg antibodies. Use of preS containing vaccine will help against such infection. Lastly, some patients just do not respond which may be because of Tcell suppression without obvious immune deficiency or they may be harboring low-grade HBV infection which goes undetected before vaccination.

8. How do you manage a newborn to HBsAg positive mother?

Ans. To protect the infant the first dose of vaccine should be given as early as possible after birth (preferably within 12 hours of birth). If affordable and available, HBIg 0.5 mL should be given IM on the other thigh within 6 hours of birth (Do not give HBIg and vaccine on the same site). Vaccination alone will bring down the chances of becoming carrier by 65–90% and if HBIg is also given it will bring it down further by another 5–10%.

9. What about immunocompromised children?

Ans. Children with leukemia, on chemotherapy, multi-transfused thalassemic and patients on hemodialysis have poor seroconversion following conventional schedule. Hence, it is recommended to double the dose of vaccine (i.e. 20 µg <10 years, and 40 µg >10 years). If antibody titers are not satisfactory after 3 doses, additional doses should be given. If still there is no response one can give HBIg passive prophylaxis. If rapid response is necessary one can use 0, 1, 2- and 12-months' schedule.

10. What is the upper age limit for HB vaccination?

Ans. As the risk of horizontal/parenteral route transmission continues throughout life, no age is late for starting HB vaccination. Response to vaccination is low after 4th decade of life. Hence earlier the better.

11. Should HB vaccine be given to a carrier or to a patient who has recovered from HBV infection?

Ans. Neither to the carrier nor to the patient who has recovered need HB vaccine. In fact, a patient of HBV infection develops protective antibodies to surface antigen (anti-HBs) on recovery. There is no risk associated with vaccination, but it becomes a wasted dose.

12. Can you use different HB vaccines interchangeably?

Ans. If there is no other option, yes, they can be interchanged. However, it is not ideal or desirable to do so. With many brands now available, it may be practically difficult, as a patient may go to a different doctor to complete the course and may get a different vaccine.

Frequently Asked Questions on Immunization

13. Can you give HB vaccine along with other vaccines?

Ans. With so many vaccines needed to be given in the first year of life, one must give more than 2 vaccines on the same day to complete all the vaccinations in time. First dose of HB vaccine can be given along with OPV zero dose/BCG. 2nd dose of HB vaccine can be given along with OPV/DPT/Hib at 6 weeks of age and 3rd dose can be given along with DPT vaccine at 14 weeks or at 6 months. The vaccines should be given on the same day but at different site using different syringes and needles.

14. What if the newborn is premature?

Ans. Newborn <2.0 kg, will have lesser seroconversion than a full-term baby. If the mother is known to be HBsAg negative, you can postpone the vaccination. But if the mother is HBsAg positive or if the status is not known, one should give first dose at birth with HBIg on the other thigh which will be mandatory. This can be followed by completion of course using birth, 6- and 14/24-weeks' schedule.

15. Hepatitis B: Pediatric dose is recommended up to 18 years by American Academy of Pediatrics (AAP) in India it is 10 years or 18 years?

Ans. Recombinant HB or Engerix B is the licensed and widely used hepatitis B vaccine in US and as per the manufacturer's recommendation based on follow-up studies the US recommendation is up to 18–20 years.

16. Are booster doses needed anymore for hepatitis B vaccine?

Ans. It has been categorically proved and documented in WHO position paper on HB vaccine recommendations 2000 that if the child responds to 3 primary doses of hepatitis B vaccine given at a minimum interval of 4 weeks and if a virus exposure occurs even after several years and even if the protective level is less, then the memory cells start acting and due to natural boosting raising the protective level for HBsAg antibodies raise to above 10 IU/mL.

17. What are the serious complications of hepatitis B immunization? Who will pay compensation to the adolescent when adverse events occur?

Ans. In the US, anaphylaxis seem to occur in 1 in 6,00,000 recipients. All other complications earlier attributable to HB vaccine have been negated because of lack of evidence for causal link. The question of compensation even for vaccine-associated paralytic polio (VAPP) has not yet been debated in India. Moreover, Government of India has introduced HB vaccine for infants at 0, 6, 10, 14 weeks. Hence, the question of compensation to hepatitis B vaccine does not arise in India. Even ethically outweighing the complications of hepatocellular carcinoma, HB vaccine is considered safe in adolescents also.

18. What advances have occurred in HB vaccine?

Ans. Two advances are of importance. First is the development of better immunogenic vaccine especially the one with the preS component and second is the combination vaccine where HB vaccine is combined with hepatitis A (hepatitis A, B) or with other vaccines such as DTwP/DTaPIPVHibHB combinations, etc. This will bring down the number of injections given to the child and may even reduce the cost.

19. How many doses of HBV can be justified using combination vaccine?

Ans. In case of use of combination vaccines, a total of four doses of HBV are justified.

DTP/DT/TT VACCINES

1. Should Tetanus toxoid (TT) be given frequently following every trauma? Any side effects if given too frequently.

Ans. No. The following table is self-explanatory. Some cases of amyloidosis of liver have been reported following too frequent administrations of tetanus toxoid.

Guide to Tetanus Prophylaxis in Routine Wound Management

History of absorbed Tetanus toxoid (doses)	Clean, minor wounds TT/Td, TIG	All other wounds TT/Td TIG
Unknown or <3	Yes, No	Yes, Yes
>3	No*, No.	No**, No

*Yes, if more than 10 years since last dose.
**Yes, if more than 5 years since last dose.

2. What is the difference between DT/Td vaccines (Dual antigen)—are they the same? For Td vaccines—0.45 mL

of TT + 0.05 mL of DT-will it dilute tetanus toxoid? Should we give dual antigen booster every 10 years in India also?

Ans. Td, Tdap or DT vaccine contains >2 Lf (flocculation units) of diphtheria toxoid per dose compared with 6.7 to 25 Lf per dose of diphtheria toxoid in DTwP. Only standard licensed preparations should be used. No extemporal mixing is permitted. The Td/Tdap vaccine is adult type of diphtheria and tetanus toxoid for maintaining diphtheria immunity whereas DTwP is meant for primary immunization series. Td must be repeated every 10 years to sustain diphtheria and tetanus immunity in adolescents and adults wherever primary immunizations has been done with DTwP or DTaP. All children must receive Tdap at least once after 4–6 year DPT booster followed by Td every 10 years.

3. Can we use DTP HB or DTP monovalent formulation as diluent for dissolving the pellet of the Hib vaccine?

Ans. Yes, provided the manufacture have conducted extensive field trials and obtained certification from Drug Controlling Authority of India or obtained certification from WHO.

4. Which vaccine provides longer protection to a child aP or wP?

Ans. The schedule of IAP provides protection for at least 6 years using wP vaccine whereas using aP vaccine protection may decline before 6 years of age.

For a person aged 7 years only aP containing vaccine should be used. Regular age-specific boosters are a must for continued protection.

5. What is the role of Td/Tdap in routine immunization?

Ans. WHO now recommends Td instead of TT in wound management prophylaxis and prophylaxis against neonatal and maternal tetanus in pregnant women. Td is to be repeated every 10 years only. Unimmunized pregnant women should receive minimum 3 doses of Td at 4–8 weeks' interval as against 2 doses in previously immunized women, with first dose being Tdap preferably. Tdap is given as a single booster at 10 years in regions endemic for adolescent and adult pertussis to affordable beneficiaries.

Hib VACCINE

1. What is the disease spectrum of Hib infection?

Ans. Hib infection usually leads to invasive diseases such as meningitis, epiglottitis, pneumonitis, cellulitis, arthritis, septicemia, etc. Of the invasive *H. influenzae* infections in children, 99% are due to type b and rarely due to type a or other nontypeable *Haemophilus* influenzae organisms. Various studies show that 15–20% of cases of ALRI and 15–25% cases of pyogenic meningitis are due to Hib infection.

2. What is the incidence of Hib in India?

Ans. Exact incidence of Hib in Indian community is not known. Looking at the world experience it is likely to be as high as the other developing countries. There are two problems to our country. First is lack of community-based data and second is lack of laboratory facilities as Hib is a fastidious organism to grow. In a study from Pune, Maharashtra it was shown that protective levels of antiPRP antibodies (>0,15 pg/mL) were present in 20% of children by 1 year of age, 35% by 3 years and 80% by 5 years. It suggests the pattern of natural, clinical or subclinical infection and immunity acquired at different ages. Yet, majority of them are not protected in the early months or years of life.

3. What is the spectrum of non-type B *H. influenzae* infections?

Ans. Non-type B non-capsulated *H. influenzae* infections commonly lead to upper respiratory tract infections, otitis media, respiratory tract infections and other noninvasive infections especially in children >7 years of age.

4. Which age group is affected by Hib infections?

Ans. Hib infection is most seen in children <5 years of age. The mean age of onset is 6–24 months after which it declines gradually till 5 years. Higher the incidence of Hib in community more is the chance of meningitis, less of epiglottitis and earlier is the age of onset. In developed countries, 10% of Hib disease occurs before 6 months of age, 40% by 1 year and 75% by 2 years. In developing countries 45% of total Hib infections occur by 6 months of age and 65–75% by 1 year. This has a bearing on the immunization strategy as earlier stage of onset (like in India), earlier should be the completion of 3 primary closes.

5. What is the severity of Hib infection?

Ans. Hib leads to very severe infections at a very young age. The case fatality rate in developed countries is 2–4% but that in developing countries it is as high as 30–40%. The long-term sequelae are also high with meningitis and epiglottitis. Post-meningitis sequelae are seen in 15–30% of cases in the form of mild sequelae such as deafness or severe sequelae such as blindness or severe neurological damage, etc.

6. What is Hib carrier state?

Ans. Newborns are protected against Hib by maternal antibodies for first few months of life. After that the child encountering Hib develops nasopharyngeal carrier state from where it can spread and lead to invasive Hib disease or spread to other susceptible hosts in community. The carrier state in developed countries is estimated to be 2–3% and in developing countries 5–10%. In daycare centers, it can reach as high as 20–30%. In family contacts of index case, it is 10–12%. After effective immunization, the carrier rate has decreased to 1.5% from 6.0% in some countries.

7. What about drug resistant Hib in India?

Ans. Before 1984, reports suggested almost 100% sensitivity of Hib to common antibiotics. Since then many reports have shown emergence of multidrug resistant strains to the tune of 40–60% of total Hib cases. However, all of them appear to be sensitive to 3rd generation cephalosporins. The drug resistance appears to be mediated by R plasmid.

8. What is the antibody response to Hib vaccine?

Ans. As discussed before, unconjugated PRP vaccine leads to IgM type antiPRP antibody and conjugate vaccine leads to IgG to type antiPRP antibody. These can be detected by Farr type RIA or ELISA.

Anti-PRP antibody levels >0.15 µg/mL are protective against Hib and levels >1.0 µg/mL suggest long-term protection.

9. What is the effect of universal Hib immunization on the community?

Ans. Efficacy of Hib vaccine in reducing Hib infection is >95% with general acceptance of vaccine by >90% of target population. In fact, by decreasing carrier state even unimmunized children are indirectly protected. Many Western countries have shown 99–100% disappearance of invasive Hib disease following mass immunization programs.

10. Are there any Indian studies on efficacy of Hib vaccine?

Ans. Both PRPT and HbOC vaccines have undergone efficacy trials in India. Trials conducted in infants have shown near 100% seroconversion to above protective levels with 98% of vaccines having achieved titers of >1.0 µg/mL after 3 doses.

11. Why is a booster of Hib required?

Ans. As we have seen before, >90% of vaccines achieve a titer of >1.0 µg/mL after 3 primary doses giving long-term protection till 15–18 months of age. In >50% of them, the titer falls to <0.15 µg/mL or the minimum protective level by 18 months. If a booster is given at 15–18 months of age the titer rises by 30–90 fold in all of them and reaches levels as high as 40 µg/mL. Hence, a booster is recommended at 15–18 months of age.

12. Can you use the vaccines interchangeably?

Ans. Studies have shown that sero-response is same when the same vaccine is used all throughout or when they are interchanged to complete the course. In fact, some studies have shown better sero-response using different vaccines one after another. As we saw before PRPOMP leads to protective antibody titer after first dose itself so that protection starts early. This is followed by 2nd and 3rd dose of PRPT/HbOC to lead to better and long-term protection at the end of 3 doses. Hence, these studies recommend using PRPOMP as first dose and PRPT/HbOC for the 2nd and 3rd doses. Again, studies have shown equal if not better response when another vaccine is used as booster as compared to original vaccine used for primary doses. In short, the vaccines can be used interchangeably both for primary as well as booster doses.

13. Can you use other vaccines together with Hib vaccine?

Ans. With need to use many vaccines during early infancy, one must use more than two vaccines together. Hib can be given along with other vaccines such as OPV/ DPT/HBV/ IPV/PCV/RVV at 6, 10 and 14 weeks of age. However, they should be given at different sites and appropriate routes using separate syringes and droppers (oral). Currently combination formulation containing DTwPHBHib (PENTAVAC) is widely practiced in India both in National Immunization Program and in office practice. Some pediatricians prefer to use acellular pertussis component containing combination formulation DTaPHBIPV along with ready to mix Hib component (PENTAXIM) in their office practice.

14. **Is there any recommendation on Hib vaccine for adolescents with asthma?**

Ans. Some practitioners claim that in children immunized with Hib vaccine the wheezing attacks are lesser in frequency and with less severity. However, this observation can be further documented only when more studies are made available with conclusive proof.

MEASLES, MMR VACCINES

1. **Should India adopt 2 doses of MMR schedule like USA? When should the 2nd dose be given?**

Ans. In USA, the 2nd dose of MMR is recommended at 5-6 years or 10-12 years depending on measles epidemiology in a region, since no monovalent Measles vaccine is licensed in USA. However certain universities in USA recommend that 2 doses of MMR vaccine should be given at 4 weeks' interval. In India, in some areas, cases of mumps and rubella due to break through infection have been reported following administration of single dose of MMR vaccines. Moreover, it is global recommendation now that for optimal protection even for measles two doses of measles component containing vaccine formulation like MMR/MR are mandatory. The Indian Academy of Pediatrics (IAP) now recommend 3 doses of MMR vaccine; first dose at 9 months, second dose at 15 months and third dose at 4-6 years. Government of India is introducing MR vaccine along with DTwP booster at 18 months apart from monovalent measles vaccine at 9 months plus in the National Immunization Schedule. In the mean-time, some states in India such as Delhi, Kerala, Tamil Nadu, etc. have already introduced immunization of adolescent girls with MMR vaccine. The National Technical Advisory Group on

Immunization (NTAGI) in 2009 has recommended the inclusion of MR vaccine (measles, rubella) in the National Immunization Program.

2. Why 2 doses are needed for control of measles/mumps/rubella? Will 3 doses of vaccine, viz a monovalent measles vaccine at 9 months followed by trivalent MMR vaccine at 15 month, and 5 years will harm/overload the immune system?

Ans. The second dose in the form of MMR vaccine is considered as an insurance dose for complete protection against measles which will cover about 15% of infants who do not sero-convert after the first dose of monovalent measles vaccine formulation administered at 9 months. For complete protection against mumps and rubella infections, also a second dose of MMR vaccine is mandatory at 4–6 years of age. However, the object of rubella immunization is different, i.e. to control the circulation of rubella virus in the community and thus protecting pregnant women from delivering babies with congenital rubella syndrome (CRS). The 3rd opportunity for measles vaccine as MMR II will not in any way overload the immune system.

3. When 2 doses of MMR are to be given to adolescents what should be the optimum interval?

Ans. A minimum of 4 weeks' interval should suffice.

4. Can MMR and chickenpox vaccines be given at the same time? If not at what interval? Why?

Ans. Yes. MMR and chickenpox vaccines can be given at the same time by subcutaneous route at two different sites. If not given on the same day, minimum 4 weeks' interval is a must, since it is feared that the measles vaccine can suppress the immunogenicity of the varicella vaccine if given at shorter intervals.

5. How to use combined MMR–Varicella vaccine in routine immunization?

Ans. With the recommendation of 3 doses for MMR and 2 doses for varicella vaccines, trivalent MMR vaccine (MMR) at 9 months followed by trivalent MMR + monovalent varicella (MMR+V) vaccines at 15 months and MMRV combo vaccine (MMR tetra) at 4–6 years will be an ideal schedule in office practice. But as the incidence of febrile seizures increases significantly with the MMRV given around 15 months, it is advisable to use this (MMRV) tetravalent vaccine at 4–6 years and avoid using it earlier.

6. Can MMR be given to adolescents if not previously immunized? Do you recommend MMR or rubella vaccine?

Ans. Yes. MMR is the ideal recommendation for both boys and girls. Two doses at 4–8 weeks' interval is presently the IAP's recommendation. It should not be given in pregnancy.

7. Rubella vaccination certificate is insisted by temple authorities at Thiruvannamalai in the famous Lord Shiva Temple (where the Lord is worshiped as AGNI), Tamil Nadu, India for performance of marriage? Why not this be practiced everywhere?

Ans. Yes, it is ideal that throughout the country the temple and school authorities must insist on MMR vaccination certificate (rather than rubella alone) though the vaccine is not included in routine immunization. IAP recommended inclusion of MMR vaccine at 15 months of age in National Immunization Schedule long back. GOI has now decided to include MR vaccine at 18 months of age along with DTP booster. Currently IAP has advanced the age of administration or the 3 doses of MMR vaccine, viz. first dose at 9 months, second dose at 15 months along with first dose of varicella vaccine and third dose of MMR and varicella vaccine at 4–6 years of age.

8. Why a female after MMR vaccine administration should wait for 28 days or more to become pregnant?

Ans. The optimum interval should be 3 months and not 28 days, because of the theoretical risk to the developing fetus (iatrogenic congenital rubella syndrome).

9. Why do American universities require MMR immunization certificate from students coming from India? Is any other vaccination certificate required?

Ans. Because, measles continues to be a problem in adolescents too in some parts of USA along with mumps and rubella infections. Though under control, they can reemerge if an unimmunized Indian/Foreign adolescent contracts the same which may cause epidemiological concern. Some universities also insist complete immunization certificate from birth and some others particularly regarding meningococcal, hepatitis A, Varicella, typhoid vaccines, etc.

10. What is "MR campaign" by Government of India?

Ans. The Measles and Rubella campaign is a public health initiative of the Government of India to eliminate measles by 2020 and control rubella. It targets children from 9 months to 15 years.

TYPHOID VACCINE

1. Why in India typhoid immunization is not given any importance as is given to hepatitis B vaccination?

Ans. World over typhoid vaccine administration is regarded only as an epidemiological need-based vaccine. Even in US and other industrialized countries typhoid vaccination is recommended only in endemic zones or as a traveler vaccine. However, IAP recommends routine typhoid immunization with conjugate or Vi antigen vaccine at the appropriate age.

2. Should typhoid vaccine be given every 3 years as booster?

Ans. A booster dose of Vi vaccine is mandatory every 3 years; however, should be restricted to G boosters only. Recently introduced typhoid conjugate vaccine (TCV) is recommended by IAP to be given at 9–12 months. This will probably protect the individual for life.

3. Can MMR and typhoid conjugate vaccine be given together?

Ans. As per recent recommendations by IAP 2018–2019, MMR and typhoid conjugate vaccine can be given together at the same time. Single dose of typhoid conjugate vaccine of 25 mg is recommended from 6 months onwards.

HEPATITIS A VACCINE

1. For which high-risk groups hepatitis A vaccine is currently recommended?

Ans. At present, we certainly recommend it for the following high-risk groups of patients.
- *Foreign traveler:* Those staying in low endemic areas do not develop natural immunity till adulthood. Such persons when they travel to areas of high endemicity develop hepatitis A, which will be very severe at that age.

If such a person is going to be exposed to risk for <3 months, hepatitis A immunoglobulin (HAIg) can be enough to prevent hepatitis A. If the stay is going to be prolonged it is better to vaccinate them as otherwise, they will need to be given large volumes of HAIg frequently.

If there are <2-4 weeks before departure one will need to use HAIg and first dose of vaccine together so that immediate protection (in 4-5 days) can be started by HAIg and vaccine can take over by 2-4 weeks. If there is >4 weeks available before departure, vaccination will be enough to protect them.

- *Patients with chronic liver disease:* Such patients can develop further liver damage if they develop superadded hepatitis A infection hence, they must be protected by vaccine.
- *During epidemics:* Vaccination by inactivated HAV of all people in an area with epidemic has been found to be nearly 100% effective in containing the epidemics.
- IV drug abusers
- Homo- and bisexual individuals
- Those who have occupation hazards such as staff working in laboratories.
- Potential indications are for those who work in daycare centers or schools or institutions for children, food handlers, health personnel, etc. They are all at high risk of exposure to hepatitis A and hence can be vaccinated.

2. Can hepatitis A vaccine be given along with other vaccines?

Ans. Yes, hepatitis A vaccine can be given along with any other vaccine provided one uses separate syringe and separate sites for different vaccines.

In fact, with more and more vaccines being advocated in first 2 years of life, one must give more than 2-4 vaccines simultaneously with combination vaccines. Once more combination vaccines are available, it will be possible to reduce the number of injections to children. Combination formulation vaccines containing hepatitis A and B vaccine is already available commercially. However, the recent recommendation is to administer hepatitis A vaccine (inactivated) at completion of 12 months of age itself due to waning of maternal antibodies in infants against hepatitis A infection followed by a booster after 6 months. Live-attenuated hepatitis A vaccine needs to be given as single dose subcutaneously after 1 year of age.

VARICELLA VACCINE

1. What is the changing epidemiology of varicella?

Ans. Varicella is a highly contagious disease with 90% secondary case attack rate. It affects almost 100% of population at some time or other during life. So far, chickenpox has been a disease with peak age at 5–9 years, or school-going preadolescent children. In the last 20 years, there has been an increase in cases of chickenpox and a shift of the peak age to older age with majority of cases occurring between 15–24 years. In many countries such as USA, UK, Singapore, as well as developing countries such as Thailand, Philippines and in India too some regions such as Kerala have peak at older age. It is common experience that nurses from Kerala working in other parts of India develop chickenpox as adults.

2. What is the problem of chickenpox occurring in adolescent or adults?

Ans. As compared to children, when adults develop chickenpox, it is more severe. Fever is higher and severity more prolonged. Rash is also more severe. Disease can spread to lungs, liver or CNS. Complications such as pneumonitis, encephalitis are more common in adults than in children.

In fact, chances of pneumonitis are 14% in adults (<10% in children), mortality rate is 25/100,000 as compared to 2/100,000 in children and 8/100,000 in infants <1 year. About 70% of total fatality is contributed by adults (<5% by children). Adults with immunocompromised state have almost 50% chances of mortality (13% in children who are immunocompromised).

Besides increased morbidity and mortality in adults and adolescents, many days of works and school days are lost in addition to cost of healthcare.

3. What about chickenpox in pregnancy?

Ans. It is rare to develop chickenpox during pregnancy as most of the women have had chickenpox as a child or as an adolescent. In fact, the chances are only 5–7/10,000 pregnancies. But once it occurs during pregnancy there are 25% chances of transmission of the virus to fetus. If it occurs in first half of pregnancy, then it will lead to fetal varicella syndrome characterized by scarred skin, limb atrophy, ophthalmic anomalies, etc. If it occurs in 2nd half of pregnancy, the newborn has chances of developing herpes zoster at an early age. If it occurs within 21 days of delivery, there are 25% chances of newborn developing chickenpox. Again, in such cases, if chickenpox occurs in newborn in first five days of life, it is likely to be mild as it means there was enough time for antibodies to develop in mother and some antibodies do pass transplacentally and partially protect the newborn. If the newborn develops chickenpox after 5–6 days, it is likely to be severe with 30% mortality as the newborn is totally unprotected and immunologically naive.

4. What if chickenpox occurs in a child?

Ans. Chickenpox is a benign disease in children. The mortality is 2/100,000 in <1-year infant. Chances of developing complications are rare. Less than 10% develop pneumonia or need hospitalization.

If it occurs in school-going child, it leads to missing school for 1–2 weeks. The parents may need to take leave. It also increases cost of treating the child with symptomatic treatment and acyclovir, if indicated. Further the chickenpox cases are source of infection to unprotected contacts and re-activation in form of Herpes zoster.

5a. Which high-risk group should receive varicella vaccine and why?

Ans. Varicella vaccine is indicated in certain high-risk groups:
- *Immunocompromised host:* Varicella can be very severe in immunocompromised host as seen before. Hence such children, except the ones with severe T cell defects, should be immunized irrespective of age. One needs to give 2 doses of vaccine. Care should be taken

to stop chemotherapy/steroids for at least 2 weeks before and after vaccination or at least for the first dose of vaccination.
- *Adults and adolescents (>13 years old):* Those with no definite history of chickenpox in the past can be assumed to be susceptible, as subclinical cases of varicella are very rare. Such patients have high morbidity and mortality, if they develop chickenpox. Ideally all such adults should be vaccinated but especially the following high-risk groups:
  - Non-pregnant women of child-bearing age.
  - Adults in contact with children who are at high risk of complications of chickenpox, e.g. family members of leukemia child.
  - Those at high-risk of exposure to chickenpox such as teachers of young children, college students, daycare nursery workers, military personnel, etc.
  - Health personnel
  - Persons with chronic heart, lung, liver, kidney diseases, diabetes mellitus, etc.

5b. If so, how many doses and in what schedule?

Ans. A two-dose schedule with first dose at 15 months and 2nd dose at 4–6 years of age are mandatory. For travelers and students travelling abroad for higher studies, where 2 doses of MMR vaccine are required, the first dose can be given on an elected date and the second dose at 4–6 weeks' interval.

6. Is any vaccine available for use commercially?

Ans. Live-attenuated vaccine containing wild Oka strain of virus is available for commercial use in India *(Refer to section on Vaccines)*.

7. What is the efficacy of vaccine?

Ans. Seroconversion is seen in 98.5% of immunocompetent hosts and in 80–90% of immunocompromised hosts. The protective antibodies are formed within 2 weeks after the first dose. There is no cut-off level of antibody titer defined as protective. It has been found effective even as post-exposure vaccine if given 72 hours after exposure/contact with the 'Index case'.

In limited studies done in Japan, the immunity was found to last at least up to 20 years in >95% of vaccines. 2% of vaccines can develop breakthrough varicella at later age which is usually mild with low fever and occasional rash (mean <10-15 vesicles). Studies done in USA have shown the immunity to last for at least 6 years in children and up to 10-13 years in adults.

8. What are the contraindications to varicella vaccine?

Ans. Firstly, it is not indicated in those who have definite history of chickenpox in the past. It is contraindicated in patients with neomycin hypersensitivity as the vaccine contains traces of neomycin. It is contraindicated in patients with immunodeficiency including HIV and severe T-cell deficiency with absolute lymphocyte count less than 1200 and in children with acute leukemia on chemotherapy. For patients undergoing chemotherapy for leukemia, vaccination is advocated 3 months after cessation of chemotherapy during remission. Similarly, patients on steroid therapy should receive the vaccine after 2 weeks of stopping steroids temporarily. Since, it may neutralize the vaccine. In immunocompromised host, it should not be given simultaneously with any other live vaccine. It is contraindicated during pregnancy and in fact pregnancy should be avoided for at least 6-8 weeks after vaccination.

PNEUMOCOCCAL VACCINE

1. In sickle cell anemia, are only 2 doses of pneumococcal vaccine appropriate or should the vaccine be repeated every 3-5 years? What is the schedule for routine immunization?

Ans. In countries where, pneumococcal vaccine is recommended routinely, a 3-dose schedule is practiced at 2, 4, 6 months followed by a booster at 18-24 months. However, in case of sickle cell disease/functional or anatomical asplenia, conditions associated with rapid antibody decline following initial immunization, such as nephrotic syndrome, renal failure or transplantation or suffering from HIV infections or other conditions associated with immunosuppression including malignant neoplasm (e.g. leukemia, lymphoma and Hodgkin's disease) reimmunization is recommended for children in '2 to 10 years' age group. For children, younger than 10 years reimmunization is recommended every 3–5 years. For older children 5 or more years and adults reimmunization once only is recommended with 23 valent polysaccharide vaccine.

2. **Pneumococcal meningitis is not uncommon. Should pneumococcal vaccine be advocated routinely or still in special circumstances only? Is currently available vaccine suitable for India?**

Ans. The pneumococcal PCV13/PCV10 valent conjugated pneumococcal infant formulation is recommended for routine immunization. The PPSV23 formulation is recommended for adults and high-risk group children. The 10 valent and the 13 valent PCVs now available in India will offer protection against 75% of serotypes contained in these vaccine formulations. Regional serotype prevalence may be considered prior to choosing a vaccine formulation. PCV13 having additional serotypes, has more protective efficacy than PCV10.

3. **What is the schedule of PCV introduced by Government of India in NIP?**

Ans. PCV will be administered in three doses 2 primary and I booster at 6 weeks and 14 weeks and 9 months of age as a part of routine vaccination.

ROTAVIRUS VACCINES

1. **Do we need to give rotavirus vaccine routinely? If so which vaccine monovalent formulation?**

Ans. Routine rotavirus vaccine in now advocated by ACIP/AAP/IAP with the currently available monovalent/ pentavalent rotavirus vaccine without fear of intussusceptions in a two/three-dose schedule if dose at 6 weeks and 2nd/3rd dose before 32 weeks of birth at an interval of 4–8 weeks. Few cases of intussusception have been reported in India even with the currently available Rotavirus vaccines and such cases should be managed in tertiary care hospitals and promptly reported to the local health authority and the vaccine manufacturer concerned. Indian RVV 116E neonatal human monovalent vaccine has now been introduced with equal or better efficacy than the existing foreign brands. RVV is now a part of NIP.

2. In case of Rotavirus vaccine which schedule is to be used—2 dose schedule or 3 dose schedule?

Ans. RV1 Rotavirus vaccine (Rotarix) only can be used in 6- and 10-weeks schedule. In rest of the RVV 3 dose schedule is recommended.

HPV VACCINES

1. What is the role of HPV vaccine in adolescent girls and women aged up to 45 years?

Ans. The HPV vaccine is found to be safe and effective against cervical cancer. Hence, it should be given as early as 9 years of age before sexual activity is established since sexual exposure can cause microepithelial abrasion in vaginal epithelium favoring human papilloma virus infection which produces 'cervical intraepithelial neoplasia' (CIN). There are 3 stages, viz. CIN1, CIN2 and CIN3. CIN3 is considered as precancerous stage and hence vaccination should be given before this stage. CIN3 is demonstrable by PAP smear. Long term efficacy trials are now available. As of now no booster dose is recommended after primary vaccination series. The bivalent vaccine is given in 0, 1- and 6-months' schedule, and the tetravalent vaccine is given in the 026 months' schedule.

Whereas the bivalent vaccine protects against cervical cancer the tetravalent vaccine offers additional protection against cervical warts and cervical dystocia. IAP now recommends ONLY 2 doses (0-6 months) of either vaccine formulation for adolescent girls aged 9-14 years. However, for older girls and women the 3-dose schedule is mandatory.

2. Is HPV vaccine recommended for boys also?

Ans. Yes. HPV vaccine is recommended in boys also as they too can suffer from HPV infections and cancers other than cervical cancers. Boys homosexual, bisexual are a source of infections to others contacts.

RABIES VACCINES

1. What are recent changes or update about rabies vaccine?

Ans. IAP endorses administration of 4 dose schedule of Rabies vaccine recommended by WHO 2018 for post-exposure prophylaxis. It also endorses the use of monoclonal antibody as an alternative to Rabies immunoglobulin for category 3 bites.

AEFI GUIDELINES

1. What are the latest guidelines by DGHS on reporting of AEFI?

Ans. *National AEFI Guidelines in India:* There are two sets of national guidelines available in India. The detailed version is called 'Operational Guidelines', and a shorter version is for 'Standard Operating Procedures'. These guidelines, based upon World Health Organization suggested framework, were developed through a consultative process with various stakeholders, including various Government departments involved in immunization program, state government program managers, academic institutions, independent subject experts, Drug Controller General of India (DCGI) officials, development partners, etc.

The AEFI reactions can broadly be classified as 'serious AEFIs' (death, disability, cluster and hospitalization) which need to be reported immediately and investigated as per the laid down procedures. The other, i.e. 'minor AEFIs' are reported through monthly reporting systems in UIP in Government of India. For the programmatic purpose, the AEFIs are classified in five broad categories of programmatic error, vaccine reaction, injection reactions, coincidental, and unknown.

Frequently Asked Questions on Immunization

AEFI Reporting Form

Section A (To be submitted by MO within 24 hours of case notification to DIO)

State	District
Block/ward	Village/urban area

Name of reporting MO (person filling this form):

Today's date:

Posted at: Designation:

Time of preparing this form: a.m./p.m.

Contact phone number:
email:

Date case visited and examined/interviewed: __/__/____

Notified by (name): Designation (please circle): health worker/government doctor/private practitioner/community/media/others (specify)

Date notified to MO: __/__/____

Patient's name

Date of birth DD/MM/YYYY   **Age** (in months): _____ months   **Sex** Male Female

Mother's name
Father's name

Complete address of the case with landmarks *(street name, house number, village, block, tehsil, pin no., telephone no.)*

P i n -   P h o n e -

Date of vaccination: __/__/____
Time of vaccination: __:__ a.m./p.m.

Address of session site:

Session: Routine (including SIW)*
Campaign (SIA)-IPPI/MR/JE/others (specify): _____
Other _____

Place of vaccination: govt health facility/outreach/private health facility/others ____

Names of vaccines received (write vaccine & diluent details in separate rows)	Dose no. (zero/first/second/etc. as applicable)	Name of manufacturer	Batch/lot No.	Expiry date	Date of opening of vial	Time of opening the vial (for reconstituted vaccine)	No. of OTHER beneficiaries who received vaccine from the SAME vial in this session

Date of first symptom		Time of first symptom
Hospitalization: No/yes – (Date)		Time of hospitalization

Name and address of hospital (if hospitalized):

*Special immunization week

Current status (encircle)	Death/still hospitalized/recovered & discharged with sequelae/recovered completely and discharged/left against medical advice (LAMA)/not hospitalized
If died, date of death	Time of death
Post mortem done? Yes/no/unknown If yes, then write date post mortem done	If not done, but planned, write date planned

Describe AEFI (signs and symptoms):

Suspected adverse event(s) (tick at least one):
- [ ] Severe local reaction
  - >3 days
  - beyond nearest joint
- [ ] Seizure
  - febrile
  - afebrile
- [ ] Abscess [ ] Sepsis [ ] Encephalopathy [ ] Toxic shock syndrome [ ] Thrombocytopenia [ ] Anaphylaxis [ ] Intussusception
- [ ] Fever≥39 °C (102 °F) [ ] Hypotonic hyporesponsive episode (HHE) [ ] Acute flaccid paralysis [ ] Sudden unexplained death syndrome
- [ ] Death due to any reason other than above – specify..........
- [ ] Hospitalization due to any reason other than above – specify.......... [ ] Disability
- [ ] Cluster – is this case part of a cluster? Yes/no/unknown
  If Yes, no of other cases in the cluster _____ (use separate form for each case in a cluster)

Signature and name of reporting medical officer:

BIBLIOGRAPHY

1. Bhave SY, Parthasarathy A. Yadav S. EPI, non-EPI vaccines. In: A Ready Reckoner for Vaccinations Adult, Adolescent and Pediatric. Swati Y Bhave, Parthasarathy A, Sangeeta Yadav (Eds). Jaypee Brothers Medical Publishers: New Delhi, 2009.
2. Centers for Disease Control and Prevention: Epidemiology and Prevention of Vaccine Preventable Diseases. Atkinson W, Wolfe S, Hamborsky J, McIntyre L (Eds), 11th edn. Washington DC: Public Health Foundation, 2009.
3. Newer vaccines your questions answered: In: Shah N, Parthasarathy A (Eds). Proceedings of the Dialogue session on "Newer Vaccines" Pedicon, IAP. Kochi; 1998:3.5
4. Vashistha V, Choudhury P, Bansal CP, Yewale VN, Agrawal R (Eds). IAP Guide Book on Immunization. Jaypee Brothers Medical Publishers: New Delhi, 2013-2014.

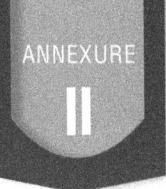

ANNEXURE II

Immunization Websites

Alok Gupta, Mohit Vohra

In these days of Internet' era several immunization resources are available is the internet with easy access both for parents and doctors. However, proper interpretation is mandatory before adapting childhood and adolescent immunization practices. A few of them are indicated below:

1. Indian Academy of Pediatrics (IAP): ***www.iapindia.org***
2. American Academy of Pediatrics: *www.aap.org*
3. Free Medical Journals: *www.freemedicaljournals.com*
4. Global Alliance for Vaccines and Immunization: *www.vaccinealliance.org*
5. Immunization Action Coalition: *www.immunize.org*
6. John Hopkins University: *www.jhuccp.org/mmc/immune*
7. Injection Safety: *http://www.injectionsafety.org*
8. International Vaccine Institute: *www.ivi.org*
9. MD Consult: *www.mdconsult.com*
10. Medscenic Mail: *www.medscenic.de/cgibin/biomail/users.pl*
11. National Network for Immunization Information: *http//www.immunizationinfo.org*
12. National Polio Surveillance Project (NPSP): *www.npspindia.org*
13. Polio Eradication: *www.polioeradication.org*
14. New Vaccines: *www.cdc.gov/nip.newrac.htm*
15. The Vaccine Page: *www.vaccines.org*
16. United Nations Children's Fund (UNICEF): *www.unicef.org*
17. Vaccine Adverse Event Reporting System: *www.vaers.org*
18. Vaccines for Children in Rich and Poor Countries: *www.thelancet.com/newlancet/reg/supplements/vol35452/article2.html*
19. Vaccine weekly: *www.newsfile.com/072699vs.htm*
20. World Health Organization (WHO): *www.who.int/vaccines*
21. NLMNIH Clinical trials: *www.clinicaltrials.gov/www.vrc.nih.gov/VRC*

22. Current Controlled Trials: *www.controlledtrials.com*
23. WHO Vaccine and Biologicals Vaccine Trials: *www.who.int/vaccine_research/trials_database/en/index.htm*
24. International Federation of Pharmaceutical Manufacturers and Associations (IFPMA) Clinical Trials Portal: *www.ifpma.org/clinicaltrials*
25. Albert B. Sabin Vaccine Institute: *www.sabin.org*
26. Vaccine: *www.elsevier.com/locate/issn/0264410X*
27. Vaccine Weekly: *www.publist.com/search/show.asp?ISSN=10742921*
28. Immunization Newsbriefs: *www.immunizationinfo.org/newsbriefs/index.cfm*
29. American Society for Microbiology: *www.asmusa.org*
30. Infectious Diseases Society of America: *www.idsociety.org*
31. National Foundation for Infectious Diseases: *www.nfid.org*
32. Pediatric Infectious Disease Society: *www.pids.org*
33. Center for Biologics Evaluation and Research: *www.fda.gov/cber/vaccines.htm*
34. Association for Professionals in Infection Control and Epidemiology: *www.apic.org*
35. Vaccine Research Center: *www.niaid.nih.gov/vrc*
36. TB—Aeras Global TB Vaccine Foundation: www.aeras.org/
37. TB Vaccine Fact Sheet: *www.cdc.gov/nchstp/tb/pubs/tbfactsheets/250120.htm*
38. Malaria Vaccine Initiative: *http://malariavaccine.org*
39. AIDS Vaccine advocacy Coalition: *www.avac.org*
40. Viral Hepatitis Prevention Board: *www.vhpb.org*
41. Meningitis Foundation of America: *www.musa.org*
42. Varicella Zoster Virus Research Foundation: *www.vzvfoundation.org*
43. Polio—Global Polio Eradication Initiative: *www.polioeradication.org*
44. Indian Pediatrics: *www.indianpediatrics.net*
45. Indian Journal of Pediatrics (IJP): *www.ijppediatricsindia.in*
46. Indian Journal of Practical Pediatrics (IJPP): *www.ijpp.in*
47. Indian Journal of Medical Research (IJMR): *www.icmr.nic.in/ijmr/ijmr.htm*
48. National Family Health Survey (NFHS): *www.nfhsindia.org*
49. Pediaindia: *www.pediaindia.net*
50. IAP Open Forum: *www.iapindia.org/cfforum*

51. Pediatriconcall: *www.pediatriconcall.coms*
52. Sanofi Aventis: *www.sanofiaventis.com*
53. Chiron Panacea: *www.chiron.com*
54. GlaxoSmithKline (GSK): *www.gskvaccines.com*
55. Merck Vaccine Division: *www.merckvaccines.com*
56. Wyeth-Lederle Vaccines: *www.vaccineworld.com*
57. *https://www.indianpediatrics.net/dec2018*
58. *https://www.cdc.gov/adult*

BIBLIOGRAPHY

1. Immunization resource on the Worldwide: https://www.google.co.in/webhp?sourceid=chrome-instant&ion=1&espv=2&ie=UTF-8#q=immunization (Accessed on Dec, 2016).

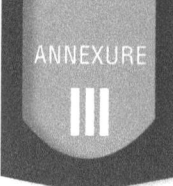

Immunization Techniques

Alok Gupta, Mohit Vohra

IMMUNIZATION TECHNIQUES FOR INTRAMUSCULAR, SUBCUTANEOUS, AND INTRADERMAL INJECTIONS

In this annexure, the correct positioning and injection techniques are depicted. It is imperative that the correct routes of administration of an antigen is adhered to, so that appropriate antibody production is achieved.

Gentle pressure for a few seconds at the site of injection is only needed. Vigorous rubbing should be avoided. Should swelling or redness appear just apply wet cloth soaked in ordinary water potable for a few seconds. No need for cold or hot water fomentation.

Intramuscular Injection

This is one of the most common procedures that any doctor carries out, yet it is surprising how often it is wrongly done.

Usual Sites

- In infants and young children, the best place is the anterolateral aspect of the mid-thigh **(Fig. AIII.1)**.
- The mid-deltoid area is used in children with well-developed muscle mass and who are cooperative.

Method

- Hold the child securely to prevent movement of the extremity.
- Thoroughly cleanse the skin with an antiseptic sponge working circularly from the center outward.
- Allow the wet cleansed skin to dry.
- Hold skin tight and insert needle quickly.

Immunization Techniques 347

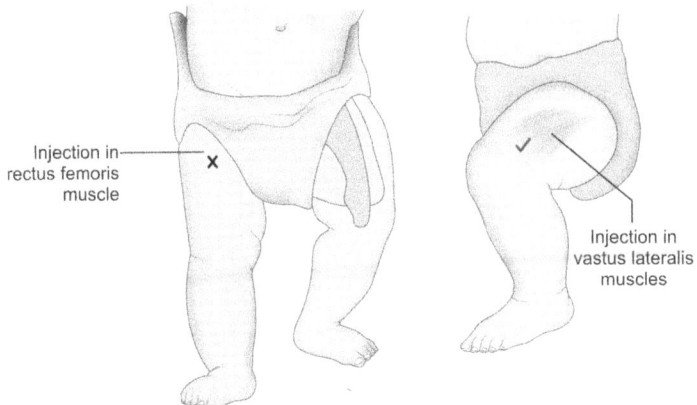

Fig. AIII.1: Site for intramuscular injections in an infant is vastus lateralis and not rectus femoris.

Special Note

- The size of the needle varies with the vaccine to be administered and the age of the child (between 22 and 24 size).
- For all intramuscular (IM) injections in children, the needle should not be more than 1" in length.
- While using the anterolateral aspect of the thigh insert the needle at an angle at 90° for IM injection **(Fig. AIII.2)**.

Subcutaneous Injection

This is a common mode of giving few vaccines such as measles, MMR (measles, mumps, and rubella), and varicella vaccines. It is preferable to use 26G needle is the mid triceps muscle area by pinching the skin fold for subcutaneous injections.

Method

- Clean the area using "appropriate" agent usually an alcohol swab.
- Pinch up the skin fold with your fingers.
- Use only a subcutaneous needle 26G 5/8" size and push it into the skin at an angle of about 45–60° **(Fig. AIII.2)**.

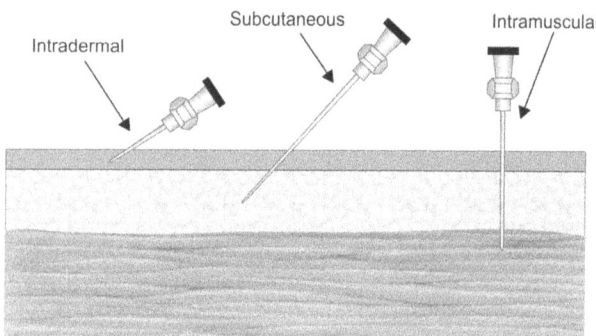

Fig. AIII.2: The position of the needle during the different ways of administering injections.

Special Note

Do not rub vigorously over the injection site.

Intradermal Injection

Intradermal injection is commonly used for giving the BCG vaccine, test dose for drug allergy and for the Mantoux test **(Fig. AIII.2)**.

Method

- Clean the area of the skin appropriately.
- Support the child's arm with your nondominant hand and use the thumb and fingers to encircle the child's arm and to stretch the skin.
- Holding the syringe in your dominant hand almost flat on the child's skin, insert the needle into the skin with the bevel of the needle facing up, taking care that only the needle tip enters the skin.
- Use your nondominant thumb to hold the syringe close to the skin while you inject the material.

Special Note

- Do not rub the site.
- After the injection there must be a clear, flat topped, raised wheal at the site.

ADMINISTERING VACCINES: DOSE, ROUTE, SITE, AND NEEDLE SIZE (TABLE AIII.1)

Table AIII.1: Administering vaccines: Dose, route, site, and needle size.

Vaccines	Dose	Route	Needle size
Diphtheria, tetanus, pertussis (DTaP, DT, Tdap, Td)	0.5 mL	IM	22–23G 1.5"
Haemophilus influenzae type b (Hib)	0.5 mL	IM	"
Hepatitis A (Hep A)	≤18 years: 0.5 mL ≥20 years: 1.0 mL	IM	"
Hepatitis B (Hep B)	≤19 years: 0.5 mL ≥20 years: 1.0 mL		
Human papillomavirus (HPV)	0.5 mL	IM	"
Live-attenuated influenza vaccine (LAIV)	0.2 mL	Intranasal spray	
Trivalent inactivated influenza vaccine (TIV)	6–35 months: 0.25 mL >3 years: 0.5 mL	IM	
Measles, mumps, and rubella (MMR)	0.5 mL	SC	26G 5/8"
Meningococcal conjugate vaccine (MCV)	0.5 mL	IM	23G 11/4"
Meningococcal polysaccharide vaccine (MPSV)	0.5 mL	SC	
Pneumococcal conjugate vaccine (PCV)	0.5 mL	IM	
Pneumococcal polysaccharide vaccine (PPSV)	0.5 mL	IM or SC	
Inactivated polio virus (IPV)	0.5 mL	IM or SC	
Rotavirus (RV)	2.0 mL	Oral	
Varicella (Var)	0.5 mL	SC	
Zoster (Zos)	0.65 mL	SC	
Combination vaccines			
DTaP + Hep B + IPV (Pediarix*) DTap + Hib + IPV (Pentacel*) DTaP + Hib (Trihibit*) DTaP + IPV (Kinrix*) Hib + Hep B (COMVAX*)	0.5 mL	IM	

Contd...

Contd...

Vaccines	Dose	Route	Needle size
MMR + Var (ProQuad*)	≤12 years: 0.5 mL	SC	
Hep A + Hep B (Twinrix*)	≥18 years: 1.0 mL	IM	

Injection site and needle size

Subcutaneous (SC) injection—Use a 26G needle. Choose the injection site that is appropriate to the person's age and body mass

Age	Needle length	Injection site
Infants (1–12 months)	5/8"	Fatty tissue over anterolateral thigh muscle
Children 12 months or older, adolescents, and adults	5/8"	Fatty tissue over anterolateral thigh muscle or fatty tissue over triceps

Intramuscular (IM) injection—Use a 22–25G needle. Choose the injection site and needle length appropriate to the person's age and body mass

Age	Needle length	Injection site
Newborns (1–18 days)	5/8"*	Anterolateral thigh muscle
Infants (1–12 months)	1"	Anterolateral thigh muscle
Toddler (1–2 years)	1–1¼" 5/6–1"	Anterolateral thigh muscle or deltoid muscle of arm
Children and teens (3–18 years)	5/3–1" 1–1¼"	Deltoid muscle of arm or anterolateral thigh muscle

Adult 19 years of older

Male or female less than 130 lbs	5/6–1"	Deltoid muscle of arm
Female: 130–200 lbs *Male:* 130–260 lbs	1–1½"	Deltoid muscle of arm
Female: 200+ lbs *Male:* 260+ lbs	1½"	Deltoid muscle of arm

*A 5/6" needle may be used only if the skin is stretched tight, subcutaneous tissue is not bunched and injection is made at a 90° angle.
Source: Centers for Disease Control and Prevention: Epidemiology and Prevention of Vaccine Preventable Diseases. In: Atkinson W, Wolfe S, Hamborsky J, McIntyre LE (Eds). 11th edition. Washington DC: Public Health Foundation; 2009.

Please note: Always refer to the package insert included with each biologic for complete vaccine administration information.

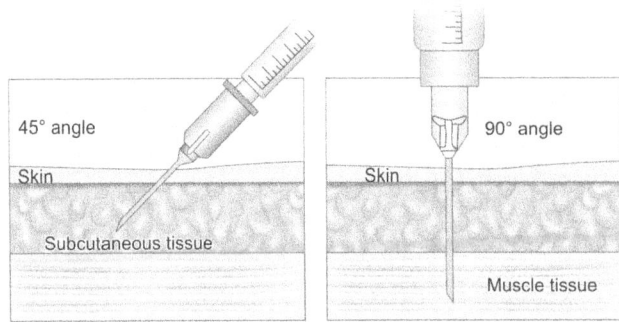

Fig. AIII.3: Angle from skin surface and depth of needle tip inserted for subcutaneous and intramuscular injections.

CDC's (Centers for Disease Control and Prevention) Advisory Committee on Immunization Practices (ACIP) recommendations for the vaccine should be reviewed as well as **Table AIII.2**.

Please note: Always refer to the package insert included with each biologic for complete vaccine administration information. CDC's Advisory Committee on Immunization Practices (ACIP) recommendations for the vaccine should be reviewed as well. Access the ACIP recommendations at www.immunize.org/acip.

- *Subcutaneous (Sub-Q or SC) injections* are administered into the fatty tissue found below the dermis and above muscle tissue.
  - *Site **(Fig. AIII.4)**:* Subcutaneous tissue can be found all over the body. The usual sites for vaccine administration are the thigh (for infants <12 months of age) and the upper outer triceps of the arm (for persons ≥12 months of age). If necessary, the upper outer triceps area can be used to administer subcutaneous injections to infants **(Fig. AIII.5)**.
  - *Needle gauge and length:* 5/8", 23–25G needle.
  - *Technique:*
    - Follow standard medication administration guidelines for site assessment/selection and site preparation.
    - To avoid reaching the muscle, pinch up the fatty tissue, insert the needle at a 45° angle and inject the vaccine into the tissue **(Fig. AIII.6)**.

Table AIII.2: Administering vaccines to adults—dose, route, site, needle size, and preparation.

Vaccine	Dose	Route	Site	Needle size	Vaccine preparation
Tetanus, diphtheria (Td) with pertussis (Tdap)	0.5 mL	IM	Deltoid muscle	22–25G, 1–1½"	Shake vial vigorously to obtain a uniform suspension prior to withdrawing each dose. Whenever solution and container permit, inspect vaccine visually for particulate matter and/or discoloration prior to administration. If problems are noted (e.g. vaccine cannot be resuspended), the vaccine should not be administered.
Hepatitis A (Hep A)	≤18 years: 0.5 mL ≥19 years: 1.0 mL	IM	Deltoid muscle	22–25G, 1–1½"	
Hepatitis B (Hep B)	≤19 years: 0.5 mL ≥20 years: 1.0 mL	IM	Deltoid muscle	22–25G, 1–1½"	
Hep A + Hep B (Twinrix)	≥18 years: 1.0 mL	IM	Deltoid muscle	22–25G, 1–1½"	
Human papillomavirus (HPV)	0.5 mL	IM	Deltoid muscle	22–25G, 1–1½"	
Trivalent inactivated influenza vaccine (TIV)	0.5 mL	IM	Deltoid muscle	22–25G, 1–1½"	
Pneumococcal polysaccharide vaccine (PPSV)	0.5 mL	SC	Fatty tissue over triceps	23–25G, 5/8"	
Meningococcal conjugated vaccine (MCV)	0.5 mL	IM	Deltoid muscle	22–25G, 1–1½"	

Contd...

Contd...

Vaccine	Dose	Route	Site	Needle size	Vaccine preparation
Meningococcal, polysaccharide vaccine (MPSV)	0.5 mL	SC	Fatty tissue over triceps	23–25G, 5/8"	Reconstitute just before using. Use only the diluent supplied with the vaccine. Inject the volume of the diluent shown on the diluent label into the vial of lyophilized vaccine and gently agitate to mix thoroughly. Withdraw the entire contents and administer immediately after reconstitution
Measles, mumps, and rubella (MMR)	0.5 mL	SC	Fatty tissue over triceps	23–25G, 5/8"	Discard single dose MPSV, varicella, and zoster vaccines if not used within 30 minutes after reconstitution
Zoster (Zos)	0.65 mL	SC	Fatty tissue over triceps	23–25G, 5/8"	*Note:* Unused reconstituted MMR vaccine and multidose MPSV vaccine may be stored at 35–46°F (2–8°C) for a limited time. The reconstituted MPSV vaccine must be used within 35 days; the reconstituted MMR vaccine must be used within 8 hours. Do not freeze either reconstituted vaccine
Varicella (VAR)	0.5 mL	SC	Fatty tissue over triceps	23–25G, 5/8"	
Live-attenuated influenza vaccine (LAIV)	0.2 mL (0.1 mL into each nostril	Intranasal spray	Intranasal	NA	Consult package insert

*When giving intramuscular (IM) injections, a ½" needle is sufficient in adults weighting <130 lbs (<60 kg); a 1" needle is sufficient in adults weighting 130–152 lbs (60–70 kg); a 1–1½" needle is recommended in women weighing 152–200 lbs (70–90 kg) and men weighing 152–260 lbs (70–118 kg); a 1.5" needle is recommended in women weighting >200 lbs (>90 kg) or men weighing >260 lbs (>118 kg). A 5/4" (16 mm) needle may be used only if the skin is stretched tight the subcutaneous tissue is not bunched and injection is made at a 90° angle.

Source: Centers for Disease Control and Prevention: Epidemiology and Prevention of Vaccine Preventable Diseases. In: Atkinson W, Wolfe S, Hamborsky J, McIntyre LE (Eds), 11th edition. Washington DC: Public Health Foundation; 2009.

354 Partha's Immunization Digest

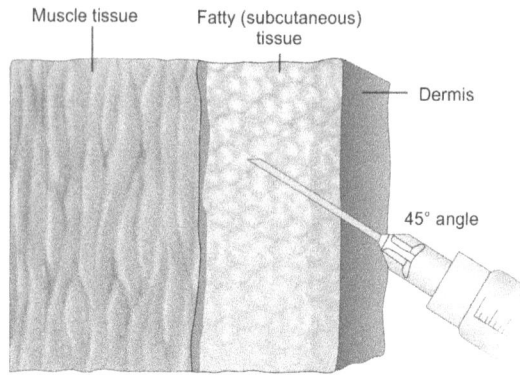

Fig. AIII.4: Subcutaneous injection.

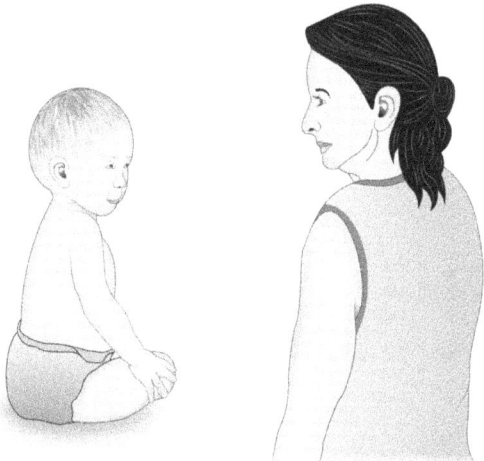

Fig. AIII.5: Arm and thigh are preferred areas for vaccine administration.

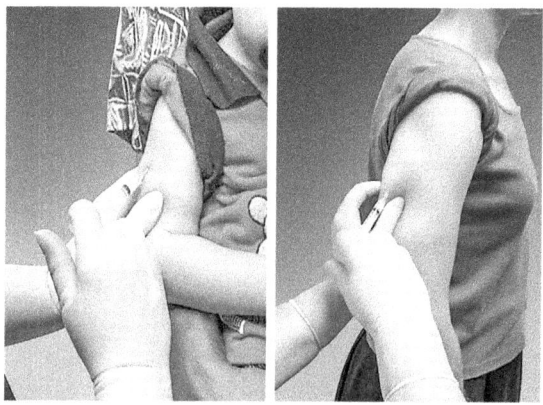

Fig. AIII.6: Subcutaneous administration techniques.

Immunization Techniques

- Withdraw the needle and apply light pressure to the injection site for several seconds with a dry cotton ball or gauze.
- *Intramuscular injections* are administered into muscle tissue below the dermis and subcutaneous tissue.
  - *Site:* Although there are several IM injection sites on the body, the recommended IM sites for vaccine administration are the vastus lateralis muscle (anterolateral thigh) and the deltoid muscle (upper arm). The site depends on the age of the individual and the degree of muscle development.
  - *Vastus lateralis for IM injection* **(Fig. AIII.7):** The vastus lateralis muscle of the upper thigh used for IM injections.
  - *Anatomy of vastus lateralis* **(Fig. AIII.8)**: The vastus lateralis site of the right thigh, used for an IM injection.
  - *Needle gauge:* 22–25G needle.
  - *Needle length:* For all IM injections, the needle should be long enough to reach the muscle mass and prevent vaccine from seeping into subcutaneous tissue, but not so long as to involve underlying nerves, blood vessels, or bone. The vaccinator should be familiar with the anatomy of the area into which the vaccine will be injected **(Fig. AIII.9)**.

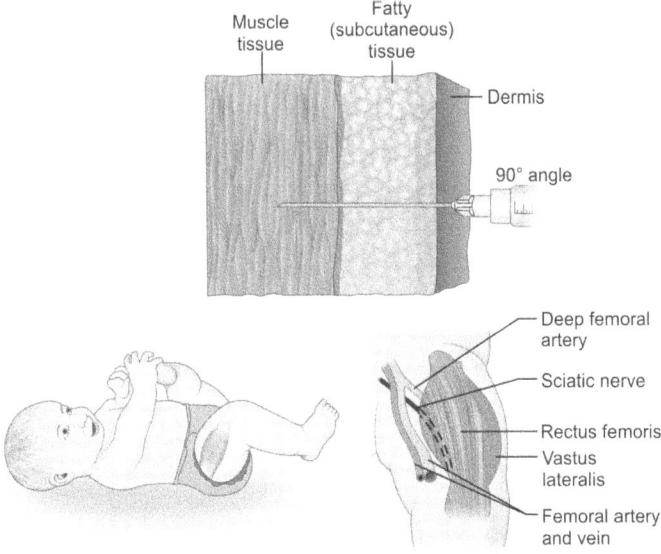

Fig. AIII.7: Vastus lateralis for intramuscular injection.

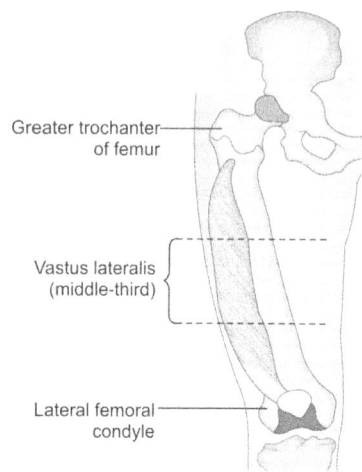

Fig. AIII.8: Anatomy of vastus lateralis.

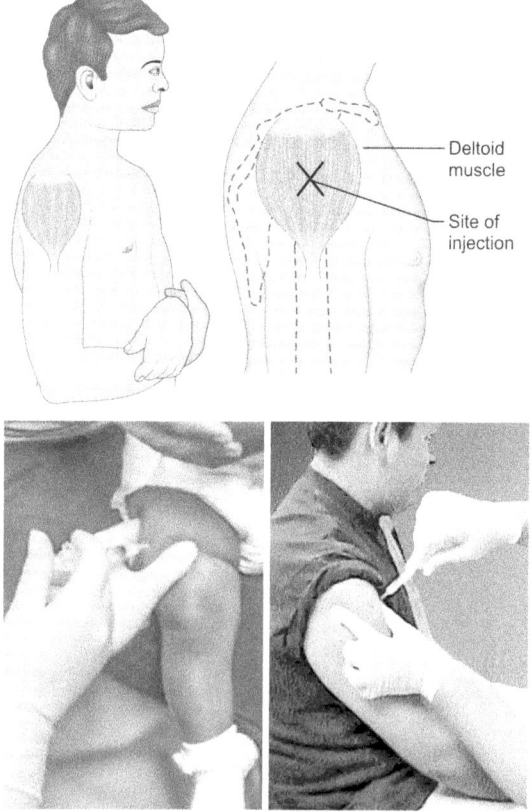

Fig. AIII.9: Intramuscular administration techniques.

Decision on needle size of injection must be made for each person based on the size of the muscle, the thickness of adipose tissue at the injection site, the volume of the materials to be administered, injection technique, and the depth below the muscle surface into which the material is to be injected.

Infants (younger than 12 months): For most infants, the anterolateral aspect of the thigh is the recommended site for injection because it provides a large muscle mass. The muscles of the buttock have not been used for administration of vaccines in infants and children because of concern about potential injury to the sciatic nerve, which is well documented after injection of antimicrobial agents into the buttock. If the gluteal muscle must be used, care should be taken to define the anatomic landmarks.*

Multiple Vaccinations

When administering multiple vaccines, never mix vaccines in the same syringe unless approved for mixing by the manufacturer. If more than one vaccine must be administered in the same limb, the injection sites should be separated by 1-2", so that any local reactions can be differentiated. Vaccine dose ranges from 0.5 mL to 1 mL. The recommended maximum volume of medication for an IM site, varies among references and depends on the muscle mass of the individual. However, administering two IM vaccines into the same muscle would not exceed any suggested volume ranges for either the vastus lateralis or the deltoid muscle in any age group. The option to also administer a subcutaneous vaccine into the same limb, if necessary, is acceptable since a different tissue site is involved.

If a vaccine and an immune globulin preparation are administered simultaneously (e.g. Td/Tdap and tetanus immune globulin (TIG) or hepatitis B vaccine and hepatitis B immune globulin (HBIG), a separate anatomic site should be chosen for each injection. The location of each injection should be documented in the patient's medical record.

---

*If the gluteal muscle is chosen, injection should be administered lateral and superior to a line between the posterior superior iliac spine and the greater trochanter or in the ventrogluteal site, the center of a triangle bounded by the anterior superior iliac spine, the tubercle of the iliac crest, and the upper border of the greater trochanter.

Nonstandard Administration

Nonstandard administration; deviation from the recommended route, site and dosage of vaccine is strongly discouraged and can result in inadequate protection. In situations where nonstandard administration has occurred, refer to the manufacture package inset.

Giving all the Doses Under 12 Months (Figs. AIII.10 and AIII.11)

- *Needle lengths:* IM— 1"; SC— 5/8"
- Using combination vaccines will decrease the number of injections
- IM injections are given in the infant's thigh

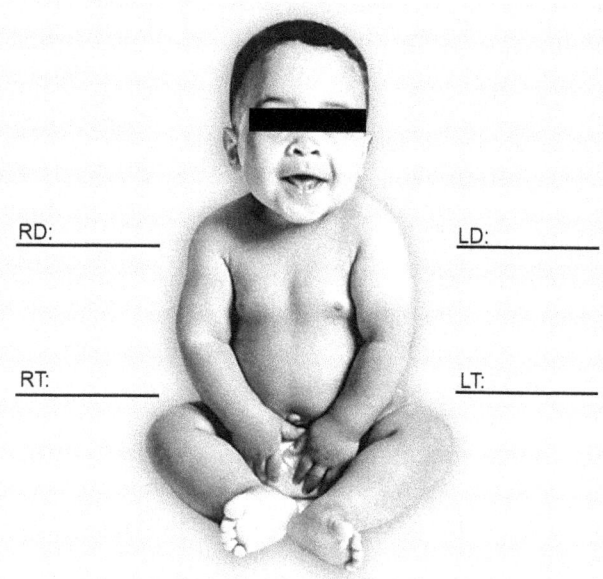

Fig. AIII.10: Suggested sites for infant immunization.
Note: RD: Right deltoid muscle (IM) or subcutaneous tissue on upper arm (SC); *RT*: Right vastus lateralis (IM) or subcutaneous tissue on thigh (SC); *LD*: Left deltoid muscle (IM) or subcutaneous tissue on upper arm (SC); *LT*: Left vastus lateralis (IM) or subcutaneous tissue on thigh (SC).

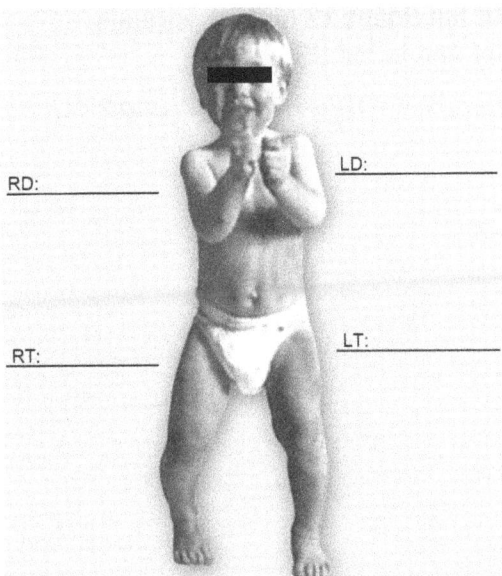

Fig. AIII.11: Suggested sites for toddler immunization.
Note: RD: Right deltoid muscle (IM) or subcutaneous tissue on upper arm (SC); *RT*: Right vastus lateralis (IM) or subcutaneous tissue on thigh (SC); *LD*: Left deltoid muscle (IM) or subcutaneous tissue on upper arm (SC); *LT*: Left vastus lateralis (IM) or subcutaneous tissue on thigh (SC).

- SC injections may be given in the arm or thigh
- Separate injection sites by 1–2".

May consider a 5/8" needle for IM injections only in newborns less than 4 weeks.

Giving All the Doses Under 12 Months and Older Children

- *Needle lengths:* IM— 1–1.5"; SC— 5/8"
- Separate injection sites by 1–2"
- Anterolateral thigh is the preferred site for multiple IM injections.
- Deltoid (upper arm) is an option for IM in children ≥18 months with adequate muscle mass.
- Using combination vaccines will decrease the number of injections needed to keep a child uptodate.
- If recommend so by the manufactures.

Giving All the Doses 12 Months Through 5 Years of Age in the US

Using Pediarix™ (DTPa/Hep B/IPV) and ProQuad® (MMRV)

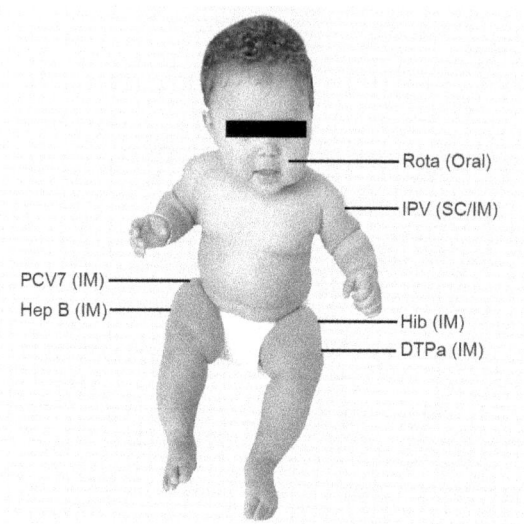

Fig. AIII.12: Vaccines and their sites of administration.

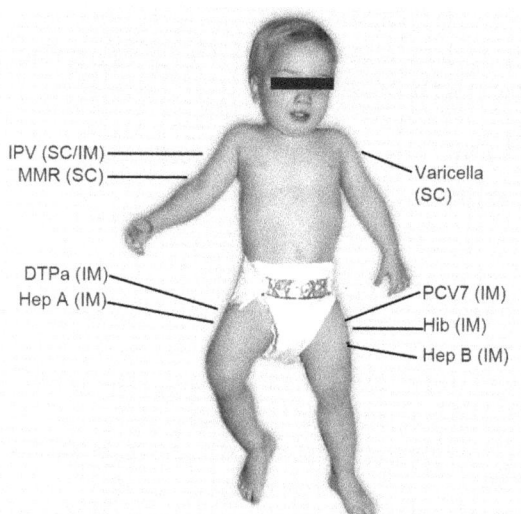

Fig. AIII.13: Vaccines and their sites of administration.
Note: In India, the preferred route of administration is IM for the currently registered IPVs except fIPV which is given ID in Government settings.

Immunization Techniques

Pediarix™ can only be used for the primary series; do not use for: 4th or 5th dose of DTPa, 4th dose of IPV

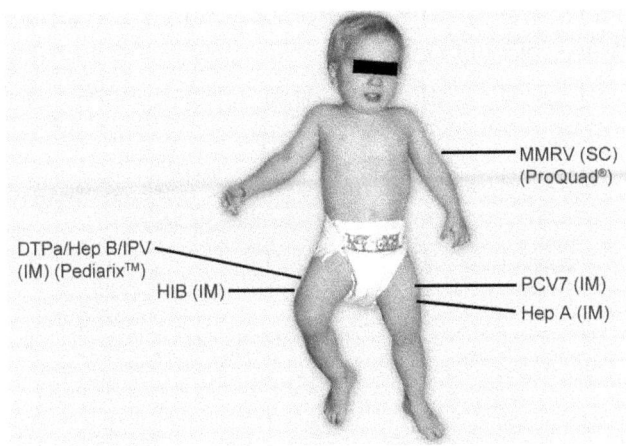

Fig. AIII.14: Vaccines and their sites of administration.

| Needle length: IM—1–1.5" SC—5/8" | Injection sites should be separated 1–2" | The anterolateral thigh is the preferred site for multiple IM injections | The deltoid (upper arm) is an option for IM in children ≥18 months with adequate muscle mass |

Using COMVAX™ (Hep B/Hib) and ProQuad® (MMRV)

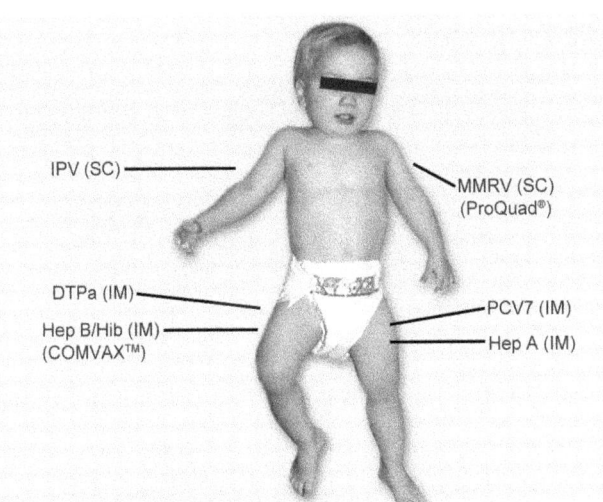

Fig. AIII.15: Vaccines and their sites of administration.

Giving All the Doses Including Influenza Vaccine (TIV) in US

Using Pediarix™ (DTaP/Hep B/IPV) and ProQuad® (MMR/Var)

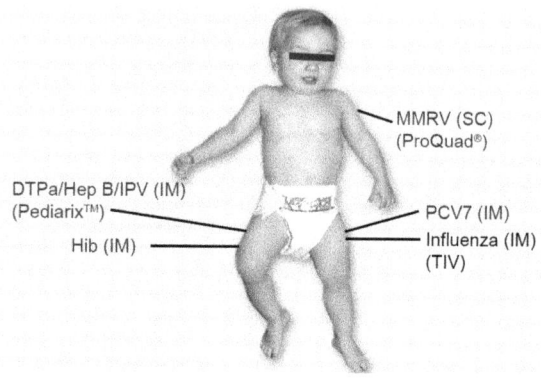

Fig. AIII.16: Vaccines and their sites of administration.

| TIV dosages:
6–35 months:
0.25 mL
3–8 years:
0.5 mL | Two doses (4 weeks apart) are recommended for children 6 months through 8 years receiving any flu vaccine for the first time | Children 6 months to 8 years who received influenza vaccine for the first time during the previous influenza season, and got only one does, should receive two doses this season separated by 4 weeks |

Using COMVAX™ (HepB/Hib) and ProQuad® (MMR/Var) in the US

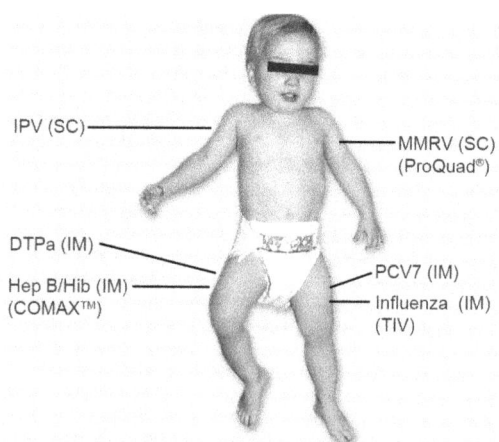

Fig. AIII.17: Vaccines and their sites of administration.

For Children

- 12 months through 4 years of age—giving all the doses.
- *11-12 years of age:*
  - *Needle lengths:* IM—1- 1.5"; SC— 5.8"
  - Separate injection sites by 1-2"
  - Professional judgment is appropriate when selecting needle length for use in all children, especially small infants or larger children.
  - Assess for other recommended vaccines that may be need MMR, polio, Hep B, Hep A, and influenza.
  - Syncope fainting after vaccination may occur in adolescents and young adults, usually within 15 minutes of vaccination.
  - When giving vaccines to teens: Have the patient sit down while you are giving vaccine(s). Consider observing patients for 15-20 minutes after vaccination.

Note: Varicella should be administered to school-age children and adolescents without:

- History of two doses of varicella vaccine.
- A healthcare provider's diagnosis of varicella disease or verification of history of typical varicella disease.
- History of shingles.

HPV4 is licensed for use in girls only 9-26 years of age MMRV (ProQuad®) is licensed for children 12 months to 12 years of age only.

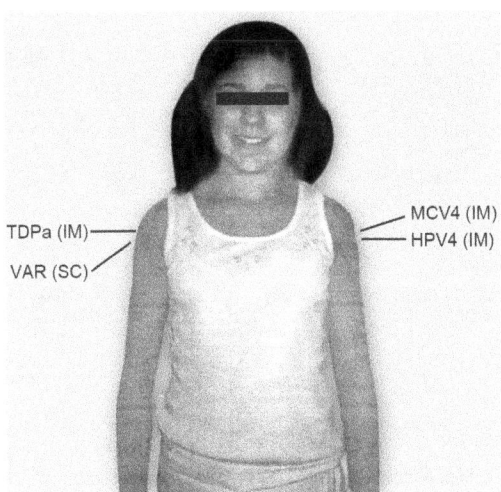

Fig. AIII.18: Vaccines and their sites of administration.

COMFORTING RESTRAINT

For Immunizations

Method

This method involves the parent in embracing the child and controlling all four limbs. It avoids *holding down* or overpowering the child, but it helps you steady and control the limb of the injection site.

For Infants and Toddlers (Fig. AIII.19)

- Have parent hold the child on parent's lap.
- One of the child's arms embraces the parents' back and is held under the parent's arm.
- The other arm is controlled by the parent's arm and hand. For infants, the parent can control both arms with one hand.
- Both legs are anchored with the child's feet held firmly between the parent's things, and controlled by parent's other arm.

For Kindergarten and Older children (Fig. AIII.20)

- Hold the child on parent's lap or have the child stand in front of the seated parent.
- Parent's arms embrace the child during the process.
- Both legs are firmly between parent's legs.

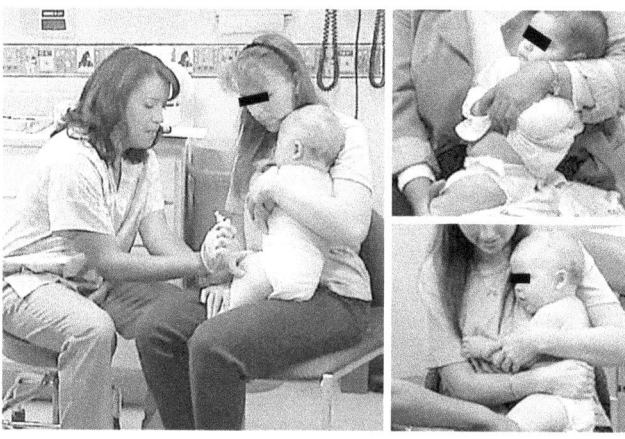

Fig. AIII.19: Restraining an infant for vaccination.

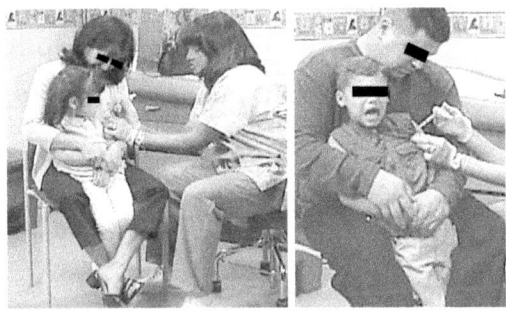

Fig. AIII.20: Restraining kindergarten and older children for vaccination.

BIBLIOGRAPHY

1. Centers for Disease Control and Prevention: Epidemiology and Prevention of Vaccine Preventable Diseases. Atkinson W, Wolfe S, Hamborsky J, McIntyre LE (Eds). 11th edition. Washington DC: Public Health Foundation; 2009
2. Parthasarathy A, Nair MKC (Eds). Partha's Immunization Digest, 2nd Edition. Jaypee Brothers Medical Publishers; 2011.

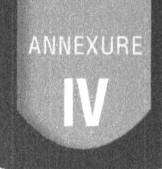

Vaccine Formulations (Brands) Commonly Available in India for Office Practice

(Vaccines in NIP—Government supply not included here)

Alok Gupta, Mohit Vohra

Sl. No.	Vaccine against	Brand name	Company	Presentation
1.	Oral polio vaccine (bOPV) (Live-attenuated vaccine, LAV)	Bio Polio B1/3	Bharat Biotech	20 doses vial with VVM (Oral containing LAPV1 and 3
2.	Tetanus toxoid	Serum Institute of India (SII) TT	SII	0.5 mL ampoule and 5.0 mL multidose vial
	Tetanus and diphtheria	SII Td vac BETd	SII Biological E	0.5 mL ampoule and 5.0 mL multidose vial (for age 7 years and above)
3.	Diphtheria tetanus and Pertussis (DTwP)	SII DTwP	SII	5.0 mL multidose vial
4.	BCG (LAV)	Tubervac	SII	Freeze dried 1 mL vial (10 doses)
		Genevac-B	SII	0.5 mL, 1 mL, 10 mL
		Revac-B	Bharat Biotech	0.5 mL, 1 mL, 10 mL
		Shanvac-B	Shantha Biotech	0.5 mL, 1 mL, 10 mL
		Biovac-B	Wockhardt Ltd	0.5 mL, 1 mL, 10 mL
		Bevac	Biological E	0.5 mL, 1 mL, 5 mL,
		Q-VAC	SII	0.5 mL, 5 mL vial
		Shan Tetra	Shantha-Merieux Ltd	0.5 mL, 5 mL vial
		Comvac-4	Bharath Biotech	0.5 mL, 5 mL vial
7.	DTwP-HIB combination	Comvac 3 + Bio Hib	Bharat Biotech	Lyophilized Hib + DTP (0.5 mL)
		Quadrovax	SII	0.5 mL PFS

Contd...

Vaccine Formulations (Brands) Commonly Available in India...

Contd...

Sl. No.	Vaccine against	Brand name	Company	Presentation
		Easy four	Chiron Panacea vaccines	Liquid 0.5 mL, vial
		Shan four	Shantha Merieux Ltd	Liquid 0.5 mL, vial
		Tripvac Hib	Biological E Ltd (Origyn)	Lyophilized HIB + DTP (0.5 mL)
8.	Hib vaccine	Stand-alone Hib vaccine not available at present		
		Pentavac	SII	0.5 mL PFS
		Easy-five liquid	Chiron Panacea	0.5 mL PFS, multidose vial
		Shan five (liquid)	Shantha Merieux Ltd	0.5 mL vial
		Comvac-4-Biohib	Bharath Biotech	0.5 mL
		Quinvaxem	Novartis Vaccines	0.5 mL vial
10.	Varicella vaccine (LAV)	Variped	MSD	Single vial dose (lyophilized) with diluent 0.5 mL
		Varilrix	GSK	Single vial dose (lyophilized) with diluent 0.5 mL
		Zuvicella	Zuventus Pharmaceuticals	Single vial dose (lyophilized) with diluent 0.5 mL
		Nexipox	Novo	Single vial dose (lyophilized) with diluent 0.5 mL
11.	Hepatitis A vaccine (Ped) (Killed)	Avaxim 80U	Sanofi Pasteur	GBM strain (0.5 mL) PFS
	Hepatitis A vaccine (LAV)	Havrix 720	GSK	HM 175 strain (0.5 mL vial)
		Biovac-A	Wockhardt Ltd	H2 strain (1 mL)
12.	Hepatitis A vaccine (adult)	Avaxim 160U	Sanofi Pasteur	GBM strain

Contd...

Contd...

Sl. No.	Vaccine against	Brand name	Company	Presentation
13.	Influenza vaccine (IIV)-Tri, or Tetravalent (NH/SH)	Fluquadri (0.25, 0.5 mL)	Sanofi Pasteur	PFS (tetravalent)
		VaxiFlu-4 (0.25, 0.5 mL)	Zydus	PFS (tetravalent)
		Zuviflu		PFS
		Fluarix	GSK	PFS
		Influvac (0.25, 0.5 mL)	Abbot	PFS
14.	Pneumococcal conjugate vaccine	Synflorix (PVC 10) Prevenar (PCV 13)	GSK Wyeth India Ltd	0.5 mL, vial
15.	Pneumococcal polysaccharide vaccine	Pneumovax-23	Merck Sharp and Dome (MSD)	0.5 mL, PFS
16.	Rabies vaccine	Rabivax-S Zuvirab	SII Zuventus	1.0 mL single dose
	Rabies human monoclonal antibody	Rabishield-100	SII	100 IU/2.5 mL (dose: 3.33 IU/kg)
17.	Rubella vaccine (LAV)	R-VAC	SII	0.5 mL amp
	Measles, rubella vaccine (LAV)	MRVac	SII	0.5 mL, 5.0 mL
	Measles, mumps, and rubella vaccine (LAV)	Tresivac Priorix	SII GSK	Freeze dried (vial, diluent PFS) Freeze dried (diluent PFS)
	MMR + Varicella vaccine (LAV)	Priorix Tetra	GSK	Single vial dose (lyophilized) with diluent 0.5 mL
18.	Hepatitis B immune globulin	Hepabig	VHB pharmaceuticals	100 IU and 200 IU, vial
19.	Tdap vaccine	Boostrix Adacel	GSK Sanofi Pasteur	0.5 mL, PFS
		Easy Six	Panacea vaccine	0.5 mL in PFS, (Prefilled syringe)

Contd...

Vaccine Formulations (Brands) Commonly Available in India...

Contd...

Sl. No.	Vaccine against	Brand name	Company	Presentation
21.	DTaP-IPV-HIB combination	Pentaxim	Sanofi Pasteur	0.5 mL, PFS
	DTaP-HB-HIB-IPV combination	Hexaxim Infanrix Hexa	Sanofi Pasteur GSK	0.5 mL, PFS DTaP-HB-IPV (liquid) + HIB (dry)
22.	Typhoid vaccine	Typbar TCV	Bharat Biotech	0.5 mL, PFS, 2.5 mL vial
		Enteroshield TCV	Abbot	0.5 mL
		VAC-T (TCV)	Zuventus	
		Typhim–Vi (ViPS)	Sanofi	0.5 mL, vial
		Zyvac TCV	Zydus	0.5 mL, vial
		Peda Typh (Conjugate typhoid vaccine)	Bio Med Pvt Ltd	0.5 mL vial single dose vial
23.	Human papillomavirus vaccine	Gardasil (4 strain)	MSD	Recombinant hHPV vaccine (types 6,11,16, and 18) 0.5 mL vial (single dose) PFS
		Cervarix (2 strain)	GSK	(types 16 and 18) 0.5 mL vial (single dose) PFS
		Nasovac	Serum Institute of India	0.25 mL spray for each nostril (children above 3 years, adolescent, adults. Pack (5 doses) with special device for intranasal spray.
25.	Oral cholera vaccine	Shanchol (killed bivalent 01 and 139)	Shantha Biotech Ltd/ Sanofi	1.5 mL orally on Day 0 and 14 2 doses
26.	Japanese encephalitis vaccine	1. Jenvac 2. Jeev	Bharat biotech BE	0.5 mL IM single dose PFS 0.25 mL IM/2 doses
27.	Meningococcal conjugate vaccine	Menactra (ACYW) Manveo (ACYW)	Sanofi GSK	0.5 mL 0.5 mL

Contd...

Contd...

Sl. No.	Vaccine against	Brand name	Company	Presentation
28.	Rotavirus vaccine (LAV)	Rotavac (116E)	Bharat Biotech	0.5 mL monovalent neonatal
		Rotasure (116E)	Abbot	Indian 116E strain
		RotaTeq	MSD	Pentavalent
		Rotarix	GSK	2 dose schedule—human monovalent
		Rotasiil	SII	Bivalent
29.	Yellow fever vaccine (LAV)	Stamaril	Sanofi	0.5 mL

Index

Page numbers followed by *f* refer to figure and *t* refer to table.

A

Abdominal discomfort 197, 296
Accelerated disease control 231
Acellular pertussis 46, 269
Acquired splenic dysfunction 49, 105
Active immunizing antigens 26
Acute flaccid paralysis surveillance 232, 241
Acute illness
  moderate 113
  severe 113
Adenovirus, non-replicating 86
Advisory Committee on Vaccines and Immunization Practices 42
Albuterol 188
Alcoholism 73
Allergic reactions 137
  severe 193, 285
Allergy, history of 180
Aluminium salts 219
Aminophylline 188
Amyloidosis 126
Anaphylaxis 137, 187
  treatment of 187
Anatomic asplenia 103
Animal bites, management of 147
Anogenital cancers 127
Anorexia 193, 296
Anthrax 3
  vaccine 222
Antibody 16, 93
Antibody-containing blood product, recent receipt of 108
Antigen 16
  presenting cells 23*f*, 25*f*
Antigenic drift 293
Antihistamines 188
Antisera 83, 84, 161, 162
Anti-snake venom 84, 161
Anti-Vaccination League of America 8
Asian Network for Surveillance of Resistant Pathogens 104
Aspiration 43
Asplenia
  acquired 49, 105
  functional 103
Asthma 73, 136, 137
Atonic cerebral palsy 232
Autism 27

B

Bacillus anthracis 222
Bacillus calmette-guérin 30, 35, 60, 84, 85, 163, 164, 201
  vaccination 3, 259, 260
  vaccine 43, 84, 185, 193, 258, 259, 315, 318
Bacterial polysaccharides 24
Bacterial vaccines, discovery of 3
Bacterial vectors 13
Bleeding disorders 180
Blood product, recent 113
B-lymphocyte 23*f*
  deficiency 73
Bordetella pertussis 153
Brain-derived vaccines 194
Breastfeeding 86, 172
Burns 159
Buruli ulcer 259

C

Canadian International Development Agency 184
Cancer precursors 127
Cardiopulmonary resuscitation 180
Cell culture 147
  Japanese encephalitis vaccine 138
  techniques, development of 215
Cell pertussis 174, 313
Cellular immune 227
Centers for Disease Control and Prevention 351
Cerebrospinal fluid
  fistula 105
  leak 48
Cervical abnormalities, low-grade 127
Cervical cancer 14, 126, 299, 300
  screening 128
Cervical intraepithelial neoplasia 131
Chemotherapy 103
  short course 85
Chicken cholera 3
Chickenpox 288, 335

problem of 334
vaccine 115, 330
Chikungunya vaccine 228
Chimeric vaccines 310
Chimeric yellow fever dengue 133
Chlamydia trachomatis 228
Cholera 36, 62, 175
vaccine 54, 56, 143
Chronic cardiac disease 105
Chronic disease 99
Cimetidine 188
Circumsporozoite protein 224
Cirrhosis 73
Civil Society Organization 241
Clostridium
difficile 216
tetani 272
tetanus 158
Cochlear implants 105
Cold chain 199, 199*f*
equipment 199, 201*t*
technical specifications of 201
maintenance 203
Combination vaccines 83, 144, 150, 152, 153, 155
benefits of 151*t*
Complement deficiencies 73
Congenital agammaglobulinemia 160
Congenital asplenia 49, 105, 179
Congenital immunodeficiency 49, 105
Congenital rubella syndrome 112, 286
Congenital splenic dysfunction 49, 105
Conjugate polysaccharide 19
Conjugate typhoid vaccine 121
Conjugate vaccine 312
Control rubella 112
Corticosteroids 188
local injections of 178
physiologic maintenance doses of 178
Corynebacterium diphtheria 267
transmission of 267
Cyanotic congenital heart disease 49
Cystic fibrosis 136, 137
Cytomegalovirus 5, 219
infection 213
vaccine 222

D

Dengue 5, 9, 63, 213
illness 228

tetravalent vaccine 132
vaccine 132, 226, 227
Diabetes mellitus 73, 105, 136, 138
Diarrhea 109, 296
severe 86, 281
Diphenhydramine 188
Diphtheria 11, 204, 213
antitoxin 84, 267
Diphtheria toxin 267
antitoxin mixture, bacterial contamination of 7
risk of 269
vaccines 266
Diphtheria toxoid 22, 26, 67, 96, 204, 206, 269, 313
containing vaccine, doses of 268
dose of 174
low-dose 267
Diphtheria, tetanus 12, 163
vaccination 301
vaccine 122
Diphtheria, tetanus pertussis 151, 189, 201, 264
vaccine 267
Diphtheria, tetanus toxoids 23*f*, 97, 125, 163, 174
and acellular pertussis 163
and pertussis 32, 163, 175
vaccine 45
Directly Observed Treatment Short Course 85
Diseases requiring long-term aspirin therapy 136, 138
DNA-BCG vaccine, new 85
Dopamine 188
Draining lymph node 220

E

Edmonston-Enders strain 111
Edmonston-Zagreb strain 110
Egg
allergy 114
antigens 26
Emphysema 73
Endgame milestones 244*f*
Endgame strategic plan 244, 245*t*
Epidemics 57
Epinephrine 187
Epstein-Barr virus 228
Erythema 118, 183
Escherichia coli 144
vaccine 228
Expanded Indian National Rotavirus Surveillance Network 251
Expanded Program on Immunization 11, 13, 29

F

Fatigue 93, 296
Febrile illness
 severe 90
  acute 115
Fever 109, 111
Flu vaccines 135
Fluid, suspending 26
Food and Drug Administration 46, 70

G

Gammaglobulin 84, 160
Gastrointestinal conditions, pre-existing chronic 108
Gastrointestinal disease, chronic 282
Gelatin 26, 285
Genetic Engineering Approval Committee 211
Genetic vaccines, characteristics of 22*t*
Genital herpes 213
Genital warts 126, 127
Gentle pressure 346
Global Advisory Committee on Vaccine Safety 184, 264
Global Alliance for Vaccines and Immunization 11, 189
Global Alliance Vaccine Initiative 7
Global Eradication of Poliomyelitis 11
Global Polio Eradication Initiative 7, 241, 242
Global Program on Vaccines 14
Global wild poliovirus 235*f*
Glycoconjugate vaccine 25, 25*f*
Glycoconjugation technology 215
Glycol conjugate vaccines 13
Granulomatous disease, chronic 73
Guillain-Barré syndrome 196, 232
Guinea pigs 9

H

Haemophilus influenzae 60, 98, 215, 274
Haemophilus influenzae B 19, 163, 176, 189, 204, 264, 274
 conjugate 22, 174
  vaccine 47, 165, 193
 immunization 327
 infections 326
  pectrum of 326
  severity of 327
 polysaccharide vaccine 99
 vaccination 78
  status 276
 vaccine 98-101, 194, 327-329
  pellet of 325
Headache 93
Heart failure, congestive 73
Helicobacter pylori 228
Hemagglutinin 293
Hematopoietic stem cell transplant 78
Hemoglobinopathy 136
Hemolytic anemia 126
Hepatitis 121, 286
 vaccination schedule 171*t*
 vaccine 172
Hepatitis A 35, 39, 40, 59, 63, 83, 153, 163, 180, 213, 297, 298
 antibody 51
 infection, immune prophylaxis of 173
 vaccination 74
 vaccine 51, 57, 58, 120, 166, 194, 295, 332, 333
  administration of 177
  dose of 297
  inactivated 51, 296
  types of 296
 virus 295
  infection 74, 177, 298
  vaccine 205
Hepatitis B 22, 30, 35, 41, 59, 60, 83, 153, 163, 164, 189, 213, 259, 313, 323
 antibody 94*f*
 immunization 24*f*
  complications of 323
  schedule of 320
 immunoglobulin 57, 84, 157, 158, 171, 172
 immunoprophylaxis 171
 natural history of 320
 prevalence of 319
 surface antigen 24*f*, 90, 172
 vaccination 75, 265, 332
 vaccine 24, 34, 41, 44, 76, 90-94, 150, 171, 194, 263, 264, 266, 319, 323
  second dose of 172
  third dose of 91, 172
 virus 93, 174, 264
  doses of 324
  maternal 171
  preventing 264
  transmission of 320
  vaccine 205

virus infection 75, 92, 322
    acute 172
    chronic 266
    prevention of perinatal 91
Hepatitis C 213, 228, 266
    virus vaccine 227
    development of 227
Hepatitis E 228
Hepatocellular carcinoma 264
Herpes simplex virus 5
    vaccines 224
Herpes zoster 115, 289
    vaccine 116, 117, 290
Hexaxim vaccines 100
High fever 86
High population immunity 246
Highly active antiretroviral therapy 283
Hodgkin's disease 49, 73, 179
Human anti-D immunoglobulin 84, 161
Human cytomegalovirus 222
Human immunodeficiency virus 105, 270
    infection 48, 73, 103, 105, 114, 136, 137, 258
    vaccine 223, 228
Human immunoglobulin 84
Human normal immunoglobulin 160
Human papillomavirus 41, 61, 126, 127
    associated disease 127
    clinical features 128
    epidemiology 128
    infection, natural history of 128
    vaccination 69, 129, 300
        routine 129
    vaccine 63, 126, 129-131, 194, 299-301, 339
        bivalent tetravalent 167
Human rabies
    immunoglobulin 159
    prevention of 305f
Hydrocortisone 188
Hydroxyzine 188
Hypersensitivity 115, 126
    history of 180
Hypertension 73
Hypogammaglobulinemia 160

I

Iatrogenic immunosuppression 73
Ideal vaccines, characteristics of 21t
Idiopathic thrombocytopenic purpura 160

Immune memory 24
Immunity 16
    active 16
    evidence of 68
    maintaining 247
Immunization 11, 29, 191, 209, 315
    activities, supplementary 241, 287
    adverse effects following 183
    childhood 178
    principles of 16
    Programs 203
    safety project 184
    schedules 29, 59t, 79, 173
    strategies 305
    stress on adolescent and adult 13
    techniques 346
    threats to 189
    timetable 60
Immunodeficiency, primary 303
Immunogenicity, reduced 126
Immunoglobulin 16, 83, 84, 157, 162, 177
    administration 316t
    intramuscular 173
    intravenous 177
Immunosuppression 103, 113
Immunosuppressive disorder 136, 137
Immunosuppressive drugs 49
Immunosuppressive therapy 105, 136, 137
Inactivated bacteria 26
Inactivated vaccines 17
    characteristics of 21t
India Experts Advisory Group 12, 232
India Polio Eradication Initiative 12
Indian Academy of Pediatrics 12, 42, 58
    Immunization Schedule 34
    immunization timetable, changes in 41t
    Infectious Disease Surveillance Program 256
Individual with cancer, vaccination of 181
Individual with chemotherapy, vaccination of 181
Infectious disease
    acute 86
    principle to 1
Influenza 22, 35, 83, 180, 189, 191, 213
    A viruses 293
        subtypes of 293
    B
        strain 294
        viruses 293

diagnosis of 293
surveillance platforms 295
vaccination 67, 295
vaccine 38, 42, 52, 56, 137, 293, 295
   inactivated 67, 78, 181
virosomes 221
virus 227
   new-generation 137
   vaccine 205, 220
Integrated Disease Surveillance Program 251, 252
Integrated Infant Immunization Strategy 157
International Certificate of Vaccination 144, 145
Intestinal malformations 282
Intradermal injection 348
Intradermal vaccination 45
Intramuscular administration techniques 356f
Intramuscular injection 346, 347f, 351f, 355, 355f
Intravenous drug usage 92
Intravenous gamma-globulin preparations 160
Invasive Bacterial Infection Surveillance Group 104

J

Japan International Cooperation Agency 184
Japanese encephalitis 22, 33, 36, 62, 83, 138, 139, 140f, 146, 228, 309
   vaccination 310
   vaccine 39, 54-56, 138, 139, 194, 309
      inactivated 138
      single dose of 34
   virus 309
Jerry-Lynn strain 190

K

Kawasaki syndrome 160

L

Laryngeal papilloma 126, 127
Lentiviruses 219
Leprosy 252, 258
Leptospirosis 228
Leukemia 49, 73, 86
Live attenuated
   bacteria 59

hepatitis A vaccines 297
influenza vaccine 52, 67, 294
rubella virus 132
vaccine 17, 86, 298, 310, 311
   characteristics of 21t
varicella virus 2 117
virus 59
Live bacteria 163
Live virus 26
   vaccine 176, 177
Liver disease, chronic 73
Liver enzymes 296
Lung disease, chronic 73
Lymphocytes 115
Lymphoma 49, 73

M

Malaise 296
Malaria vaccine 224, 228
Mass vaccination 6
Maternal and neonatal tetanus 14, 272
   elimination 274
Measles 8, 11, 61, 213
   and mumps vaccines 114
   component 70
   immunization 316t
   vaccination 183, 285
   vaccine 110, 111, 114, 282
      second dose of 113
   virus 219
      vaccine 205
Measles-containing vaccine 42
   combinations 283
   dose of 282
Measles-mumps-rubella 41, 189
   vaccine 8, 111-114, 42, 50, 70, 175, 195, 331
   varicella vaccine 111, 115, 154, 330
   viruses, live 163, 174
Measles-rubella 41
   vaccination 112
      campaign 112
   vaccine 12, 29, 42
Measles-vaccine delivery 287
Meningitis 101
Meningococcal
   conjugate vaccine 141, 144
   disease 146, 213
   polysaccharide vaccine 141, 144
   vaccination 76
   vaccine 54, 56, 79, 140, 142, 144, 181, 195, 312
Meningococcus 215

Meningoencephalitis 286
Metabolic disease, chronic 136, 138
Methylprednisolone 188
Military recruits 78, 142
Ministry of Health and Family Welfare 252
Modern medicine 1
Molecular genetics 4
Monoclonal antibody 17
Morbidity weekly report 9
Mortality weekly report 9
Mosquito-borne viral disease 301
Mucosal immunization 222
Multidrug-resistant tuberculosis 258
Multiple myeloma 73
Multiple vaccinations 357
Multiple vaccines
   administration of 175
   simultaneous administration of 175
Mumps 63, 213
   and rubella 112
   component 70
   virus vaccine, live 205
Mycobacterium
   bovis 259
   leprae 258
   ulcerans 259
Myelitis, transverse 232

N

Nasopharyngeal carriage 279
National immunization 58
   Program 12, 283
National immunization schedule 12, 29, 81
   and strategies 12
   for infants, children and pregnant women 30*t*
National passive surveillance 231
National Polio Surveillance Project 232
National Regulatory Authority 211
National Technical Advisory Group on Immunization 12, 34, 81
National Tuberculosis Control Program 255
   revised 85, 255
National Vaccine Injury Compensation Program 8
Natural measles infection 190*t*
Needle-free vaccine delivery 221
Neisseria meningitidis 77, 140, 142, 228
Neomycin 87, 285
Nephrotic syndrome 73, 103, 105, 315
Neuraminidase activity 293
Next generation technologies 216
Nontuberculous mycobacterial infections 259
Notorious vaccine controversies 8
Nucleotide-binding oligomerization domain 219

O

Obstructive lung disease, chronic 73
Older age groups, vaccination of 260
Oligodeoxynucleotides 221
Oral cholera vaccine 79, 143
   new 228
Oral polio vaccine 31, 41, 42, 86, 87, 164, 201, 304, 318
   birth dose of 44
   bivalent 42, 241
   booster 32
   doses of 318
      routine 58
   role of 88
Oral poliovirus 163
   vaccine 175, 261
      type 2 244
Oral typhoid vaccine 181
Organ transplant
   individuals 180
   recipient 105

P

Pain 118
   at injection site 93
Parainfluenza 226
Paralytic polio, vaccine associated 44, 87, 106, 190, 318
Paralytic poliomyelitis 87
   vaccine-associated 195, 243, 261
Passive immunity 16
   sources of 17
Pediatric and adolescent immunization 13
Pediatric formulation 122
Pediatric vaccines, characteristics of 22*t*
Pentavalent human-bovine vaccine, re-assorted 110
Pentavalent reconstituted vaccine 152
Pentaxim vaccines 100

Index

Persistent infection 299
Persons with high-risk conditions, vaccination of 48
Pertussis 11, 269
   acellular 22
   vaccine 269
      component 96
      inactivated 96
      whole- cell 22
Phagocytic disorders 73
Pipeline vaccines 228
Plague 175
Plan polio's legacy 243
Plant vaccines 5
Plasmodium falciparum
   infection 225
   sporozoites 225
Pneumococcal
   conjugate vaccine 12, 31, 41, 47, 57, 71, 102, 103, 276, 277
   immunization 105
   infection 213, 277
   meningitis 338
   polysaccharide vaccine 48, 56, 102, 103
   vaccination 71, 73
   vaccine 31, 38, 101, 102, 104, 105, 167, 195, 205, 337, 338
Pneumococcus 4, 215
Pneumonia 101
Polio 35, 37, 60, 252, 318
   elimination, progress of 6f
   endgame strategic plan 240, 242f, 245
   eradication 87, 203
      initiative 233f
   history of 238f
   vaccination 7
      schedule 107
Polio vaccine 41, 195, 261, 263
   adverse reactions 87
   contraindications 90, 107
   enhanced potency inactivated 86
   fractional inactivated 31
   inactivated 22, 41, 44, 86, 89, 106, 174, 189, 201
   injectable 42
   precautions 90, 107
   role of inactivated 88
Polio virus 7, 86, 87
   containment 246
   inactivated 163
   infection 6
   live 174
   location of 236f
   seroprevalence against 247t
   serotype 89, 261
   type 2 vaccine-derived 261
   vaccine-derived 88, 237f
   vaccines 44, 206
      inactivated 245, 261
      types of 261
Poliomyelitis 11, 14, 86, 213, 261
   controlling 261
   incidence of 261
Polysaccharide 13, 16, 25f
   conjugate vaccines 99
   protein conjugate
      diphtheria toxin 163
      tetanus toxoid 163
      vaccines 277
   pure 19
   typhoid vaccine 121
   vaccines 19, 54, 99, 276
      pure 20
      response to 24
Population immunity 245
Postexposure immune prophylaxis of hepatitis A infection 173t
Post-exposure prophylaxis 56, 93, 148-150, 305f, 306
   vaccines 147
Post-polio scenario 88
Pre-exposure Universal Immunization 172
Pregnancy 113, 178
   vaccination during 130
Pregnant household contacts 109
Preterm infants 91
   born 171
Prevaccination serologic testing 91
Preventable diseases 253
Prophylactic human papillomavirus vaccines 299
Prophylaxis, pre-exposure 55, 79, 305f, 309
Protective antibody titers 90
Protein 16
   molecules 16
   vaccines 23, 23f
Provocative polio 319
Public Health Programme 6
Public Resistance to Immunization Programmes 7
Public-sector Program 252
Pulmonary diseases, chronic 136, 137
Pulmonary tuberculosis 260
Pulse polio immunization 318

Q

Quadrivalent polysaccharide vaccine 141
Quality control 255
Queensland disaster 7

R

Rabies 63, 83, 146
   human monoclonal antibody 159
   immunoglobulin 84, 159, 160, 177, 196, 305
      administration 308
   vaccine 42, 55, 56, 79, 147, 196, 305, 308, 340
      administration of 306
   virus 306
Radiation therapy 49, 73
Ranitidine 188
Rash 111
   generalized 118
Rectus femoris 347*f*
Refrigerator 200
   ice-lined 201
Renal disease, end-stage 225
Renal dysfunction, chronic 136, 138
Renal failure, chronic 73, 103
Researcher's point of view 151
Respiratory diseases vaccine 253
Respiratory papillomatosis, recurrent 127, 299
Respiratory syncytial virus 5, 226
Respiratory vaccines 226
Reverse vaccinology 215
Rotarix 49
Rotavirus 35, 38, 61, 280
   disease 281
   gastroenteritis episodes 280
Rotavirus vaccine 29, 42, 49, 107, 108, 110, 167, 196, 201, 280-282, 314, 338, 339
   adverse reactions 109
   and intussusception 109
   and preterm infants 109
   dose of 282
   effectiveness 108
   recipients 109
      immunosuppressed household contacts of 109
   storage and handling 109
   types of 107
Routine immunization 60*t*
Routine Immunization Program 313
Rubella 61, 189, 213, 285
   component 71
   containing vaccines 286
   vaccine 132, 285, 286, 331
      during pregnancy 187
      dose of 286

S

Sabin polio vaccine 4
Salk polio vaccine 4
Salmonella 215
   enteric serovar typhi 290
   typhi 19, 187, 290
Schistosomiasis 228
Schwartz strain 110
Seasonal flu vaccine, dose of inactivated 137
Seasonal influenza 63
Seizures 193
Sendai virus 219
Sentinel sites, reporting format for 254
Severe systemic reactions 93
Sexually transmitted disease 75
Shigella 5
   vaccine 228
Shock, anaphylactic 183
Sickle cell
   anemia 136, 138, 337
   disease 48, 105, 179
Smallpox 1, 2, 6, 8, 213, 214
   eradication of 11
   vaccine 11
      discovery of 11
Snake bite 1
   management of 162
Snake venom 1
Solid organ transplant 49, 73, 266
Splenectomy 179
Staphylococcal vaccine 225
Staphylococci vaccines 225
Staphylococcus 5
   aureus 191, 197, 216, 225
      bacteremia 225
Steroid 103, 178
   therapy 315
Streptococcal
   disease, group B 213
   vaccine, group B 223
Streptococcus
   group A 228
   group B 223, 228
   pneumonia 101
      serotypes of 277
   pyogenes 5
Streptomycin 87
Structural vaccinology 216

Subcutaneous administration 187
  techniques 354f
Subcutaneous injections 347, 351, 354f
Sudden infant death syndrome 27
Symptomatic human immunodeficiency viruses infection 303
Systemic complaints, mild 93
Systemic corticosteroids 178
  high doses of 178, 179
  long-term 73
Systemic reactions 118, 193

T

Tabletop simulation 248
Takeda's dengue vaccine 226
Tetanus 26, 206
  and diphtheria
    acellular pertussis 267
    and acellular pertussis vaccination 67
    toxoids 46, 58, 67
    toxoids booster doses 47
  immunoglobulin 84, 158
  maternal 14
  neonatal 11, 14
  prophylaxis 324
  toxin 4
  toxoid 20, 22, 96, 123, 124, 174, 201
    vaccines 272
  vaccine 272
    dose of 293
Tetravalent rotavirus vaccine 107
T-helper cell 24
Thrombocytopenia 286
Thymus disorder 303
Tick-borne encephalitis 62
Tissue culture-derived antigens 26
T-lymphocyte deficiency 73
Toddler immunization 359t
Towne strain 223
Toxic shock syndrome 183, 191, 197
Toxins 4
Toxoids 163
  and inactivated bacteria 163
    components 163
  discovery of 4
Transcutaneous vaccines 13
Traumatic neuritis 232
Travel related vaccines 79, 83, 135
  schedule 79t
Trivalent inactivated influenza vaccines 294
Tuberculin skin testing 114, 259
Tuberculin syringe 84
Tuberculosis 213, 252, 258
  epidemiology of 259
  vaccines 224
Tuberculosis Control Program 255
Typhoid 35, 59, 62, 83
  conjugate vaccine 39, 52, 176, 291, 292, 332
  fever 146, 290
  immunization 332
  polysaccharide antigen vaccine 166
  vaccination 292
    programs 291
  vaccine 42, 52, 121, 197, 290, 332
    administration of 292
    parenteral 175

U

United Nations Children's Fund 184
Universal Child Immunization 11
Urticaria 197
US Agency for International Development 184

V

Vaccination 315
  administration of 183
  program 289
  risks of 303
  routine 43, 44, 45, 46, 47, 49, 50, 51, 52, 54
  scares 189t
  schedule 52
Vaccine 29-33, 37-41, 83, 119-121, 123, 155, 162-167, 360-363f
  adverse event reporting system 184
  characteristics of 21
  childhood 186
  classification of 17, 18, 19f
  cold chain for 199
  components 137
  composition of 26
  derived polioviruses, emergence of 261
  determining efficacy of 3
  doses 23, 64t
  efficacy of 336
  failure 321
  fractional 18
  immunogenicity 211
  licensed 162

live 181, 317
    further attenuated 111
    recombinant 310, 311
reactions, prevention of acute 185
ready reckoner for 164t
safety 183
select 222
setbacks and disasters from 7
status of combination 155t
storage of 200f, 202
supply gaps, mitigating risk of 249
timeline 1, 5f, 228
vial monitors 201, 202f
virus, serotypes of 87
Vaccine development 209
    clinical development 210
    exploratory stage 210
    newer technologies in 213
    preclinical stage 210
    process 209, 209t
    systems biology approach to 217
Vaccine for Children Program 207
Vaccine formulations 366
    single-antigen 74
Vaccine preventable disease 11, 231, 241
    surveillance 231
        types of 231
Vaccinia Ankara, modified 86
Vaccinia virus 218, 219
Varicella 35, 40, 63, 115, 146, 174, 180, 288
    and herpes zoster vaccination 288
    breakthrough infection 116
    containing vaccine 115, 118, 119
    epidemiology of 334
    immunity 177
    vaccination 68
        absence of 290
    vaccine 50, 57, 115, 116, 118, 119, 166, 334, 335, 337
        immunogenicity and efficacy 116
        post-exposure prophylaxis 118
    virus 206
    zoster vaccine 197
    zoster virus 181, 288
        vaccination 290
Vastus lateralis 347f, 355f
    anatomy of 356f
Vector-borne disease 253
Vero cell
    culture 55
    inactivated 55, 311
Vesicular stomatitis virus 219
Vibrio cholera 54
Viral antigen, inactivated 163
Viral subunit, inactivated 163
Viral vaccines 5
Viral vector 5
    ineffective 218
    replication deficient 218
    vaccines 218
Viral zoonotic disease 305
Virosomes 220
Virus vaccine development 226
Vitamin A 32, 33
Vomiting 109, 193, 296

W

Water-borne disease 253
West Nile virus 218
Whole cell
    pertussis 189
    vaccines 18
Whooping cough 269
Wild poliovirus 236f, 261
    eradication and containment, certification of 232, 248
    location of 238f
World Health Organization 5, 29, 144, 183, 231
World Tuberculosis Day 85
Wound management, routine 324

Y

Yellow fever 62, 79, 83, 146, 301
    vaccination against 301
    vaccine 56, 144, 181, 302-304

Z

Zoster vaccination 70
Zoster vaccine 118

EU GSPR Authorised Reprsentative
Logos Europe, 9 rue Nicolas Poussin
1700, La Rochelle, France
Phone: +33 (0) 6 67 93 73 78
E-mail: contact@logoseurope.eu

www.ingramcontent.com/pod-product-compliance
Ingram Content Group UK Ltd.
Pitfield, Milton Keynes, MK11 3LW, UK
UKHW021829140426
5217IPUK00021B/1350